Manual of HIV Therapeutics

Second Edition

Manual of HIV Therapeutics

Second Edition

Edited by

William G. Powderly, M.D., F.R.C.P.I.
Professor of Medicine
Chief, Division of Infectious Diseases
Department of Internal Medicine
Washington University School of Medicine
St. Louis, Missouri

LIPPINCOTT WILLIAMS & WILKINS
A **Wolters Kluwer** Company
Philadelphia · Baltimore · New York · London
Buenos Aires · Hong Kong · Sydney · Tokyo

Acquisitions Editor: Jonathan Pine
Developmental Editor: Julia Seto
Production Editor: Emily Lerman
Manufacturing Manager: Benjamin Rivera
Cover Designer: Patricia Gast
Compositor: Circle Graphics
Printer: R.R. Donnelley—Crawfordsville

© 2001 by LIPPINCOTT WILLIAMS & WILKINS
530 Walnut Street
Philadelphia, PA 19106 USA
LWW.com

Printed in the USA

Library of Congress Cataloging-in-Publication Data

Manual of HIV therapeutics / edited by William G. Powderly.—2nd ed.
        p. ; cm.
    Includes bibliographical references and index.
    ISBN 0-7817-3011-2 (alk. paper)
    1. AIDS (Disease)—Treatment. 2. AIDS (Disease)—Complications—Treatment. I. Powderly, William G.
    [DNLM: 1. HIV Infections—therapy. 2. AIDS-Related Opportunistic Infections—therapy. 3. Acquired Immunodeficiency Syndrome—complications. 4. Anti-HIV Agents—therapeutic use. WC 503.2 M294 2001]
    RC607.A26 M3475 2001
    616.97'9206—dc21   00-042824

Care has been taken to confirm the accuracy of the information presented and to describe generally accepted practices. However, the authors, editor, and publisher are not responsible for errors or omissions or for any consequences from application of the information in this book and make no warranty, expressed or implied, with respect to the currency, completeness, or accuracy of the contents of the publication. Application of this information in a particular situation remains the professional responsibility of the practitioner.

The authors, editor, and publisher have exerted every effort to ensure that drug selection and dosage set forth in this text are in accordance with current recommendations and practice at the time of publication. However, in view of ongoing research, changes in government regulations, and the constant flow of information relating to drug therapy and drug reactions, the reader is urged to check the package insert for each drug for any change in indications and dosage and for added warnings and precautions. This is particularly important when the recommended agent is a new or infrequently employed drug.

Some drugs and medical devices presented in this publication have Food and Drug Administration (FDA) clearance for limited use in restricted research settings. It is the responsibility of the health care provider to ascertain the FDA status of each drug or device planned for use in their clinical practice.

10 9 8 7 6 5 4 3 2 1

To Betsy Keath, for her constant support,
and to Niall and Ailis for inspiration.

ACKNOWLEDGMENTS

I express my appreciation to Julia Seto and Jonathan Pine of Lippincott Williams & Wilkins for helping to bring this edition to fruition. I thank the faculty and fellows of the Division of Infectious Diseases at Washington University and the staff at the AIDS Clinical Trials Unit for their help and support. I am particularly grateful for the assistance of Cindy Waterman. But above all, I once again acknowledge the many patients with HIV whose paths have crossed mine in the last eighteen years. Their courage in the face of this illness and its changing burdens has added to my humility and humanity in ways that cannot be described. I can only hope that future editions of this manual will bring even better and more successful therapeutics.

CONTENTS

Acknowledgments vi

Contributing Authors ix

Preface xi

1. The Pathogenesis of HIV-1 Infection 1

2. Acute HIV Infection 6

3. Natural History 14

4. Primary Care 20

5. Antiretroviral Agents 33
   David J. Ritchie

6. Antiretroviral Therapy 48

7. Overview of Pediatric Infection 60

8. HIV Disease and Women 70

9. HIV in Pregnant Women 77

10. Management of the Terminally Ill AIDS Patient 84
    John D. Stansell and William G. Powderly

11. Pulmonary Aspects 94

12. Dermatologic Manifestations 107

13. Neurologic and Psychiatric Complications 113

14. Gastrointestinal Aspects 123

15. The Kidney in HIV Disease 130

16. Ophthalmologic Aspects 135

17. Cardiovascular Aspects 144

18. Rheumatic Aspects 149

19.   Endocrine, Metabolic, and Body Composition Disorders   154
      Kevin E. Yarasheski, Donna Marin, Sheri Claxton,
      and William G. Powderly

20.   Oral and ENT Problems   168

21.   Hematologic Problems   175

22.   Protozoan Infections   182

23.   Mycobacterial Infections   194

24.   Management of Mycoses   206

25.   Viral Infections   212

26.   Pyogenic Infections   224

27.   Treponemal Infection in HIV Disease   229

28.   Kaposi's Sarcoma   239

29.   Lymphomas   248

Appendix 1.   Available Antiretroviral Therapy with Usual Doses
              and Costs   258

Appendix 2.   Dose Modifications: Dual Protease Therapies   260

Appendix 3.   Dose Modifications: PI/NNRTI Combination Therapies   261

Appendix 4.   Dose Modifications of Antiretroviral Agents:
              Effects of Renal Failure and Hemodialysis   262
              Michael Royal and William G. Powderly

Subject Index   263

CONTRIBUTING AUTHORS

Sheri Claxton, M.S., R.D.
*AIDS Clinical Trials Unit, Washington University School of Medicine,
St. Louis, Missouri*

Donna Marin, R.N.
*AIDS Clinical Trials Unit, Washington University School of Medicine,
St. Louis, Missouri*

William G. Powderly, M.D., F.R.C.P.I.
*Professor of Medicine and Chief, Division of Infectious Diseases,
Department of Internal Medicine, Washington University School of Medicine,
St. Louis, Missouri*

David J. Ritchie, Pharm.D., B.C.P.S.
*Clinical Pharmacist, Infectious Diseases, Barnes-Jewish Hospital;
Associate Professor of Pharmacy Practice, St. Louis College of Pharmacy,
St. Louis, Missouri*

Michael Royal, R.Ph.
*Research Pharmacist, AIDS Clinical Trials Unit,
Washington University School of Medicine, St. Louis, Missouri*

Kevin E. Yarasheski, Ph.D.
*Associate Professor, Division of Metabolism, Endocrinology, and Diabetes,
Washington University School of Medicine, St. Louis, Missouri*

PREFACE

The scientific advances in HIV disease continue to proceed at a dizzying speed. Since the first edition of this manual only three years ago, there has been a staggering change in the treatment of HIV infection in the developed world with consequent implications for care of patients. Death rates from AIDS have fallen dramatically, and opportunistic infections and other complications of advanced HIV disease have become less frequent. HIV-infected patients and their providers have witnessed, over the space of a few years, a change in the disease, from one that was almost assuredly fatal to a chronic medically manageable condition. With the advent of new agents to treat HIV infection, and new strategies to use these agents, new issues related to toxicity, recovery of the immune system, and long-term complications of disease and treatment have emerged.

As we noted in the first edition, one of the challenges facing practitioners caring for patients is that the increased therapeutic knowledge is often not readily available from single sources. In perhaps no other field does material published in the classical medical literature become less relevant to practice by the time that it is published. This book attempts to remedy this problem by assembling most aspects of therapeutics for HIV into a single, manageable source, building upon the successful style of the *Washington University Manual of Medical Therapeutics*. As such, we have attempted to provide a logical approach to diagnostic evaluation and therapeutics, but this manual is not intended as a comprehensive reference on HIV disease. Discussions of pathophysiology and differential diagnoses are limited. The issue of relevance and timeliness also offers a challenge, and most chapters were revised and updated in the spring of 2000 to attempt to keep information at its most current.

Manual of HIV Therapeutics
Second Edition

1. THE PATHOGENESIS OF HIV-1 INFECTION

Human immunodeficiency virus-type 1 (HIV-1) is a retrovirus that infects human cells bearing the CD4$^+$ surface marker and causes, usually over many years, gradual loss of immune system function. A hallmark of this process is the depletion of CD4$^+$ lymphocytes, and this and other complex immune alterations predispose to the opportunistic infections and neoplasms of the **acquired immunodeficiency syndrome (AIDS).** HIV-1 is transmitted primarily through sexual (heterosexual or homosexual), parenteral, or maternal/fetal exposures. More than 40 million people worldwide are infected with HIV-1, making it a major contribution to worldwide morbidity and mortality.

I. **General characteristics of HIV-1.** HIV-1 is one of several human retroviruses. HIV-2, a related virus that is an important cause of AIDS in areas of western Africa, is transmitted in a similar fashion to that of HIV-1, yet is generally less virulent. **Human T-cell lymphotropic viruses I and II (HTLV-I and HTLV-II)** do not cause AIDS, but may be associated with rare neoplastic and neurologic conditions in humans.
   A. **Virion structure.** The **lentiviruses** (HIV-1 and HIV-2) share a common structure: two copies of a single-stranded ribonucleic acid (RNA) genome located inside a conical core, which in turn is surrounded by a lipid envelope (Fig. 1). Each virion is 100 to 120 nm in diameter. The envelope is studded with glycoproteins (**gp120** and **gp41**) that are important for invasion of cells, interactions with the immune system, and also induce antibody responses integral to diagnostic testing and vaccine development. Critical viral enzymes—**reverse transcriptase (RT), protease, and integrase**—are contained inside the virion and are the principal targets of existing antiretroviral drugs. The nucleocapsid includes a major protein, **p24 antigen,** which is sometimes assayed for diagnostic purposes.
   B. The **HIV-1 genome** is ~9.7 kb long and complex in its organization, using overlapping reading frames to encode messages for both **structural** and **regulatory** proteins.
      1. The "early" gene products (regulatory proteins) derive primarily from multiply spliced RNA transcripts, whereas the "late" products come from unspliced or single-spliced messages.
         a. One of the critical regulatory genes, **Rev**, regulates viral replication by signaling the transition from the early to late gene products.
         b. Tat, the other key regulatory gene, binds to a specific site on the HIV-1 genome and is a potent stimulus of HIV transcription.
      2. Three **structural genes** encode the virion particle itself.
         a. The **Gag** gene product forms the viral capsid proteins, including the **p24 antigen.**
         b. The **Env** gene products encode the outer glycoproteins contained in the envelope of the virus.
         c. The **Pol**-encoded proteins are produced as a precursor polyprotein, which is processed into the enzymes necessary for viral replication (RT, protease, and integrase). The viral **protease**, which is contained in the polyprotein complex itself, is responsible for cleaving the viral capsid proteins and transcriptional enzymes into functional products.
      3. The exact roles of other late regulatory or accessory gene products (**Vpr, Vif, Vpu, Nef**) are under investigation.
II. **HIV-1 life cycle and gene regulation**
   A. Specific sequences of the **gp120** envelope glycoprotein are folded together to form a binding site for the human **CD4$^+$ receptor**, which normally functions as a receptor for the major histocompatibility complex class II (**MHC-II**) molecules. The CD4$^+$ receptor alone is not sufficient for HIV-1 entry into cells. Two additional co-receptors–the C-C chemokine receptor CCR5 and

1

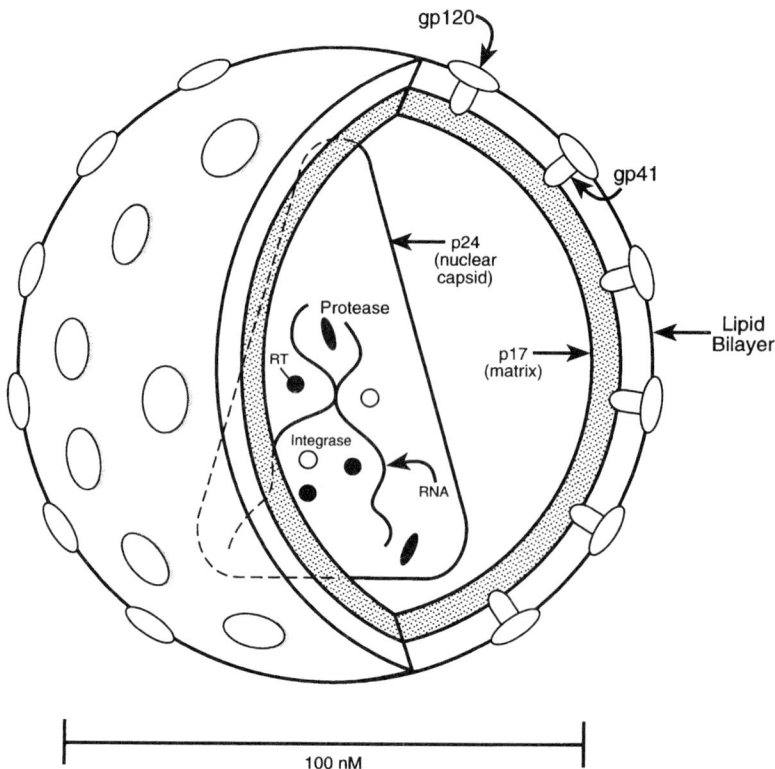

gp120

gp41

p24
(nuclear
capsid)

Protease

Lipid
Bilayer

RT

p17
(matrix)

Integrase

RNA

100 nM

FIG. 1. Structure of the HIV-1 virion. A cone-shaped nucleocapsid containing two strands of RNA and essential replication enzymes is revealed by a "cutaway" of the outer envelope, which is studded with glycoproteins derived from the cellular membrane. gp, glycoprotein; p, protein; RT, reverse transcriptase. (Reproduced with permission from Root RK, Stamm W, Waldvogel F, Corey L, eds. *Clinical infectious diseases: a practical approach.* 1st ed. New York: Oxford University Press, 1998.)

the C-X-C chemokine receptor, CXCR4–have been identified more recently. (Feng et al. *Science* 1996;272:872; Alkhalib et al. *Science* 1996;272:1955). The CCR5 receptor is expressed on monocytes and lymphocytes. The CXCR4 receptor is expressed only on T lymphocytes.

B. Once inside the cell, HIV-1 is uncoated, releasing the genome and multiple copies of RT and integrase into the cytoplasm. Reverse transcription is an ongoing process, likely initiated before cell invasion. RT has multiple functions: RNA-dependent deoxyribonucleic acid (DNA) polymerization, DNA polymerization from a single-stranded DNA intermediate, and RNAse H activity, which degrades the RNA intermediates of reverse transcription. The viral reverse transcriptase is an important target of many agents used for the treatment of HIV-1 infections (see Chapters 5 and 6). Through this complex RT process, a DNA copy of the viral genome is formed and transported into the host-cell nucleus and integrated into the host genome as a **provirus** by the actions of the **integrase** enzyme. The provirus then subverts the cellular machinery to reproduce itself.

C. Gene regulation of proviral transcription involves a complex interplay between viral and cellular signals. For example, **TAT** binds at a specific site of the provirus to upregulate HIV transcription while host cytokines, such as tumor necrosis factorα (**TNF-α**), stimulate pathways leading to increased expression of cellular immune activation factors, which in turn upregulate HIV replication. Host-cellular RNA polymerases form viral messenger RNA (**mRNA**), which is translated by ribosomes into viral proteins. These new viral components, along with RNA copies of the HIV genome, array themselves along the cellular membrane and bud out, forming new infectious progeny.

III. **Virology**

    A. The early characterization of HIV was possible because of the development of culture techniques involving special T-cell lines stimulated by interleukin-2 (IL-2); (Barre-Sinoussi et al. *Science* 1983;220:868), although these methods are often insensitive and inefficient (particularly in asymptomatic patients). Later improvements using activated peripheral blood mononuclear cells (**PBMCs**) demonstrated that infectious virions were present in virtually all patients tested, regardless of disease stage. End-point dilution methods allowed the quantification of virus isolates, which is typically greater by several orders of magnitude in late-stage AIDS cases (viral titers of ~1 in 400 PBMCs or 1 in 40 CD4+ cells) compared with early asymptomatic HIV infection (1 in 50,000 PBMCs; Ho et al. *N Engl J Med* 1989;321:1621). Quantification of infectious virus from plasma, which is generally undetectable in early stages of disease, also demonstrates higher viral burden in later stages of disease and correlates with clinical progression (Coombs et al. *N Engl J Med* 1989;321:1626). HIV-1 culture methods also have been used to develop drug **susceptibility assays** for clinical isolates. Ideally, such techniques should be applicable to a broad range of viral subtypes without providing a clear selective advantage for certain viral subtypes.

    B. HIV-1 isolates are able to bind to the CD4+ receptors of a variety of cells, but productive infection is more narrowly restricted to certain cell types. In fact, different HIV-1 strains have distinct **cell tropisms** that can be characterized along a spectrum from selective **T-cell tropism** (utilizing the CXCR4 co-receptor) to selective **macrophage tropism** (CCR5 co-receptor).[1] Cell tropism may be associated with clinical manifestations; for example, monocyte-tropic HIV-1 subtypes may be more likely to lead to central nervous system complications and may be the predominant variant transmitted from person to person.

    C. Syncytium induction, or the formation of multinucleated giant cells as HIV-1–infected T cells fuse with uninfected cells in culture media, is a distinctive laboratory feature of HIV-1 cellular infection in some cell preparations. There is a trend toward isolation of viruses that do not readily form syncytia [**non–syncytium-inducing (NSI)** viruses] from asymptomatic patients. These viruses are macrophage-tropic. These isolates frequently demonstrate relatively slow, low-level replication *in vitro* and are generally more monocyte-tropic. In contrast, some patients who have more rapid progression to AIDS have a shift in phenotype to the more T lymphocyte-tropic, **syncytium-inducing (SI)** viral isolates that replicate rapidly and to higher levels in culture. Newborn babies exposed to mixed populations of SI and NSI HIV-1 may be more likely to be infected initially with NSI viruses, suggesting that NSI variants have a selective advantage in primary infection. However, some patients are initially infected with SI virus, whereas others seem to have rapidly progressive disease without ever undergoing the NSI-to-SI phenotypic switch, demonstrating that the clinical correlates of viral laboratory characteristics are by no means absolute.

IV. **Molecular biology and viral dynamics**

    A. Molecular virologic techniques have been used to describe the global genetic diversity of HIV-1 isolates. The greatest variability in the HIV-1 genome occurs in the Env gene. Isolates from geographically separated areas may vary by >25% in the envelope sequence. Such differences allow categorization of worldwide HIV-1 isolates into genetic subtypes or **clades,** and studies of the genetic relatedness of viral subtypes contribute to the development of **phylogenetic trees** describing the evolution of viral diversity and the history of the HIV-1 epidemic. Viral diversity is critically important in global research efforts such as vaccine development and diagnostic testing.

B. Molecular methods also have demonstrated that individual patients are infected with a highly related, yet genetically distinct pool of viruses, or **quasispecies.** The coexistence of multiple viral genotypes and the rapid evolution of viral subtypes within a single individual have been well described. Because of the very high rates of viral replication and high frequency of errors during the RT process, the dynamic and complex population of HIV-1, within an individual patient, shifts in response to selective pressures exerted by antiretroviral therapy and immune-system responses. One important example of this genetic diversity is the rapid development of viral resistance to certain antiviral drugs, which correlates with the selection for specific resistance-conferring mutations in the targeted HIV-1 molecular sequence (for example, the RT or protease genes).

C. Highly sensitive, quantitative assays based on the **polymerase chain reaction (PCR)** reveal that high levels of plasma HIV-1 RNA are present at all stages of infection, even at stages of disease when attempts to culture HIV-1 are usually unsuccessful (Piatak et al. *Science* 1993;259:1749). In general, patients recently exposed to HIV-1 have very high **virus load** by PCR (>2 million copies/mL), which decreases by several orders of magnitude concurrent with the development of host-humoral and cellular immune responses; yet circulating virus remains detectable, at lower levels (100 to 50,000 copies/mL), throughout the period of **clinical latency,** which may persist for years. As disease progression ensues, viral burden increases proportionately, reaching levels comparable to acute primary infection in late-stage disease (100,000 to >2 million copies/mL; see Fig. 2). Another technique, the **branched chain DNA (bDNA)** method, is also a sensitive assay for HIV-1 RNA in plasma. The bDNA technique uses amplification of an enzyme-linked immunosorbent

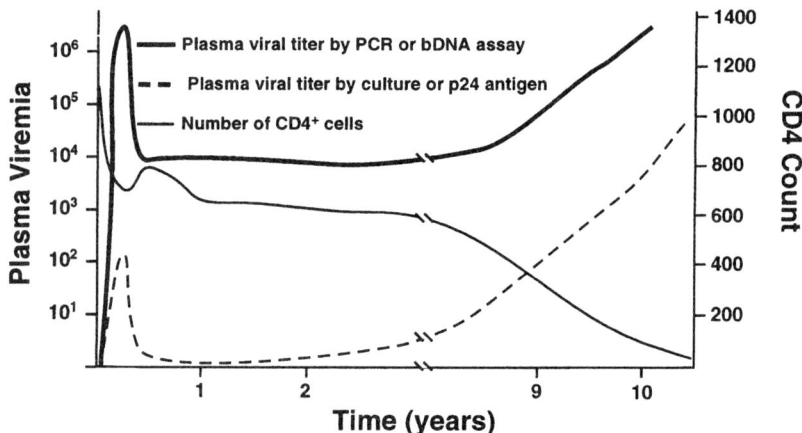

FIG. 2. Changes in viral load (expressed in $\log_{10}$ form on left side of figure from zero to >10⁶ virus copies per milliliter of plasma) and CD4⁺ lymphocyte count (expressed on right side of figure in cells/mm³) over time (years after initial exposure). Note that dotted line approximates the less sensitive, less dynamic assays (culturable virus titer or p24 antigen) previously used as research tools to monitor disease progression.

assay (ELISA) signal from captured viral RNA rather than amplification of the molecular RNA itself (as in PCR techniques). Despite determination of viral load through dramatically different means, the PCR-based and bDNA methods provide remarkably similar results. These dynamic assays reflect the immediate ("real time") status of ongoing viral replication within infected individuals. They are of great value in determining the relative effectiveness of antiretroviral therapy and the relative risk of clinical progression. As a result, the assays facilitate short-term evaluations of therapeutic strategies in both research and clinical practice.

D. Studies involving patients given potent antiretroviral therapies reveal an exponential decrease in plasma HIV-1 RNA during the initial days to weeks of therapy (Wei et al. *Nature* 1995;373:117; Ho et al. *Nature* 1995;373:123). Some patients treated with antiretroviral drugs develop rapid selection for resistant viral variants, and an exponential proliferation of resistant viral variants results in a rapid return to high levels of plasma viremia within weeks of initiating therapy. Mathematical modeling of both the clearance and the reappearance of plasma viral RNA shows that the half-life of plasma HIV-1 is <2 days. This demonstrates that there is ongoing viral replication, even in asymptomatic patients, and that the majority of free virus in the blood derives from de novo cellular infection. The rapid fluctuations in CD4+ cell counts that occur reciprocally with changes in virus load suggest a high degree of CD4+ cell turnover is occurring even in the latest stages of HIV-1 infection. Little is known about the kinetics of CD4+ cell production and destruction, and the rapid increases seen in CD4+ cell counts seen in some patients receiving antiretroviral therapy could result from peripheral proliferation, continual replenishment from a precursor pool, or mobilization of cells from other tissues (i.e., the lymphoreticular system) to the peripheral blood. Peripheral lymphocytes reflect only ~2% of total body lymphocyte pools. Viral replication is ongoing and destructive in the peripheral lymph nodes of patients who are asymptomatic and have low levels of infectious virus in the plasma (Pantaleo et al. *Nature* 1995;362:355–358).

E. With potent therapy, there is rapid clearance of most of the plasma virus; however, a second slower phase of viral decay becomes evident. This phase is believed to represent the more gradual decay of long-lived cells, such as macrophages,[2] as well as latently infected lymphocytes that may become activated to produce virus. Mathematical modeling of this phase suggest that these long-lived cells decay with a half-life of 14 days.

F. Evidence for two phases with relatively short half lives raised hopes that prolonged treatment could potentially completely eliminate virus from cellular compartments and thus potentially cure infection. However, more recent data have confirmed that HIV-1 is **latent** within **long-lived memory T cells**, and that this pool of cells is not affected by currently available treatment. Thus, this compartment can serve as a source of virus over a long period of time, making it highly unlikely that current treatment strategies can be administered long enough to completely eradicate HIV-1 from infected persons.

V. Mechanisms of immunosuppression in HIV-1 infection. Although CD4+ depletion is the most clinically familiar laboratory finding in AIDS, diverse qualitative and quantitative effects of HIV-1 can be found in the humoral and cellular immune responses. Many HIV-1–infected individuals with relatively high CD4+ cell counts are anergic to skin testing, suggesting that cellular immune defects are more complex than a simple decrease in T-helper cell numbers. Antibody responses, to vaccinations for example, are frequently suboptimal even before AIDS develops in patients infected with HIV-1. Surprisingly, little is known about the pathogenic pathway that leads to CD4+ depletion during HIV-1 infection. **Apoptosis,** or programmed cell death, can be triggered by the binding of a primed T cell to **gp120**, and this mechanism is a potential explanation for the rapid loss of CD4+ cells when virus load increases in plasma (Newell et al. *Nature* 1990;347:286; Meyaard et al. *Science* 1992;257:217). CD4+ cell counts may be maintained for many years because of ongoing repletion of the continuously destroyed cells and not because of latent or nonpathogenic infection.

2. ACUTE HIV INFECTION

The majority of individuals with human immunodeficiency virus (HIV) infection are diagnosed years after acquiring the retrovirus. However, the clinician may encounter a patient who, by virtue of the presenting symptoms or after a potential exposure, may be acutely infected with HIV. Recognition of the clinical presentation of primary HIV infection and understanding the management of those potentially exposed to HIV are essential if attempts at early medical intervention and counseling are to be initiated.

I. **Primary HIV infection** may be symptomatic in as many as 50% to 90% of persons after initial exposure to HIV. The constellation of clinical manifestations associated with acquisition of HIV are often described as "flu-like" and usually occur 2 to 4 weeks after infection, coinciding with the acute widespread dissemination of the retrovirus. Symptoms persist for 2 to 4 weeks and begin to resolve with the decline in HIV viral load after the development of cytotoxic T lymphocytes and HIV-specific antibodies. As the clinical presentation is often nonspecific, **the diagnosis of primary HIV infection requires a high index of suspicion and must be considered in any person with an acute febrile illness and a history of recent potential HIV exposure.**

A. **Diagnosis**

1. The **clinical manifestations** of symptomatic primary HIV infection are myriad and most often include the acute onset of fever, generalized lymphadenopathy, pharyngitis, erythematous maculopapular rash, arthralgias, myalgias, retroorbital headache, malaise, diarrhea, nausea, and vomiting. **Oral or genital ulceration**, or both, are diagnostically valuable, but are detected in fewer than 40% of patients with clinical illness (Kinloch-de Loes S, et al. *Clin Infect Dis* 1993;17:59). Severe neurologic manifestations including aseptic meningitis, encephalitis, the Guillain–Barré syndrome, facial palsy, cauda equina syndrome, brachial neuritis, and peripheral neuropathy may occur, demonstrating the neurotropism of HIV. In contrast to mononucleosis, with which it is often confused, **primary HIV infection typically occurs acutely** and, in over half of cases, without atypical lymphocytosis or exudative pharyngitis (Tindall B, Cooper DA. *AIDS* 1991;5:1). **Opportunistic infections** have been reported rarely during acute HIV infection and include oral and esophageal candidiasis, cerebral toxoplasmosis, and *Pneumocystis carinii* pneumonia. During the history, recent potential HIV exposures such as unprotected sex with a new partner or needle sharing may be obtained. Health-care workers may relate a history of recent percutaneous injury or mucous membrane exposure involving blood.

2. **Laboratory evaluation** within the first 2 weeks of acute HIV infection is characterized by **lymphopenia** with reduction of both the CD4$^+$ and CD8$^+$ cell subsets. Total lymphocyte counts decrease to <1,000 cells/mm^3 a median of 9 days after the onset of symptoms (*Br Med J* 1988;297:1363). A complete blood count (CBC) with differential and lymphocyte-subset analysis should be obtained at the time of presentation. The CD4$^+$ cell count during this period may decrease to <200 cells/mm^3. Three to 4 weeks after HIV infection, lymphocytosis develops, reflecting a dramatic increase in CD8$^+$ lymphocytes and, to a lesser extent, CD4$^+$ cells, leading to sustained inversion of the CD4$^+$:CD8$^+$ ratio. CD4$^+$ counts typically recover to within 200 cells/mm^3 of preinfection levels, but begin a gradual decline over the ensuing months to years. **Mild thrombocytopenia** can be seen after acute HIV infection, but rarely leads to clinically significant bleeding. Reports of increased creatine phosphokinase and even rhabdomyolysis have been described during acute HIV infection.

a. **HIV-specific antibody** screening should be performed whenever HIV infection is suspected; however, during the first weeks after acute HIV infection, HIV antibodies are usually not detectable by standard enzyme-linked immunosorbent assay (ELISA) or Western blot. Serial HIV-antibody testing should be performed to confirm seroconversion 6 weeks, 3 months, and 6 months after presentation.

b. **Serum HIV p24 antigen** detection is currently the most widely used and cheapest laboratory method to diagnose primary HIV infection prior to seroconversion. High levels of p24 antigenemia can be present as early as 24 hours following exposure (Kessler HA, et al. *JAMA* 1987;258:1196). During seroconversion, immune complexes form, lowering p24 antigen levels as antibody titers rise. Therefore, HIV p24 antigen may be undetectable in as many as 20% to 40 % of individuals with acute symptomatic HIV infection (Kinloch-de Loes S, et al. *Clin Infect Dis* 1993;17:59). If HIV infection is strongly suspected, despite lack of p24 antigenemia, qualitative HIV RNA by PCR should be performed. False positive p24 antigen detection can occur, especially in persons with connective tissue disorders and organ transplant recipients.

c. **HIV RNA** or **branched DNA (bDNA) polymerase chain reaction (PCR)** or branched DNA signal amplification may reveal high levels of HIV genomes in plasma prior to seroconversion and may have superior sensitivity compared to p24 antigen detection. HIV RNA PCR is widely used to predict HIV disease progression and assess antiretroviral activity, but is not approved by the FDA for use in the diagnosis of HIV infection. HIV RNA and DNA levels which initially, after acute infection, may be measured in the millions per milliliter can decline dramatically during seroconversion. It is important to note that all quantitative methods for measuring HIV RNA or DNA have a lower limit of detection below which the test can not yield a quantitative result.

d. **Screening for sexually or parenterally transmitted diseases** (or both) must be performed during the initial assessment and should include **hepatitis B, hepatitis C,** and **syphilis** serology. Culture for gonorrhea and screening for other sexually transmitted diseases should be performed if indicated by either the history or physical examination. Conversely, individuals with these sexually transmitted diseases should be screened for HIV infection.

3. **Differential diagnoses of primary HIV infection** include viral hepatitis, toxoplasmosis, rubella, infectious mononucleosis caused by Epstein–Barr virus (EBV) or cytomegalovirus (CMV), disseminated gonococcal infection, secondary syphilis, herpes simplex virus infection, Lyme disease, drug reactions, and connective tissue diseases.

4. **Management of primary HIV infection.** The most essential element in the management of acute HIV infection is its early recognition. Therapeutic interventions and counseling can be undertaken only if the diagnosis is considered.

a. **Medical intervention** with combination antiretroviral therapy can be considered. Several studies using antiretroviral therapy, initiated at the time of or shortly after the diagnosis of seroconversion, have indicated that treatment will slow progression of HIV disease and delay the onset of symptoms (including relatively minor problems such as shingles or thrush). Enthusiasm for initial treatment has also been engendered by preliminary studies that suggest that potent antiretroviral therapy may preserve immune responses to HIV-1 that tend to be lost early in infection, again potentially slowing disease progression. However, most patients with acute HIV-1 infection will have a relatively slow progression to AIDS (median time of 10 years) even in the absence of therapy. A small percentage, 5% to 8%, will have little or no progression in the absence of therapy.

Combination antiretroviral therapy is complicated, requires strict adherence, and has both short-term and long-term side effects (see Chapter 6). Furthermore, treatment is almost certainly for life, which may be a daunting prospect given that most acute infections occur in adolescents and young adults. It should also be noted that, to date, no study has shown that starting treatment immediately at diagnosis is a better strategy than waiting sometime later in the infection, e.g., 5 to 10 years later when the rate of progression is more clearly established. **The decision to initiate treatment should not be undertaken lightly.** Given the complexity of the management of acute HIV infection, the rapidity with which new data are generated regarding antiretroviral therapies, and the potential for clinical trial enrollment, all patients with acute HIV infection should ideally be referred to a practitioner who specializes in HIV/AIDS care or a tertiary care facility with an AIDS center.

If treatment is started, a potent combination regimen designed to completely suppress viral replication should be used (see Chapter 6). Recent studies have shown a relatively high rate of resistance to one or more antiretroviral agents among patients with acute infection. Therefore, **genotypic or phenotypic testing** of the viral isolate for evidence of resistance should be done to guide optimal therapy.

   b. **Counseling** is an integral part of the care of patients with acute HIV infection. The diagnosis of HIV infection for many patients may precipitate an **emotional crisis** characterized by anxiety, depression, adjustment disorder, suicidal ideation, or brief reactive psychosis. The assistance of a mental health professional may be necessary in cases of severe depression or when the patient is suicidal. Psychoeducational interventions consisting of individual training sessions aimed at stress reduction have been an effective method of reducing patient distress after HIV testing (Perry S, et al. *Arch Gen Psychiatry* 1991;48:143). In addition to stress control and personal support, patients require guidance concerning the variable natural history of HIV infection, partner-notification responsibilities, financial assistance, informational resources, substance-abuse counseling when indicated, and **safer sex** and **injecting practices**. In some states, health-care providers are mandated by law to advise HIV-seropositive patients of safer sex and injecting procedures. Given the chronic nature of HIV infection and the establishment of early medical care, a hopeful outlook can be presented to the patient. Scheduled medical follow-up also provides opportunities to reinforce early counseling and to offer the reassurance of continued care.

II. Occupational HIV exposure is a rare but much feared hazard to health-care personnel. The majority of infections acquired as a result of occupational exposure occurred percutaneously through **needlesticks** or other instruments contaminated with blood; however, **mucocutaneous transmission** of HIV also has been documented. The risk of HIV infection after percutaneous injury is estimated to be 0.25% and is dramatically less for mucocutaneous exposure (Gerberding JL. *N Engl J Med* 1995;332:444). To date, all exposures resulting in HIV infection of health-care clinicians have involved blood or blood-containing fluids. The decision to recommend HIV postexposure prophylaxis must take into account the nature of the exposure and the amount of blood or body fluid involved in the exposure (Table 1). Other considerations include the potential for exposure to virus known or suspected to be resistant to antiretroviral drugs. If postexposure prophylaxis is to be successful, health care facilities must have systems in place for the timely evaluation and management of exposed health-care workers and for consultation with experts in the treatment of HIV.

   A. Risk assessment. Exposures posing risks to health-care providers include percutaneous injuries with sharp objects contaminated with blood or blood-

Table 2-1 Recommendations for prophylaxis for occupational exposure to HIV disease

Type of Injury	Status of source patient		
	Asymptomatic	Symptomatic	Acute infection Advanced AIDS High viral load
PERCUTANEOUS INJURIES			
Superficial injury	Offer	Recommend	Strongly encourage
Visible blood Used in artery or vein	Recommend	Recommend	Strongly encourage
Deep IM exposure; injection	Strongly encourage	Strongly encourage	Strongly encourage
MUCOSAL EXPOSURE			
Small volume Brief duration	Offer	Offer	Offer
Large volume OR long duration	Recommend	Recommend	Recommend
Large volume AND long duration	Recommend	Recommend	Strongly encourage

containing fluids and mucous membrane or cutaneous contact with blood, tissues, or other body fluids to which universal precautions apply (*MMWR* 1998;47:RR-7).

1. **Percutaneous HIV exposures,** with large inoculum volumes of blood or bloody fluid, increase the risk of HIV transmission. Factors associated with an increased risk of HIV acquisition following percutaneous exposure to HIV-infected blood identified in a multinational case-control study of health care workers included depth of tissue penetration, the presence of visible blood on the penetrating device, injuries occurring with devices previously in the vein or artery of the source patient (hollow bore needles), and advanced HIV disease of the source patient (Cardo DM, et al. *N Engl J Med* 1997;337:1485). The use of latex gloves during simulated needlesticks has been demonstrated to reduce transferred blood volume by 46% to 86% (Mast ST, et al. *J Infect Dis* 1993;168:1589). Following potential percutaneous HIV exposure, information regarding the needle gauge and type, degree of penetration, injection of contaminated fluid, clinical stage of the source patient, and use of gloves should be obtained. These are used in combination to assess the risk of true exposure and the need for prophylaxis (Table 1)

2. **Mucocutaneous HIV exposure** presents a substantially lower risk of HIV transmission than does percutaneous exposure (Gerberding JL. *N Engl J Med* 1995;332:444). Factors associated with the few instances of mucocutaneous HIV transmission include contamination of open wounds, mucous membrane splashes, and prolonged physical contact with infected blood. HIV infection through intact skin has not been documented.

B. **Management of exposures to HIV** should be initiated as promptly as possible after potential inoculation.

1. **First aid** for needle-stick or other contaminated cutaneous wounds consists of washing the area with soap and clean water. Open wounds should be irrigated with sterile saline. Mucous membranes should be flushed with copious amounts of water, and eyes irrigated with clean water, sterile saline, or eyewash preparations (Gerberding JL, Henderson DK. *Clin*

Infect Dis 1992;14:1179). No data exist to support the use of bleach, iodophors, peroxides, or other germicidal preparations for wound care in preventing HIV transmission. The use of antiseptics is not contraindicated; however, the application of caustic agents (e.g., bleach) is not recommended.

2. **Documentation** of the circumstances of the exposure is essential and required if claims for Worker's Compensation or other benefits are to be made by the exposed health-care worker. Such reporting may also help identify deficiencies in infection-control procedures. The **confidentiality of the exposed health-care provider should be protected** during the initial evaluation and at all phases of follow-up. This may require the filing of the exposed provider's records separately from the general medical record and the labeling of laboratory samples without data that could directly identify the employee.

3. **Laboratory evaluation** after occupational HIV exposure entails the screening of both the source individual and the exposed health-care worker for HIV and other blood-borne infections including hepatitis B and C.

   a. **The source individual** should be evaluated for HIV infection.
      (1) If the source is known to have HIV infection, available information about the stage of infection (i.e., asymptomatic or AIDS), CD4+ cell count, results of viral load testing, and current and previous antiretroviral therapy, should be obtained if available.
      (2) If the HIV status of the source individual at the time of the exposure is unknown, HIV-antibody testing of this individual should be performed once informed consent has been obtained and pretest counseling completed. If the source individual is unwilling or unable to consent to HIV testing, institution policies and state and local laws regarding HIV testing should be adhered to and the confidentiality of the source individual protected.
         (a) A rapid HIV antibody test may be particularly useful in this setting.
         (b) The nature of the exposure, the conditions of the exposure (e.g., a nursing home for the elderly as opposed to a drug rehabilitation center) and the prevalence of HIV infection in the community may be factors in allowing an assessment of possibility of exposure to HIV.

   b. **The exposed health-care provider** should undergo baseline HIV-antibody testing when the source patient is HIV seropositive or of unknown HIV status. If HIV testing is deferred, the employee should have serum banked in case future testing is desired. If the health-care worker is HIV seronegative at baseline, HIV testing should be repeated at 6 weeks, 3 months, and 6 months after exposure. No health-care worker has been reported to seroconvert beyond 6 months after exposure. Exposed individuals must be advised to return if symptoms of primary HIV infection develop so that repeated HIV serology and HIV p24 antigen detection can be obtained.

4. **Other blood-borne pathogens** including **hepatitis B** and **hepatitis C** can be occupationally acquired with or without concomitant HIV transmission. The source patient should be evaluated for the presence of hepatitis B surface antigen and hepatitis C antibody. Health-care providers not known to be immune to hepatitis B (through natural infection or documented adequate immunization response) should have hepatitis B surface antibody (anti-HBs) titers and baseline hepatitis B surface antigen (HBsAg) drawn, and be administered hepatitis B vaccine if there is no serologic evidence of hepatitis B immunity. Hepatitis B immune globulin (HBIG) is recommended when the source patient is HBsAg positive and the exposed person does not have protective anti-HBs titers. Hepatitis C antibody testing is indicated in all exposed health-

care workers when the hepatitis C antibody status of the source patient is positive or unknown. There is no effective prophylaxis for hepatitis C.
5. **Postexposure prophylaxis.** The ideal prophylactic agent should have potent antiretroviral effect, be distributed throughout the body, have no toxicity as most of those receiving the drug will not be infected and must act rapidly to prevent disseminated infection. Due to the relatively low incidence of occupationally acquired HIV infection, controlled trials of antiretroviral postexposure prophylaxis have been limited. No randomized controlled trial has been undertaken and it is very unlikely that one ever will. However, studies demonstrating the ability of antiretroviral therapy to significantly decrease maternal-fetal HIV transmission and the effectiveness of the treatment during primary HIV infection bolster arguments favoring its use as a postexposure prophylaxis agent. A retrospective case-controlled study of 700 health-care workers exposed to HIV infected blood has also demonstrated a protective effect of antiretroviral therapy (in this case, zidovudine, ZDV). Of those health-care workers who did not seroconvert following exposure to HIV, 247 (36%) used ZDV prophylactically. In this study, the risk of HIV infection among health-care workers who used ZDV was reduced by approximately 79% (Cardo DM, et al. *N Engl J Med*, 1997;337:1485).
   a. The decision to use antiretroviral therapy can be based on the nature of exposure and assessment of the risk (Table 1). In general, a percutaneous injury that involves an exposure to a patient with advanced disease or one known to have a high viral load, should lead to a strong recommendation for initiation of prophylaxis. Where there is doubt, the initial reaction ought to be to start prophylaxis as reassessment of its need can follow later.
   b. The U.S. Public Health Service has formulated guidelines for the management of occupational exposure to HIV *(MMWR* 1998;47:RR-7). Most exposures that warrant postexposure prophylaxis need only a two-drug regimen—the **combination of ZDV (300 mg b.i.d.), and 3TC (150 mg b.i.d). The addition of a protease inhibitor (nelfinavir 1250 mg b.i.d. or indinavir, 800 mg t.i.d.)** is recommended, according to these guidelines, for health-care workers with the highest risk HIV exposures, such as those sustaining deep-penetrating injuries with hollow bore needles visibly contaminated with a large volume of blood from a patient with advanced AIDS. Postexposure antiretroviral prophylaxis for exposures involving intact skin or non-bloody body fluids other than semen; vaginal secretions; cerebrospinal, synovial, pleural, peritoneal, pericardial and amniotic fluid is not justified.
   c. The **optimal duration** of postexposure treatment is currently unknown. As 4 weeks of ZDV administration appears to be effective, postexposure prophylaxis should be continued for 4 weeks, if tolerated.
   d. Postexposure prophylaxis should be **initiated as soon as possible** following the exposure and **ideally within 1 to 2 hours**. There is no outside time limit for initiating therapy, however, treatment delayed more than 24 hours is not likely to be effective in aborting infection. As a result, it is usually prudent to start prophylaxis soon after the exposure, while gathering information. If circumstances become clearer and it becomes apparent that prophylaxis is not necessary, it can be readily discontinued.
   e. **Other antiretroviral agents.** Concern that HIV transmitted from patients being treated with antiretroviral therapy may be antiretroviral resistant has prompted some to recommend that postexposure prophylaxis regimens contain, when possible, two agents not used by the source patient. Many also advocate the substitution of the protease inhibitor in the above postexposure "cocktail" with the non-nucleoside reverse transcriptase inhibitor, nevirapine, which has

been demonstrated to dramatically and rapidly decrease HIV viral load in those infected with the virus and has been shown to be highly effective in prevention of perinatal transmission.

f. Adverse effects. All persons receiving prophylactic antiretroviral therapy should receive information regarding the efficacy of these medications in this setting and of the **potential toxicities** associated with these agents (see Chapter 5). Close clinical monitoring should be part of any postexposure protocol. Women should have pregnancy tests, and if pregnant, counseling about the potential risk to the fetus from antiretroviral agents (see Chapter 9).

g. Establishment of a postexposure protocol is essential for optimal management of occupational exposures to HIV and should be implemented in all cases of exposure. In most institutions postexposure management decisions are made by an occupational health service. Such a service should be accessible 24 hours a day, be staffed by personnel familiar with the latest information concerning exposure to blood-borne pathogens, and be dedicated to protecting the confidentiality of the health-care worker and the source patient.

6. **Counseling of health-care workers exposed to HIV** must include advice concerning the risk of transmission for a given exposure, postexposure prophylaxis, follow-up medical and laboratory evaluations, and assurances of confidentiality. Exposed workers must also be informed regarding the necessity of practicing safer sex during the 6-month HIV antibody–testing period. Likewise, women should defer pregnancy and breastfeeding, and all employees must be advised to refrain from semen, blood, or organ donation until HIV infection has been ruled out. Counseling of exposed workers, their families, and their sexual partners may require the assistance of mental health professionals well versed in the psychological dynamics of occupational HIV exposure.

C. Universal precautions reduce the risk of occupational HIV exposure. Use of barrier protection during procedures in which there is a risk of contact with potentially infectious body fluids is the mainstay of universal precautions and includes the wearing of gloves, gowns, masks, and protective eyewear when appropriate. The avoidance of situations in which penetrating injuries with contaminated instruments are possible, such as **needle recapping**, the adoption of **double gloving** during surgical procedures, and the development of **proper sharps disposal systems** further decrease the occupational hazard of HIV infection. Devices designed to reduce the risk of needlestick accidents have been developed and include blunted suture needles and sleeved phlebotomy needles, both of which have been found to reduce the incidence of percutaneous injuries.

III. **Nonoccupational exposure to HIV** is obviously more common than occupational and is increasingly coming to medical attention. The success of postexposure prophylaxis for occupational injury has led some clinicians to offer antiretroviral drugs to persons with unanticipated sexual or injecting-drug-use HIV exposure to prevent transmission. However, no data exist regarding the efficacy of this therapy for persons with nonoccupational HIV exposure, and as yet this strategy remains unproven. If antiretroviral drugs are used after nonoccupational HIV exposures that carry a high risk for infection, it should be done in the context of appropriate counseling of the patient, not only about the uncertainties of the treatment, but also advice concerning the circumstances in which the exposure occurred [*MMWR* 1998; 47(No. RR-17)].

A. Exposed individuals should be evaluated for **sexually transmitted diseases (STDs) and substance abuse.** If victims of sexual assault, they should receive additional evaluation and counseling. Women at risk for unintended pregnancy should be offered emergency contraception. Persons with possible HIV exposure through percutaneous routes from sharing syringes or needles should be assessed for hepatitis B and hepatitis C virus infections and considered for hepatitis B virus vaccination.

B. Persons with nonoccupational HIV exposures should receive medical evaluations, including HIV-antibody tests at baseline and periodically for at least 6 months after exposure (e.g., at 4 to 6 weeks, 12 weeks, and 6 months). They should be counseled regarding protective behaviors to prevent additional exposure and to prevent possible secondary transmission if they become infected while receiving antiretroviral therapy.

C. If antiretroviral therapy is being given, it needs to be **prompt**. Animal studies indicate that antiretroviral agents are most effective within 1 to 2 hours of exposure and probably not effective when started later than 24 to 36 hours after exposure.

D. The choice of **antiretroviral therapy** should be made based on the nature of exposure and the likelihood of resistance. Regimens similar to those used in occupational exposure (II.B.5 above) can be used. Follow-up for side effects and additional counseling about risk avoidance is essential.

3. NATURAL HISTORY

The human immunodeficiency virus-1 (HIV-1) causes a chronic infection that leads to profound immunosuppression. The course of the infection may vary somewhat, with some individuals developing immunodeficiency within 2 to 3 years and others remaining acquired immunodeficiency syndrome (AIDS) free for 10 to 15 years. This appears to be influenced by host and viral factors. A common clinical pattern is well recognized. The virus is transmitted, and acute symptomatic HIV infection may occur. This is typically followed by a period of clinical latency of varying duration. Eventually the infected individual develops early symptomatic HIV, which progresses to AIDS and its associated opportunistic infections and malignancies. The definition of AIDS is based on the revised 1993 Centers for Disease Control (CDC) classification (CDC. *MMWR* 1992;41:RR-17). This course is paralleled by ongoing viral replication during all stages of the infection (Fig. 1). It is estimated that half of the virus population is cleared and replenished every 2 days (Ho DD. *Nature* 1995;373:123–126). The level of plasma viremia during primary infection is high, and the virus population is relatively homogeneous. Viral replication continues in the lymphoid tissue during the stages of clinical latency and early symptomatic disease, as evidenced by the progressive decline in CD4+ T cells. In late-stage disease, there is a high level of plasma viremia and, in contrast to that in the primary infection, the population of virions is diverse. The high level of viral replication, combined with the spontaneous rate of mutation of essential genes, such as HIV-1 reverse transcriptase, gives rise to the diversity. This results in rapid development of resistance to single-agent therapy with nucleoside analog reverse transcriptase inhibitors such as zidovudine. Combination antiviral therapy may be more effective as it will force the virus to mutate simultaneously at two or more sites on any given viral genome, possibly delaying resistance. The CDC classification of HIV disease is based on CD4+ cell counts and the presence of constitutional symptoms, opportunistic infections, and neoplasia (Table 1). The CD4+ cell count is the best predictive marker for the risk of developing HIV-related complications. The natural history can be divided into the initial infection and four other categories based on the CD4+ cell count: primary HIV infection (acute HIV seroconverting illness); asymptomatic disease (CD4+ count >500 cells/mm³); early symptomatic disease (CD4+ count between 200 and 500 cells/mm³); late symptomatic disease (CD4+ cell count between 50 and 200 cells/mm³); and advanced disease (CD4+ count <50 cells/mm³).

I. **Acquisition of infection.** The major routes of transmission of HIV-1 are sexual contact, parenteral exposure to blood and blood products, and vertical transmission during pregnancy (*MMWR* 1992;41:RR-18). The rate of progression of the infection depends on a number of factors, including the route of transmission. Time to development of AIDS appears to be most rapid in recipients of blood transfusion at 7 years, compared with an average of 10 years in hemophiliacs and 10 to 12 years in homosexual men. HIV-2 has the same route of infection as HIV-1, but appears to be transmitted at a lower rate and to have a slower rate of progression.

II. Primary HIV infection (see Chapter 2).

III. **Asymptomatic HIV infection** (early-stage disease; CD4+, >500 cells/mm³).
  A. **Clinical features.** As the stage implies, the patient does not have any HIV-related symptoms. Clinical manifestations include persistent generalized lymphadenopathy (PGL), involving two or more sites, and skin manifestations such as seborrheic dermatitis. Even though this is a period of clinical latency, there is a high rate of viral replication in lymphatic tissue, as reflected by a gradual decrease in the CD4+ cell count (Fig. 1).
  B. **Duration.** May depend on the route of acquisition of the infection, the age of the patient, the virulence of the virus, and other unidentified factors. It may range from 2 to >15 years, with an average of 7 to 10 years.
  C. **Laboratory tests.** The CD4+ cell count is usually >500 cells/mm³. The rate of decline of the CD4+ cell count is 40 to 80 cells/mm³ per year on average

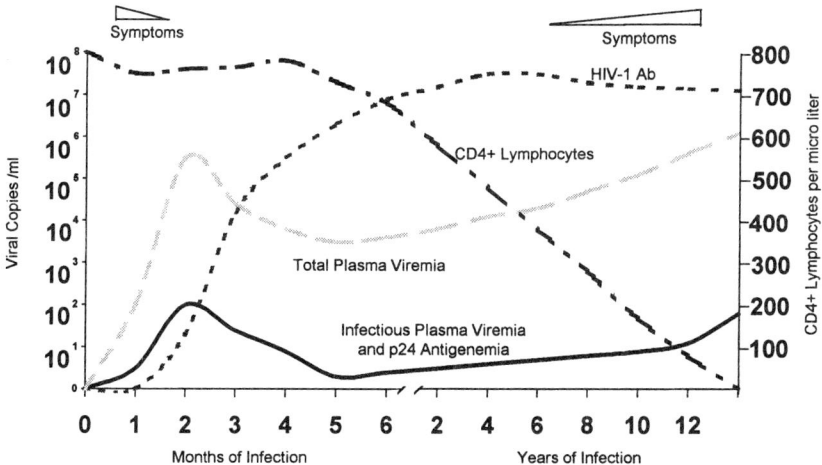

FIG. 1. Natural history of human immunodeficiency virus-1 infection.

without antiretroviral therapy. Mild abnormalities in complete blood count (CBC) and increases in transaminases may be seen. Free virus in the plasma is detected by polymerase chain reaction (PCR) or branched DNA signal amplification.

    D. Management. CBC, CD4+ cell count, and HIV RNA viral load should be obtained every 6 months to look for evidence of disease progression. Toxoplasma immunoglobulin G (IgG), syphilis serology (VDRL/RPR), and tuberculin skin test should be obtained yearly. The patient should be educated on the future use of antiretroviral therapies (see Chapter 6). In some circumstances, where the plasma HIV RNA is very high (>30,000 copies/mL) and the rate of fall of CD4+ lymphocytes is more rapid than usual, consideration can be given to initiation of antiviral therapy even at CD4+ counts > 500 cells/mm³. Nutrition counseling and daily multivitamins are recommended.

IV. Early symptomatic HIV disease (CD4+, 200 to 500/mm³)

    A. Clinical features. Most patients remain asymptomatic or have mild features of disease. Clinical manifestations, previously known as AIDS-related complex (ARC), and more recently referred to as "B symptoms" (Table 1), may start to appear. These are not AIDS-indicator conditions, but represent disease progression and may be more common in patients with higher viral loads. **Constitutional symptoms** include fever, unexplained weight loss, recurrent diarrhea, fatigue, and headache. **Cutaneous manifestations** include seborrheic dermatitis, folliculitis, recurrent vulvovaginal candidiasis, oral candidiasis, herpes zoster, recurrent herpes simplex infection, and oral hairy leukoplakia. Sinusitis, bronchitis, and pneumonia caused by community-acquired organisms such as *Streptococcus pneumoniae*, *Haemophilus influenzae*, and *Mycoplasma pneumonia* may occur. Idiopathic thrombocytopenic purpura, Kaposi's sarcoma, pulmonary tuberculosis, and cervical dysplasia may be seen at this stage. PGL (see IIIa), described previously, may be found, but it is not predictive of disease progression.

    B. Laboratory tests. CD4+ cell counts should be performed every 3 to 6 months. The trend is downward with counts <200 cells/mm³ representing increased risk for developing opportunistic infections and malignancies. HIV viral load should be measured with CD4+ counts. Blood-count abnormalities such as

Table 3-1 1993 revised classification for HIV infection and expanded case definition for AIDS in adolescents and adults

CD4 cell count	A	B	C
>500/mm^3 (>29%)	A1	B1	C1
200 to 499/mm^3 (14% to 28%)	A2	B2	C2
<200/mm^3 (<14%)	A3	B3	C3

CATEGORY A
Asymptomatic HIV infection
Persistent generalized lymphadenopathy
Acute retroviral syndrome

CATEGORY B
Bacillary angiomatosis
Oral or recurrent vulvovaginal candidiasis
Cervical dysplasia
Constitutional symptoms (fever of 38.5°C, diarrhea >1 month)
Oral hairy leukoplakia
Herpes zoster
Idiopathic thrombocytopenic purpura (ITP)
Listeriosis
Pelvic inflammatory disease (PID)
Peripheral neuropathy

CATEGORY C (AIDS-DEFINING CONDITIONS)
CD4 count <200 cells/mm^3
Candidiasis of esophagus, pulmonary
Cervical cancer^a
Coccidioidomycosis
Cryptococcosis, extrapulmonary
Cryptosporidosis
Cytomegalovirus infection
Herpes simplex with esophageal, pulmonary, or mucocutaneous involvement
    of >1 month
Histoplasmosis
HIV encephalopathy
Isosporiasis
Kaposi's sarcoma
Lymphoma
Mycobacterium avium complex or *M. kansasii*
Mycobacterium tuberculosis^a
Pneumocystis carinii pneumonia
Pneumonia, recurrent with more than two episodes in 12 months^a
Progressive multifocal encephalopathy
Salmonellosis
Toxoplasmosis

^{a} Added in the 1993 Centers for Disease Control revised case definition.

anemia, leukopenia, thrombocytopenia, and mild elevations in transaminases are seen. Hypergammaglobulinemia, reflecting polyclonal B cell activation, can occur.

C. **Management**

1. **Antiviral therapy.** Institution of antiretroviral therapy is often recommended whether the patient is symptomatic or not. Most experts favor treating all patients with plasma HIV RNA levels >30,000 copies/mL and all patients with CD4+ counts <350 cells/mm³. Patients with lower viral loads and higher CD4+ counts may be considered for treatment. It should be recognized however, that, to date, no studies have demonstrated that starting patients on treatment is superior in clinical outcome to a policy of waiting until the CD4+ count is lower. Approach to antiviral therapy is discussed in Chapter 6.

2. The presence of oropharyngeal candidiasis or an unexplained fever for >2 weeks is an indication to begin antibiotic prophylaxis against *Pneumocystis carinii* pneumonia (PCP). Primary prophylaxis of opportunistic infections is discussed in Chapter 4.

D. **Prognosis.** An infected individual has a 20% to 30% chance of developing an AIDS-defining illness within the next 18 to 24 months if not receiving antiviral therapy. With treatment the risk of progressing is reduced by at least 50%.

V. **Late symptomatic HIV disease** (CD4+ count, 50 to 200/mm³)

A. **Clinical features.** The risk of developing an AIDS-related opportunistic infection or malignancy substantially increases with a CD4+ cell <200 cells/mm³ (Table 1). Common examples are PCP, *Toxoplasma gondii* encephalitis, disseminated *Mycobacterium avium* complex infection, esophageal candidiasis, lymphoma, and Kaposi's sarcoma. Persistent or progressive constitutional symptoms may occur, as described in early symptomatic infection. Fever may indicate the presence of an underlying opportunistic infection and may be associated with other features that may help focus an evaluation. Other features of late disease are AIDS-related wasting, neurologic disease such as peripheral neuropathy, and AIDS dementia complex.

B. **Laboratory tests** are characterized by:

1. Declining CD4+ count <200 cells/mm³.

2. Anemia, leukopenia, and thrombocytopenia. This may be drug-related or reflect underlying infection or malignancy.

3. Isolated elevation of lactate dehydrogenase (LDH) and globulin may be seen.

4. An elevation in creatinine with proteinuria may result from HIV-associated nephropathy.

C. **Management** should be directed toward prevention, diagnosis, and treatment of opportunistic infections. Antiretroviral therapy is **indicated in all patients** who have never received therapy. Potent antiretroviral therapy that suppresses viral replication has been shown to dramatically decrease mortality in patients with AIDS. Many patients have significant rises in CD4+ lymphocyte counts with reversal of immunodeficiency.

1. Current recommendations for primary and secondary prophylaxis against opportunistic infections based on CDC/IDSA recommendations are discussed in Chapter 4.

2. Early diagnosis of opportunistic infections and malignancies such as cervical and rectal neoplasia, lymphoma, and Kaposi's sarcoma may depend on careful periodic examination, as discussed in Chapter 29.

3. Antiretroviral therapy is recommended, as discussed in Chapters 5 and 6. The goal of therapy is to maintain viral replication below detectable levels. Many studies have demonstrated continued clinical and immunological benefit in patients receiving potent antiretroviral therapy, even when viral replication is not completely suppressed.

4. Symptomatic treatment of diarrhea and other constitutional symptoms may be indicated. Management of weight loss is crucial to the patient's future well-being.

D. **Prognosis.** One half to 75% of patients will develop an AIDS-related condition within 18 to 24 months in the absence of treatment. Weight loss, history of oral candidiasis, and lower hemoglobin levels were independent predictors of progression to AIDS. Overall survival has improved since the introduction of antibiotic prophylaxis against opportunistic infections (Hoover DR et al. *N Engl J Med* 1993;329:1922–1926) and the use of potent antiretroviral therapy.

VI. **Advanced HIV disease** (CD4$^+$ count, <50 cells/mm^3)

A. **Clinical features.** As in late symptomatic HIV infection, this includes all AIDS-defining opportunistic infections and malignancies. Certain opportunistic infections are more likely to occur with profound immunosuppression such as disseminated *M. avium* complex infection, cytomegalovirus (CMV) retinitis, cryptococcal meningitis, disseminated histoplasmosis, progressive multifocal leukoencephalopathy (PML), and cervical dysplasia. Typically the patient may develop coexisting infections. Neurologic disease is more prevalent at this stage of the infection and may manifest as AIDS dementia complex, primary CNS lymphoma, or infections such as PML and CMV. AIDS wasting syndrome with a weight loss of >10% of ideal body weight is common. The origin is often multifactorial and may reflect a combination of decreased caloric intake, increased catabolism, and malabsorption.

B. **Laboratory tests** (see Section V.b.).

C. **Management.** Each specific opportunistic infection requires appropriate treatment. Life-long suppressive therapy is the rule because of the high relapse rate even in those successfully treated. **Antiretroviral therapy is indicated** in all patients. Patients who are naive to the drugs may experience dramatic benefit and reversal of immunodeficiency. Long-term control may be more difficult in patients who have received prior therapy, because of the presence of resistant HIV.

D. **Prognosis.** With increased use of antiretroviral agents, earlier identification, and more effective treatment of certain opportunistic infections, survival among patients with advanced HIV disease has substantially improved.

VII. **Predictors of HIV-disease progression**

A. The median time from the acquisition of infection to the development of AIDS is 10 to 12 years. Without therapy, the CD4$^+$ count declines 40 to 80 cells/mm^3 each year. The rate of progression of HIV infection varies considerably. It is difficult to predict the course in any individual. Certain clinical features and laboratory tests may help predict the rate of disease progression in a patient.

1. **Risk factors for acquiring the infection.** Transfusion recipients progress to AIDS more rapidly than do hemophiliacs, injecting drug users, or homosexual men, based on the 1987 CDC classification. This factor is often not helpful, as the patient may not recall the time of seroconversion.

2. **Age at onset of infection.** The rate of progression appears to be more rapid if acquisition of the infection occurs after age 35 years.

3. **Clinical indicators.** Symptomatic primary HIV infection is associated with a more rapid course. Development of oral candidiasis, oral hairy leukoplakia, herpes zoster (shingles), constitutional symptoms, and weight loss are all signs of progression to varying degrees.

4. **Laboratory factors.**

   a. Plasma **HIV RNA viral load** correlates well with infectious virus titers. Plasma HIV RNA levels are highest in acute infection and late-stage disease and are intermediate in asymptomatic infection. A single measurement of viral load provides information on the relative risk of progression of the infection; higher viral loads are associated with more rapid disease progression. A plasma HIV RNA level below 10,000 copies/mL in early HIV disease is associated with a decreased likelihood of early progression to AIDS.

   b. **CD4$^+$ cell count** and percentage and the trend over time provide crucial information as to the degree of immunodeficiency. On average, the CD4$^+$ count decreases 40 to 80 cells/mm^3 each year. Patients should have CD4+ cell counts performed at least every 6 months to monitor trends.

   c. Combined use of plasma HIV RNA and CD4+ count allows the best predictor of an individual patient's prognosis. Higher viral loads and lower CD4+ counts indicate a patient with more advanced disease with a greater risk of more rapid progression.

VIII. Long-term survivors. About 5% of infected individuals have long-term non-progressive disease. The definition may vary, but usually the patient has documented infection for >10 years, is asymptomatic with a stable CD4+ count of >500 cells/mm³, and is receiving no antiretroviral therapy. It is most likely a heterogeneous group, with some individuals manifesting a normal, but delayed response to HIV infection, and others infected with a genetically unique virus or displaying a highly effective immune response to an ordinary strain of the virus (Kirchoff F. *N Engl J Med* 1995;332:228–232). HIV-1 replication is present but is many magnitudes lower than that in individuals with progressive disease (Pantaleo G. *N Engl J Med* 1995;332:209–216). Lymphoid architecture and immune function remain intact. This group remains at a clinically latent stage, as described previously (see III). It is unclear at this point whether therapy offers any advantage to such patients.

4. PRIMARY CARE

I. Introduction. Approximately 900,000 Americans are already infected with the human immunodeficiency virus (HIV). The epidemic is taking a disproportionate toll among the poor and minorities. As with all chronic diseases, the role of the primary care provider is essential. He or she coordinates care of the patient by providing comprehensive medical care and addressing any active social and psychological issues. Health maintenance and primary prevention of disease are important aspects of HIV care.

II. Diagnosis of HIV infection
  A. Current recommendations for HIV testing are
   1. Persons with sexually transmitted diseases (STDs).
   2. Patients identified as being in high-risk categories:
     a. Intravenous drug users.
     b. Homosexual and bisexual males.
     c. Hemophiliacs.
     d. Regular sexual partners of the previously listed patients.
     e. Sexual partners of a known HIV patient.
     f. Prostitutes and their sexual partners.
     g. Persons receiving blood products between 1977 and 1985.
     h. Heterosexual persons with multiple sexual partners or unprotected intercourse.
   3. Persons who consider themselves at risk.
   4. Pregnant women.
   5. Patients with active TB.
   6. Recipient and source of occupational exposures.
   7. Hospital admissions between age 15 and 54 years if the seroprevalence rate exceeds 1% or the number of acquired immunodeficiency syndrome (AIDS) cases exceeds 1/1,000 discharges.
   8. Health-care workers who perform invasive procedures (depending on the policy of the institution in which they work).
   9. Donors of blood, semen, and organs.
   10. Medical evaluation of diseases with findings suggestive of HIV infection.
  B. Informed consent is required in most states and countries and is always recommended. Pretest and posttest counseling should be available. The individual undergoing testing should be made aware of the possibility of discrimination in medical and life insurance and at the work place, and the implications on personal relationships. If an individual tests positive, he or she should be evaluated according to these guidelines.
  C. Testing
   1. Serology
     a. Enzyme-linked immunosorbent assay (ELISA) is a screening assay for HIV antibodies. It has a sensitivity >99.7% and a specificity >98.5%. Specimens that are repeatedly reactive by ELISA should be confirmed by Western blot. An isolated ELISA result should not be reported to the patient without a confirmatory Western blot.
     b. Western blot (WB) detects HIV antibodies and the specific antigen against which the antibody is directed. The results may be positive, negative, or indeterminate.
       (1) Positive WB is determined by the presence of two of the following bands: p24, gp41, or gp 120/160.
       (2) Negative test is the absence of such bands.

The author acknowledges the contribution of Pablo Tebas and Mary M. Horgan to the previous edition of this chapter.

(3) **Indeterminate test** is one that does not fulfill the criteria for a positive WB.

   c. As in any test, the **predictive value** varies with prevalence of disease in the population considered. An indeterminate test should be evaluated according to the risk factors of the patient. Patients with no identifiable risk factors usually have false-positive results caused by cross-reacting antibodies elicited by nonretroviral antigens. The patient should be reassured, and the test repeated in 3 months. Patients from high-risk categories may be seroconverting, and the test should be repeated in 1 month. Alternatively an antigen-detection test, p24, or polymerase chain reaction (PCR) should be sent (see section II.C.2.d).

2. **Other methods** include antigen detection **(p24 assay)**, **PCR**, and **viral culture**. These tests are rarely used in diagnosis, but can be used in the following situations:

   a. To confirm infection in individuals if the regular serology is inadequate (e.g., infants, patients with agammaglobulinemia and acute infection). Detection of **p24 antigen** is the most effective way to diagnose acute infection (see Chapter 2).

   b. To clarify indeterminate WB (see Section II.C.1.b).

   c. To monitor drug trials.

   d. In the case of PCR-based tests, to plan and monitor antiretroviral therapy.

III. The HIV-infected patient

A. **General issues.** This chapter is written mainly for the care of the HIV-positive patient whose infection has recently been diagnosed. The approach is similar if the patient has been referred after an initial complication or has recently moved from the care of another physician, but every effort should be made to recover all records from previous medical providers, to avoid duplication and unnecessary, expensive testing.

B. **Patients with special needs.** HIV care should be individualized as each patient has special needs. Special considerations apply to the following groups:

1. **Substance abusers.** Early diagnosis and treatment of addictions (alcohol and drugs) are important. Open discussion between patient and caregiver on approach to management of addiction and physician concerns about prescribing controlled substances helps to improve compliance and outcome.

2. **The female patient.** The number of women infected with AIDS has increased steadily. The majority of newly diagnosed cases are acquired by heterosexual transmission. More than three-fourths of cases occur in African-Americans and Hispanics.

   a. Infected women are less likely to seek medical attention for many reasons:

      (1) Lack of health insurance;
      (2) Distrust of the medical profession;
      (3) Women are very often the main providers and caregivers of children, some of whom may be infected, and whose health and social needs are given a greater priority;
      (4) Many infected women have a myriad of other social problems including homelessness and poverty;
      (5) Lack of transportation; or
      (6) Ongoing substance abuse.

   b. A **"one-stop shop,"** combining adult and pediatric services, at a clinic that caters to the needs of the infected women (medical, OB/GYN, etc.) and her infected children has proven to increase compliance (see Chapter 8).

3. **The pregnant woman.** Vertical transmission ranges from 13% to 39%. HIV testing should be offered early in pregnancy to identify and treat those infected (see Chapter 9).

4. The adolescent. The incidence of HIV infection is increasing among teenagers, especially in minorities.

   a. This population represents unique challenges to the health-care provider for the following reasons: it is a difficult population to reach and to enroll in clinical trials; consent and confidentiality issues are complicated; and few clinical data are available on management of the adolescent HIV-infected patient.

   b. A useful, practical approach to **dose adjustment** for the adolescent is to begin with pediatric dose schedules for adolescents who are Tanner stage I or II and adult doses for adolescents who are Tanner stage IV or V. Stage III needs close monitoring, as this is the phase of rapid growth.

   c. Education stressing the need for condom use and reduction in the number of sexual partners is especially important in this group to prevent further spread of the infection among peers. A "one-stop shop" catering to all health-care needs of the adolescent may help compliance.

IV. The initial office visit

A. The interview. The initial office visit is crucial in establishing a good relationship with patients. The interview should be open and nonjudgmental. This visit gives the patient an opportunity to verbalize concerns about his or her health and the future. Typically the patient will have been tested positive before the referral. A history of when he or she tested positive, where the test was performed, and why it was done are all important. Previous medical records should be obtained if possible. Any infectious or neoplastic complication should be documented, as well as vaccination history. Although a complete evaluation and physical examination are necessary, sometimes those can be postponed for a second visit in 1 or 2 weeks. This short period helps to improve confidence and compliance and gives the patient time to develop further questions for his provider and to have some laboratory results that will help in making further therapeutic decisions, especially in the asymptomatic or paucisymptomatic patient.

B. Current symptoms. HIV and the immunodeficiency it produces affect every system of the body. The history taking should be complete and systematic, focusing on any current symptoms suggestive of an HIV complication.

C. Medical history should be taken, with special emphasis on areas like tuberculosis, STDs, and drug abuse. A travel history also is important because it helps to identify risks for certain endemic infections like Histoplasma (Midwestern states, South America), Isospora (Caribbean islands), Coccidioides, and Leishmania. This is also a good opportunity to start education to prevent as much as possible new exposures and transmission. History of other infections, including STDs and viral hepatitis is important to elicit.

D. Family history helps to identify genetic or environmental problems that can affect the course of the disease, like hemophilia or glucose-6-phosphate dehydrogenase (G6PD) deficiency. Family history of some infectious diseases like TB also is important to determine the risk of the patient and the need for prophylaxis. Family history of cardiovascular disease, diabetes mellitus, or hyperlipidemia may assume greater importance in patients needing long-term antiretroviral therapy.

E. Social history, including social support, family knowledge of the disease and disclosed diagnosis, sexual preference and practices, drug use, smoking habits, occupation, health-care coverage, housing situation, children, and diet helps to identify in advance areas of future problems (especially regarding support). It also helps to focus the education intervention in areas in which it is probably going to be more useful.

F. Medications. All medications, including over-the-counter and "herbal" preparations, should be recorded. Interactions are very frequent, and the physician should be aware of them. The patient should be instructed to bring all active medications to each office visit. This helps to streamline the medication, educate the patient about the therapy, and improve compliance.

G. Allergies are more frequent among HIV-infected patients, with skin rashes being the most frequent manifestation. Sulfonamides and aminopenicillins are the most frequent drugs implicated. All drug allergies and type of reaction should be recorded.

H. Physical examination is important to establish a baseline. Routine examination thereafter may detect changes, especially those resulting in subclinical manifestations of HIV-related conditions. Knowledge of the degree of immunosuppression and the "expected" findings and possible complications associated with them is helpful.

1. **Weight** should be documented at each office visit. It is an important marker of progression. An unexplained 10% weight loss defines the AIDS wasting syndrome. Nutritional support and counseling to maximize caloric intake and to modify diet should be offered as soon as possible after diagnosis, irrespective of the stage of the infection. Nutritional supplements may be required with advancing disease, with or without gastrointestinal complications. The roles of enteral and parenteral nutrition are unclear.

2. **Temperature.** Fever can be an early sign of infection or neoplasia. It should be recorded at all visits. In patients with advanced disease, fever of unknown origin is a common presentation of opportunistic illness, and fever should not be assumed to result from HIV infection itself without a thorough diagnostic evaluation. Blood cultures and serum cryptococcal antigen are useful diagnostic studies in this setting. In many cases, an abdominal computed tomography (CT) scan and a biopsy of the liver or bone marrow may be needed to rule out infection or malignancy. HIV-positive patients are also more likely to develop drug reactions, and fever may result from the institution of new medications.

3. **Oral cavity.** The oral mucosal surfaces should be examined carefully. The patient should be informed of the importance of oral care and educated about common HIV-related oral lesions and associated symptoms. HIV-infected individuals should have a dental examination performed by a dentist twice a year. Oral manifestations of the HIV infection are discussed in Chapter 20.

4. **Eyes.** A careful history of visual disturbances should be obtained at each visit. Patients should be educated about the symptoms of cytomegalovirus (CMV) retinitis: floaters and blurred vision. Manifestations of HIV infection in the eye are discussed in Chapter 16.

5. **Neck/lymph nodes**
   a. Regional or generalized lymphadenopathy is common. If rapid changes in the size or characteristics of the lymphadenopathy appear, a biopsy is indicated. Fine-needle aspiration may be diagnostic in almost 50% of the cases. Lymphadenopathy may be related to
      (1) HIV (persistent generalized lymphadenopathy),
      (2) Infection (e.g., tuberculosis, syphilis, atypical mycobacteria), or
      (3) Neoplasm (Hodgkin's and non-Hodgkin's lymphoma).
   b. Bilateral salivary gland enlargement is seen occasionally and is a more common manifestation in children. No infectious cause has been found (see Chapter 18).

6. **Lungs.** Pulmonary problems are very common in HIV disease. *Pneumocystis carinii* pneumonia is still the most frequent opportunistic infection. It usually is seen as dyspnea, with low-grade fever and nonproductive cough, although it can be fulminant. A normal examination or rales are the most frequent findings. Many other opportunistic infections (e.g., TB, recurrent bacterial pneumonias, aspergillosis) and neoplasms (Kaposi's sarcoma, lymphoma) involve the lungs (see Chapter 11).

7. **Cardiovascular.** Dilated cardiomyopathy is a frequent complication of advanced HIV disease and is seen as chronic heart failure. Intravenous (i.v.) drug abusers are at risk for bacterial endocarditis, so new cardiac murmurs should be sought (see Chapter 17).

8. **Abdomen.** Gastrointestinal complaints are common (see Chapter 14).

   a. Nausea can be related to medication or be a manifestation of gastrointestinal or central nervous system disease.

   b. Dysphagia and odynophagia are most frequently caused by *Candida* esophagitis. Cytomegalovirus (CMV), herpes simplex virus, and idiopathic ulcers are similarly seen.

   c. Diarrhea may be infectious in origin or caused by an infiltrative process, drugs (especially the protease inhibitors), or lactose intolerance.

   d. Hepatomegaly and splenomegaly are signs of many opportunistic infections such as TB, *Mycobacterium avium*, histoplasmosis, and neoplasia.

   e. Cholangitis and acalculous cholecystitis are common and can be caused by Cryptosporidium, Microsporidia, CMV, or *M. avium* complex (MAC).

9. **Rectal.** Rectal problems are very prevalent, especially among sexually active homosexual/bisexual male and heterosexual female patients. HIV infection frequently coexists with other STDs. A rectal examination is part of a complete physical examination and should be repeated every 6 months or more frequently if symptoms appear. Complications to look for include infections herpes simplex virus [(HSV), gonorrhea], neoplasia [epidermoid carcinoma associated with human papillomavirus (HPV)], hemorrhoids, and anal fissures.

10. **Pelvic examination, Pap smear, and gonococcal and *Chlamydia* probes.** HIV-infected women have an increased prevalence and severity of cervical disease and a more rapid progression of untreated cervical dysplasia to more advanced stages of cervical disease. A Pap smear should be performed as part of the complete initial gynecologic examination in all HIV-infected women. A complete gynecologic examination, including Pap smear, should be repeated every 6 months. Individuals with a Pap smear that demonstrates atypical cells of undetermined significance, cervical intraepithelial neoplasia (CIN), or carcinoma should be referred for a colposcopic evaluation by an experienced gynecologist. Wet preps, KOH preps, and DNA probes for gonococcus (GC) and *Chlamydia* infection should be sent as a part of the initial examination. More frequent examination is indicated for new-onset vaginal discharges (see Chapter 8).

11. **Extremities.** Leg edema is a manifestation of heart or renal failure. Many skin lesions appear in the extremities. Neuropathy is a frequent complication of HIV infection and its treatment.

12. **Skin.** Complete examination of the tegument is essential because of the high frequency of skin rashes in this population (see Chapter 12).

13. **Neurologic.** Neurologic complications of HIV infection are common, especially late in the disease (see Chapter 13).

I. **Psychiatric evaluation** is an intrinsic part of the primary care of any HIV-infected individual. As with any other chronic disease, HIV infection is frequently associated with psychiatric manifestations (*AIDS Clinical Care* 1994;6:64–66, 71–78). The most frequent problems a primary care doctor will find are the following (see also Chapter 13).

   1. **Depression** affects ~20% of HIV-infected patients and is usually underdiagnosed.

      a. Depression should be suspected in patients with decreased mood, decreased interest in day-to-day activities, significant weight loss, motor agitation or retardation, sleep disturbances, or feelings of guilt and worthlessness.

      b. Treatment requires a combination of support therapy and medication. Drugs are selected based on their side-effects profile, using nortriptyline or desipramine if some sedation is desired. In more chronic cases or when the risk of suicide is higher, fluoxetine, 10 to 20 mg per day p.o., or sertraline, 50 to 200 mg per day p.o., are recommended. Half the daily dose is recommended initially, with dose adjustment after 2 weeks as required. Referral to a psychiatrist is often necessary (see also Chapter 13).

2. **Bipolar disorders with mania.** The treatment of mania in AIDS patients can be more complicated than in the general population. This problem is frequently associated with dementia (see Chapter 13).

3. **Generalized anxiety/panic disorders.** A complete evaluation is required. Acute situations should be managed with short-acting benzodiazepines such as lorazepam (Ativan), 0.5 to 2 mg p.o., every 8 hours, or alprazolam (Xanax), 0.25 to 2 mg p.o., every 8 hours. Clonazepam, 0.5 mg p.o., every 12 hours, may be used for long-term management of anxiety. The overuse of benzodiazepines should be discouraged. It should be made clear to the patient that the anxiolytic agents help alleviate symptoms but do not resolve the precipitating event. Buspirone, 10 to 15 mg p.o., 3 times daily, is sometimes effective and has the advantage of not producing addiction or sedation. For the chronic management of panic disorder, long-term treatment with an antidepressant is preferred, frequently at lower doses than those required for depression.

4. **Insomnia** should be thoroughly evaluated. It may be a symptom of an underlying mental or physical problem. Short-term diphenhydramine (Benadryl), 25 mg p.o., at bedtime, or trazodone, 25 to 50 mg p.o., at bedtime can be used and are usually effective.

5. **Disorders of temperament and personality** with high risk-behavior and poor compliance with medication or scheduled visits are frequent (e.g., drug addicts). They usually respond to a good relationship with the primary care provider, plus the definition of specific therapeutic goals with clear rewards (rather than punishment) if results are obtained and contingency plans if goals are not met.

6. **Substance-abuse** patients should be offered detoxification in a specialized setting as either inpatients or outpatients.

7. **Organic brain disease/dementia.** AIDS dementia complex is especially frequent in advanced HIV infection and can be devastating for the patient and the family. It is more common in patients who have had little or no exposure to antiretroviral therapy. Some reversal may be seen with antiretroviral therapy (see Chapter 13).

8. **Grief** is very frequent and usually results from external circumstances. Treatment is more supportive than pharmacologic. The primary care provider needs to provide support. If the patient does not improve with supportive therapy, major depression (that requires pharmacologic treatment) should be ruled out.

V. **Laboratory tests**
  A. **Hematology.** Anemia, leukopenia, and thrombocytopenia are frequent complications of HIV infection, opportunistic infections, or their treatment and prophylaxis.
   1. **A complete blood count** should be checked every 3 to 6 months in asymptomatic patients or more frequently in patients with more advanced disease or who are receiving myelotoxic drugs. Although mild anemia is common in HIV infection and worsens as the disease advances (especially with myelosuppressive therapy), sudden severe anemia is unusual and should raise the suspicion of an infiltrative process in the bone marrow (see Chapter 21).
   2. **A lymphocyte count** can be used as a surrogate marker for CD4$^+$, if this test is not readily available. A CD4$^+$ count >200 cells/mm^3 is usually associated with a lymphocyte count >1,500 cells/mm^3. A CD4$^+$ count <200 cells/mm^3 is generally associated with a lymphocyte count <1,000 cells/mm^3.

B. Serum chemistry (electrolytes and liver-function tests) should be assessed at baseline and repeated annually in asymptomatic patients who are not receiving therapy. Occasionally these tests may help to identify patients with an infiltrative/infectious process of the liver or renal insufficiency. More regular monitoring is required for potential toxic effects of many of the medications used in the treatment of HIV-infected patients. Hepatotoxicity from antiretroviral drugs is particularly more likely to occur in patients with concomitant viral hepatitis - either B or C.

C. CD4+ cell counts (*MMWR* 1994;43:RR-3). Many of the complications of HIV infection appear only when the CD4+ cell count reaches a certain level. The cell count is used as a guideline for recommending institution of antiretroviral therapy and especially prophylaxis of opportunistic infections. The absolute number of CD4+ T cells is a calculated number [white blood cell (WBC) $\times$ lymphocyte% $\times$ CD4%] and because of that is subject to many variations. A trend is more indicative than an isolated value. Measurement of the number of CD4+ cells should be done once every 6 months with a CD4+ count >600 cells/mm^3 and at least every 3 months with a CD4+ count between 200 and 600 cells/mm^3. They may be obtained more frequently if there is evidence of rapid decline or with increasing symptoms. The CD4+ cell count should be used to educate the patient on the stage of his or her disease. It should be emphasized that the numbers are used as a guide, because some patients attribute excessive value to this measurement and become obsessed and depressed with fluctuations in this number.

D. β₂-Microglobulin, neopterin, p24 antigenemia. These are markers of uncertain value that provide little information in addition of the CD4+ count, and their use is not recommended.

E. Plasma viral RNA levels and their changes **predict clinical outcome** in patient cohorts and, when used in combination with CD4+ counts, provide a better picture of the patient status. Interpreting the result of viral load must be done with caution. The intraassay variability is ~0.2 logs, and the biologic variability of the tests is ~0.3 logs; therefore only sustained changes in the plasma HIV RNA levels >0.5 log (i.e., greater than threefold) are considered significant. One isolated value is difficult to interpret. Tests should be repeated by using a single method, as comparison of results between different methods is not valid.

1. Plasma HIV RNA levels >5,000 to 10,000 copies/ml, in addition to CD4+ cell count and clinical status suggestive of progression, warrant consideration of the initiation of antiretroviral therapy. In the opinion of many experts, an HIV RNA level >30,000 copies warrants the institution of therapy regardless of the CD4+ count.

2. Maximal clinical efficacy appears to be obtained by maintaining plasma levels **below the limit of detection**, although that goal may be difficult to achieve in many patients.

3. Initially two measurements should be obtained 2 to 4 weeks apart as a baseline and after that every 3 to 4 months, together with CD4+ counts.

4. Plasma HIV RNA levels should be measured 3 to 4 weeks after **initiating** or **changing antiretroviral therapy** to determine the magnitude of the response, if any, and the need for changes. Thereafter, viral load should be measured every 4 to 8 weeks until the maximal response to treatment is determined. If patients are clinically stable and have achieved undetectable plasma HIV RNA levels on effective therapy, viral load measurement can be repeated every 2 to 3 months.

5. A threefold (>0.5 log) or greater sustained reduction of plasma levels should be used as the minimal response indicative of an antiviral effect.

6. The confirmed return to baseline value of the HIV RNA level or the reemergence of detectable HIV RNA in a patient whose viral load was previously undetectable is suggestive of drug failure and an indication for alternative treatment regimens.

F. **Tuberculin skin test.** An HIV-infected patient coinfected with *M. tuberculosis* has a 10% annual risk of developing active tuberculosis. TB is preventable and curable in this population if detected promptly. Exposure history and risk factors such as foreign born in an endemic area and homelessness should be included in the patient's history. All patients should have a tuberculin skin test (TST) during their initial visit regardless of the bacille Calmette-Guérin (BCG) vaccination status. A chest radiograph is indicated if the patient has respiratory symptoms or symptoms suggestive of TB or a positive TST. Prophylaxis with Isoniazid (INH) should be given if the TST is positive (>5 mm of induration in this population) and if active tuberculosis is ruled out. The TST should be repeated yearly until the patient becomes anergic or after exposures to known cases of tuberculosis. INH, 300 mg per day p.o. (10 mg per kg, per day, for children), with pyridoxine, 50 mg p.o., every day for 12 months is the usual prophylactic regimen. The main complication of prophylactic therapy is hepatitis. Baseline liver-enzyme levels should be checked. INH prophylaxis is not contraindicated by minor elevations of liver function tests (LFTs). Compliance may be an issue in certain patients, and directly observed therapy should be strongly considered. If the patient is exposed to a known multidrug-resistant organism, it is necessary to tailor the prophylactic regimen, and it is better to consult an infectious disease specialist (see also Chapter 23).

G. **Syphilis serology.** HIV infection alters the natural history, laboratory diagnosis, and response to therapy of syphilis. Patients with syphilis are at increased risk of HIV infection, and HIV infection complicates the management of syphilis because of frequent treatment failures. An adequate history and a Venereal Disease Research Laboratory (VDRL) or rapid plasma reagent (RPR) test should be part of the initial assessment and should be repeated yearly if the patient is sexually active. All reactive nontreponemal tests should be confirmed by a specific treponemal assay [fluorescent treponemal antibody absorption (FTA-ABS) or microhemagglutination assay for *Treponema pallidum* (MHA-TP)]. A lumbar puncture is recommended in all HIV patients with positive treponemal serologies. This recommendation is based on the higher incidence of neurosyphilis in this population. Management of syphilis is discussed in Chapter 27.

H. **Toxoplasma serology.** The incidence of toxoplasmosis in HIV infection varies greatly with geographic areas. Seroprevalence is higher in mainland Europe (70% to 90%) than the United States (30%), but is greater in minorities than in whites within the United States.
   1. Toxoplasmosis is the most frequent cause of intracranial lesions and occurs usually with $CD4^+$ cell counts of <100 cells/mm^3. Reactivation rather than primary infection is the usual pattern. On this basis, serology [i.e., Toxoplasma immunoglobulin G (IgG)] is helpful in identifying those who have been exposed. About one-third of all seropositive patients will eventually develop the disease, and prophylaxis is recommended for patients who are seropositive when the $CD4^+$ count decreases to <100 cells/mm^3 (see section **VI.B** and Chapter 22).
   2. All HIV-infected persons, particularly those who lack IgG antibody to Toxoplasma, should be counseled about potential exposure to toxoplasmosis. They should be advised not to eat raw or undercooked meat, particularly undercooked pork, lamb, or venison. If the patient owns a cat, the litter box should be changed daily, preferably by an HIV-negative, nonpregnant person; alternatively, the patient should wash the hands thoroughly after changing the litter box. Patients should be encouraged to keep their cats inside and not to adopt or handle stray cats.

I. **Hepatitis B and C serology.** There is a higher incidence of hepatitis B and C seropositivity in HIV-infected patients. If an individual acquires hepatitis B virus (HBV), there is an increased incidence of carriage. Hepatitis B vaccina-

tion is recommended for all HIV-positive patients who have not been infected with HBV. HBsAg and Anti-HBc should be checked to confirm prior infection.
VI. **Immunizations.** (*MMWR* 1993;42:RR-4). In general, live attenuated vaccines are contraindicated in HIV-infected patients. The only exception is measles-mumps-rubella (MMR) for HIV-infected children. Response to vaccination is poor with worsening immunosuppression.
   A. **Pneumococcal vaccine.** Efficacy has not been clearly established in this population, but vaccination is recommended because of the higher prevalence of pneumococcal infections. Antibody responses are better early in the disease when CD4+ counts are >350. Revaccination after 5 years should be considered.
   B. **Hepatitis B.** HIV-infected patients are at higher risk of becoming chronic carriers of HBV after having acute hepatitis B infection. This vaccine is expensive and requires a previous serology. If anti-Hbc and HbsAg are negative, vaccination is indicated. Doses are given at 0, 1, and 6 months. If the patient has abnormal LFTs, complete HBV serologic studies should be done to rule out the possibility of chronic carriage or chronic active disease.
   C. **Influenza.** The use of this vaccine is controversial. Influenza vaccination has been recommended in patients infected with HIV, although there is little information on the incidence and severity of influenza in this population. Recent studies showed evidence that influenza vaccination promotes HIV replication and produces a transient increase in the viral copy number for up to 3 months after vaccination. The long-term consequences of this are unknown.
   D. **Other**
      1. **Tetanus/diphtheria.** The current recommendation for the adult general population (vaccination every 10 years) applies to HIV-infected patients.
      2. *Haemophilus.* Patients with HIV infection are at increased risk of *Haemophilus influenzae* pneumonia. The value of vaccination has not been clearly established, but this vaccine should be considered for this group of patients. It is indicated in HIV-infected children.
      3. **Hepatitis A vaccine** is indicated for sexually active homosexual men.
VII. **Miscellaneous issues**
   A. **Contraception.** Counseling HIV-infected women regarding reproductive issues and options should be part of the initial visit. This counseling should be done in a nondirective manner, with a clear and understandable language. Pregnancy per se does not seem to alter the course of HIV infection in the mother. Breastfeeding is contraindicated. Contraception should be individualized in each patient, and this issue is discussed in Chapters 8 and 9. Independent of the method used, the continued use of condoms should be strongly encouraged.
   B. **Safer sex and other education issues.** Every patient should be educated at the initial office visit about methods of HIV transmission and the risk involved in **sexual practices**. The use of condoms should be encouraged to reduce the risk of acquisition of other STDs and the transmission of HIV to others. Patients should avoid sexual practices (oroanal contact) that will result in exposure to feces because of the increased risk of infection with enteric pathogens.
   C. **Detoxification.** If the patient is a injecting drug user, access to a detoxification program should be facilitated. Patients should be encouraged to use new needles and participate in needle-exchange programs when available. Several studies have shown a decreased rate of transmission if the sales of syringes are deregulated and needle-exchange programs are established in the community.
   D. **Pets.** HIV patients should avoid exposure to sick pets, especially those with diarrhea. Patients should wash their hands after handling them and should avoid contact with young animals (younger than 6 months). Ownership of cats probably increases the risk of toxoplasmosis and bartonellosis, and pre-

cautions should be undertaken (Section **IV.G.8**). Patient should use gloves if cleaning aquariums to prevent exposure to *Mycobacterium marinum*. Exposure to reptiles increases the risk of salmonellosis. Exposure to other exotic pets is discouraged.

E. **Diet.** Eating undercooked meat and eggs should be discouraged. In areas with high incidence of Cryptosporidium or during epidemics, tap water should be boiled. Water from rivers and lakes should not be drunk.

F. **Travel.** Travel to developing countries places HIV-infected individuals at risk of exposure to opportunistic pathogens and food-borne diseases. The rules for chemoprophylaxis for infections like malaria, traveler's diarrhea, arthropod vectors, as well as general and specific measures for certain geographic areas are similar to those for immunocompetent patients. Live-virus vaccines, such as yellow fever and oral polio vaccines, should be avoided. Killed vaccines are safe and should be used if required.

G. **Social-worker and case-manager referral.** The HIV-infected population, as a group, has more limited access to private, employment-based insurance. This is particularly true for patients with symptomatic disease who are unable to continue work or in poorer populations with no access to employment-based health care. The primary care provider should facilitate access to the financial and support services to which the HIV-positive patient is entitled. These services vary from state to state and from country to country. Each provider should be aware of the resources available for the patient.

H. **Power of attorney.** HIV infection is an incurable disease, and eventually many patients will die of its complications. It is important for the primary care provider to make the patient aware of the prognosis and to address issues such as advance directives and durable power of attorney. Terminal care should be addressed at an early stage so that the patient's wishes are fulfilled. The degree of medical intervention, intubation, and other extraordinary measures should be outlined, and comfort measures in the hospital or nursing home setting or hospice care should be discussed with the patient. The patient also can designate an individual, durable power of attorney, to make decisions when he or she is unable to do so. All decisions, after discussion with physician, family members, and loved ones, can be written in a legal document ("living will" or "advance directive"). For patients with children, it is very important to discuss who is going to raise them and to address all the legal implications of these decisions sooner rather than later in the disease.

VIII. **Follow-up visits and institution of therapy.** A return visit should be scheduled 2 to 4 weeks after the initial office visit. Subsequent scheduling depends on the stage of illness, the institution of therapy, and the needs of the patient. In general, even asymptomatic patients who are not being treated should be seen at least every 6 months with CD4$^+$ cell count and viral load repeated at those visits. As the disease advances, more frequent visits are needed. Two therapeutic decisions should be discussed with the patient after a complete initial evaluation.

A. **Initiation of antiretroviral therapy.** The primary care physician should offer the patient the most effective antiretroviral therapy available and provide access to clinical trials, if available. Multiple studies have shown the benefits of antiretroviral therapy, but also their complexity and toxicity, and it is important that physicians taking care of patients with HIV infection attempt to stay as current as possible with recommendations for treatment. Currently available antiretroviral agents are discussed in Chapter 5, and their use is outlined in Chapter 6.

B. **Initiation of prophylaxis against opportunistic infections** (Table 1) Guidelines have been established by the U.S. Public Health Service and the Infectious Diseases Society of America for primary prophylaxis in HIV-infected patients.

1. Initiation of **PCP prophylaxis** is indicated when CD4$^+$ counts decrease to <200 cells/mm^3 or when the patient has unexplained fever for >2 weeks or had a previous episode of oral candidiasis.

Table 4-1 Prophylaxis for first episode of opportunistic disease in HIV-infected
adults and adolescents

Pathogen	Indication	Preventive regimens	
		First choice	Alternatives
Strongly recommended as standard of care			
Pneumocystis carinii	CD4⁺ count of <200/µl or unexplained fever for >2 wk or oropharyngeal candidiasis	TMP-SMZ, 1 DS/d p.o.	TMP-SMZ, 1 SS/d p.o., or 1 DS p.o., t.i.w.; dapsone, 50 mg p.o., b.i.d., or 100 mg/d p.o.; dapsone, 50 mg/d p.o., plus pyrimethamine, 50 mg/wk p.o., plus leucovorin, 25 mg/wk p.o.; aerosolized pentamidine, 300 mg morning by Respirgard II nebulizer
Mycobacterium tuberculosis			
Isoniazid-sensitive	TST reaction of ≥5 mm or prior positive TST result without treatment or contact with case of active tuberculosis	Isoniazid, 300 mg p.o., plus pyridoxine, 50 mg/d p.o. × 12 mo; or isoniazid, 900 mg p.o., plus pyridoxine, 50 mg p.o. b.i.w. × 9 mo	Rifampin, 600 mg/d p.o. plus pyrazinamide, 20 mg/kg × 2 mo
Isoniazid-resistant	Same as preceding; high probability of exposure to multidrug-resistant tuberculosis	Rifampin, 600 mg/d p.o. × 12 mo plus pyrazinamide 20 mg/kg × 2 mo	Rifabutin, 300 mg/d p.o. × 12 mo plus pyrazinamide 20 mg/kg × 2 mo
Multidrug-resistant (isoniazid and rifampin)	Same as preceding; high probability of exposure to multidrug-resistant tuberculosis	Choice of drugs requires consultation with public health authorities	None
Toxoplasma gondii	IgG antibody to *Toxoplasma* and CD4⁺ count of <100/µl	TMP-SMZ, 1 DS/d p.o.	TMP-SMZ, 1 SS/d p.o. or 1 DS p.o. t.i.w.; dapsone, 50 mg/d p.o., plus pyrimethamine, 50 mg/wk p.o., plus leucovorin, 25 mg/wk p.o.

Table 4-1 *Continued*

Preventive regimens

Pathogen	Indication	First choice	Alternatives
Streptococcus pneumoniae	All patients	Pneumococcal vaccine, 0.5 mL i.m. × 1	None
Mycobacterium avium complex	CD4⁺ count of <50/μl	Clarithromycin, 500 mg p.o., b.i.d.; azithromycin, 1,200 mg/wk p.o.	Rifabutin, 300 mg/d p.o.

TMP-SMZ, trimethoprim-sulfamethoxazole; TST, tuberculin skin test; IgG, immunoglobulin G. Modified from: *MMWR* 1999;48(RR–10).

    a. Trimethoprim-sulfamethoxazole (TMP-SMZ) DS, 1 tablet daily, is the prophylaxis of choice. TMP-SMZ 1 SS tablet daily or 1 DS tablet p.o., 3 times a week are alternatives.
    b. Although ~40% of patients are intolerant to TMP/SMZ (skin rash, fever, gastrointestinal upset), as many as 50% of such intolerant patients will tolerate a rechallenge with the drug, especially if it is gradually reintroduced over a period of 7 to 14 days.
    c. If TMP-SMZ cannot be tolerated, dapsone, 100 mg per day p.o., is favored. Pentamidine by aerosol, 300 mg once a month, is an alternative for patients intolerant of standard systemic prophylaxis. Atovaquone, 750 mg p.o., twice daily appears to be as effective as dapsone. Less well-studied options include pentamidine, 4 mg per kg, i.v., once monthly.
  2. **Tuberculosis prophylaxis** is recommended in HIV-positive patients with a positive tuberculin skin test (<5 mm of induration), history of a previously untreated positive TST, or recent contact with an active TB case. INH, 300 mg per day p.o., plus pyridoxine, 50 mg/day p.o., for 12 months, is recommended (see also Chapter 23).
  3. **Antitoxoplasma prophylaxis** for patients seropositive for prior exposure to Toxoplasma is indicated when the CD4⁺ count is <100 cells/mm³. TMP-SMZ, 1 DS per day, is the preferred regimen. The combination of dapsone, 100 mg per day p.o., and pyrimethamine, 50 mg per week p.o., and folinic acid, 25 mg per week p.o., should be used in patients intolerant of TMP-SMZ.
  4. **Prophylaxis against M. avium** complex (MAC) infection should be initiated with CD4⁺ counts <50 cells/mm³ in patients with a prior AIDS-defining opportunistic infection. Options include clarithromycin, 500 mg p.o., twice daily, azithromycin, 1,200 mg per week p.o., or rifabutin, 300 mg per day p.o., (see Chapter 23).
  5. Prophylaxis is **not recommended** for most patients, for the following opportunistic infections: recurrent bacterial pneumonia, mucosal candidiasis, herpesvirus, and the endemic fungal infections, histoplasmosis, and coccidioidomycosis. Prophylaxis has been shown to be effective for the prevention of cryptococcal infection (fluconazole), histoplasmosis (itraconazole), and CMV disease (oral ganciclovir), but is not generally recommended for all patients because of concerns about the development of resistance, drug interactions, and cost.
  6. **Secondary prophylaxis** is instituted after an episode of infection that has been adequately treated; it is specifically addressed in the corresponding chapters. Most opportunistic infections in AIDS are incurable

as long as the patient remains immunosuppressed. Therefore the patient will require a treatment regimen for the rest of his or her life, unless effective antiretroviral therapy is accomplished and immune recovery occurs.

7. **Prophylaxis in patients receiving potent antiretroviral therapy.** Effective antiretroviral therapy may increase the CD4+ count to levels above the threshold where prophylaxis had been started. In such patients, it is safe to stop primary prophylaxis for PCP and MAC. Patients whose viral replication is not completely suppressed should be monitored carefully because sustained increases in CD4+ counts may not be maintained in such patients and it may be necessary to resume prophylaxis. Secondary prophylaxis for CMV can also be discontinued if the CD4+ count rises to levels > 100 to 150 cells/mm^3 (see Chapter 25). Such patients need to be monitored carefully as relapses occur if the CD4+ count falls again. Although there has been insufficient information to make definitive conclusions about secondary prophylaxis for other opportunistic infections, it is very likely that long-term treatment will not be needed for any infection in patients who have sustained immune recovery.

5. ANTIRETROVIRAL AGENTS

David J. Ritchie

Currently, available antiviral agents act by inhibiting the activity of two major viral enzymes - reverse transcriptase (RT) and the HIV protease (see Chapter 1). Other targets under active investigation include the integrase, viral entry (especially fusion) and viral activation. Although drugs targeting these areas are being developed, and some are in early clinical studies, only agents approved by the United States Food and Drug Administration in 2000, or agents in late phase of development and available through expanded investigational protocols will be discussed in this chapter. Significant drug-drug interactions and general guidelines for dosing in renal disease can be found in this chapter, but are also included in the appendices.

I. **Reverse transcriptase inhibitors.** The reverse transcriptase inhibitors (RTIs) are antiretroviral agents that act via inhibition of HIV reverse transcriptase, the enzyme that catalyzes the conversion of HIV RNA into double-stranded DNA. Inhibition of reverse transcriptase results in DNA chain termination and reduced viral replication. This class of agents is further subdivided into nucleoside RTIs, non-nucleoside RTIs, and nucleotide RTIs.

A. **Nucleoside reverse transcriptase inhibitors.** The nucleoside reverse transcriptase inhibitors currently approved by the FDA for clinical use are zidovudine, didanosine, zalcitabine, stavudine, lamivudine, and abacavir. These agents exert their antiretroviral activity after intracellular conversion to their active triphosphate moieties. The nucleoside drugs are not active against most human DNA polymerases—the one exception is DNA polymerase gamma—which is found in mitochondria. Nucleoside inhibition of mitochondrial DNA polymerase is believed to be the cause of much of the long-term toxicity seen with these agents (see below and Chapter 17). In general, resistance to this class of antiretrovirals is associated with the development of mutations in codons of the reverse transciptase gene. In general, each drug is associated with a typical, and often unique, initial mutation pattern. These initial mutations may not lead to complete cross-resistance to other nucleoside drugs. Over time, the virus may accumulate multiple mutations in the reverse transcriptase gene. In this circumstance, broader cross-resistance among the drugs of this class is likely.

1. **Zidovudine (ZDV) or azidothymidine (AZT)**

a. **Pharmacokinetics.** ZDV has an oral bioavailability of 65%. Peak serum levels are decreased in the presence of food. ZDV is about 35% plasma protein bound with a volume of distribution of 1.4 L per kg. The majority of the drug is glucuronidated in the liver to an inactive metabolite that is excreted by the kidneys. Only 15% to 20% of ZDV is excreted unchanged by the kidneys. The drug has a serum half-life of about 1 hour, but the half-life of the active intracellular triphosphate moiety, zidovudine triphosphate, is 3 hours.

b. **Adverse effects.** Common side effects of ZDV are headache, nausea, and gastrointestinal disturbances. Other common and potentially therapy-limiting effects include anemia and leukopenia, which may require exogenous administration of erythropoietin and/or filgrastim or sargramostim. A reversible myopathy associated with elevations in creatine kinase may also occur with prolonged use (>6 months) of ZDV. Other potential effects of ZDV include seizures, rash, lactic acidosis with or without hepatomegaly, and steatosis (see Chapter 17).

c. **Drug interactions.** Probenecid decreases the renal excretion and/or inhibits the metabolism of ZDV, resulting in an increased bioavailability of ZDV. However, concomitant administration of these agents may result in a high incidence of flu-like symptoms. Concomitant administration of ZDV with other myelosuppressive agents (e.g., flucytosine, doxorubicin, vinblastine, ganciclovir, interferon-α, adriamycin, vincristine) should be carried out with caution since the risk of toxicity may be increased. Valproic acid increases, whereas rifampin and rifabutin may decrease the bioavailability of ZDV.

d. **Dose and administration.** ZDV is available in 100mg capsules, 50 mg per 5mL syrup, and a 10 mg per mL injection. The recommended **adult dose** is 600 mg per day, either as 200 mg every 8 hours, or, more commonly, 300 mg every 12 hours. The dose for **children** aged 3 months to 12 years is 180 mg/m2 every 6 hours, not to exceed 200 mg every 6 hours. For prevention of maternal-fetal transmission (see Chapter 9), the following dosing schedule is recommended: 100 mg orally 5 times daily for the mother until the start of labor, followed by intravenous (IV) ZDV at a dose of 2 mg per kg over 1 hour followed by 1 mg per kg per hour (total body weight) during labor and delivery until cord clamping. The infant dose starting within 12 hours after birth is 2 mg per kg orally (or 1.5 mg per kg i.v.) every 6 hours continued through 6 weeks of age. ZDV is not significantly removed by **hemodialysis or peritoneal dialysis**; however, the daily dose should be reduced to 300–400 mg per day in patients with severe renal dysfunction. The effect of hepatic dysfunction on ZDV dosing has not been clearly established; however, dose reduction should be considered.

e. **Patient information.** Patients should be instructed to contact their physician if they experience any unexpected reactions. They should also be informed that headache and nausea are common and occur in a majority of patients taking the drug. If possible, the capsules should be taken with food to maintain peak levels. Patients should also be informed about medications that could increase the risk of myelosuppression when taken with ZDV.

f. **Resistance.** High-level resistance to ZDV requires mutations at reverse transcriptase codons 41, 67, 70, 215, and 219. These mutations usually emerge in an ordered fashion. The K70R mutation usually is the first mutational change in HIV-1 RT to emerge during ZDV therapy. Subsequently, variants with mutations at codon 215 and 41 emerge and replace the K70R mutants. The combined presence of mutations at these two codons confers a 60-fold increase in the IC50 for zidovudine.

2. **Didanosine (ddI)**

a. **Pharmacokinetics.** The oral bioavailability of ddI is decreased in the presence of food. The drug is acid labile and is formulated with buffering agents to increase its bioavailability. When taken with food and buffering agents (in the product) the bioavailability of ddI is about 40%. The drug is <5% plasma protein bound with a volume of distribution of about 1 ddIL per kg. ddI and is extensively metabolized in the liver to uric acid, hypoxanthine, and other purine metabolites. About 20% of ddI is eliminated unchanged by the kidneys. The serum half-life is about 1 hour, although the intracellular half-life of the active moiety, dideoxyadenosine triphosphate, is ≥12 hours.

b. **Adverse effects.** The major therapy-limiting side effects of ddI are reversible peripheral neuropathy in approximately 10% of patients (characterized by distal extremity numbness, pain, and tingling) and pancreatitis in 1% to 2%. Didanosine-associated pancreatitis may be severe and fatal. Headache, insomnia, gastrointestinal disturbances, uric acid elevations, rash, hepatitis, and seizures may also occur. Lactic acidosis with or without hepatomegaly and steatosis, may also occur. In contrast to ZDV, ddI is not commonly associated with myelosuppressive side effects.

  c. **Drug interactions.** Concomitant administration of ddI with drugs
     that require gastric acid for absorption (ketoconazole, itraconazole,
     dapsone) can result in decreased bioavailability of these agents.
     Bioavailability of fluoroquinolones and tetracyclines is also decreased
     when taken concurrently with ddI. To minimize the possibility of
     these interactions, ddI should be staggered by at least 2 hours with
     doses of these agents. ddI should be used cautiously in combination
     with other agents that may cause pancreatitis (e.g., pentamidine,
     valproic acid, co-trimoxazole, and in patients who have heavy use of
     alcohol) or peripheral neuropathy (e.g., isoniazid, metronidazole, vin-
     cristine) due to a possible increased toxicity risk.
  d. **Dose and administration.** ddI is available as chewable/dispersible
     tablets (25, 50, 100, 150, and 200 mg), a powder for oral solution (100,
     167, 250, and 375 mg), and as a pediatric powder for oral solution
     (2 and 4 g). The usual **adult** dosage of ddI tablets is 200 mg every
     12 hours (250 mg every 12 hours for the oral solution) or 400 mg p.o.
     qd for patients weighing ≥60 kg and 125 mg every 12 hours (167 mg
     every 12 hours for the oral solution) for those weighing <60 kg. Each
     dose should consist of 2 tablets to ensure adequate acid buffering.
     The **pediatric** dosage for ddI tablets is 100 mg b.i.d., 75 mg b.i.d.,
     50 mg b.i.d., and 25 mg b.i.d. for patients with body surface areas
     of 1.1 to 1.4, 0.8 to 1.0, 0.5 to 0.7, and ≤0.4 m2, respectively. The
     effects of renal and hepatic failure on ddI dosing have not been fully
     determined; however, reduced doses should be considered. About
     20% of ddI is removed by hemodialysis; therefore daily doses should
     be administered after dialysis on dialysis days. The effects of peri-
     toneal dialysis on ddI dosing have not been determined.
  e. **Patient information.** Patients should be reminded that each ddI
     dose should contain 2 tablets. The tablets should either be thor-
     oughly chewed or dispersed in at least 1 ounce of water and ingested
     on an empty stomach. Patients should also be instructed to report
     any new and unusual symptoms, particularly symptoms of periph-
     eral neuropathy or pancreatitis, and should consult with their
     physician or pharmacist prior to taking any new medications.
  f. **Resistance.** Mutations at codon 74 emerge after 6 to 12 months of
     monotherapy with ddI and correlate with a reduction in antiviral
     activity of ddI, The L74V mutation also confers cross-resistance to
     zalcitabine (ddC). Didanosine rarely can select for the M184V muta-
     tion, which also confers resistance to 3TC (see below); the clinical
     significance of this pathway is doubtful. Emergence of the codon
     74 mutation is prevented or delayed in patients treated with ddI
     in combination with ZDV.
3. **Zalcitabine (ddC)**
  a. **Pharmacokinetics.** The oral bioavailability of ddC is ≥80% and is
     decreased in the presence of food. ddC is <4% plasma protein bound
     with a volume of distribution of about 0.5 L per kg. ddC is not appre-
     ciably metabolized by the liver and the majority (60% to 80%) of the
     drug is eliminated unchanged by the kidneys. The serum half-life of
     ddC is about 20 minutes, but the intracellular half-life of the active
     moiety, dideoxycytidine triphosphate, is about 2.5 hours.
  b. **Adverse effects.** The major therapy-limiting adverse effect of ddC
     is peripheral neuropathy, usually associated with burning sensations
     and pain in the distal extremities. Pancreatitis is rare with ddC, but
     may be fatal when it occurs. Rash and stomatitis are common side
     effects occurring early in therapy with ddC. Anemia, leukopenia, and
     thrombocytopenia may occur, but less commonly than with ZDV.
     Other possible effects include ototoxicity, fever, malaise, hepatic fail-
     ure, myalgias, and pruritis. Lactic acidosis, with or without hepato-
     megaly and steatosis, may also occur.

   c. **Drug interactions.** ddC should be used cautiously in combination
      with other agents that can cause peripheral neuropathy (e.g., isoni-
      azid, metronidazole, vincristine) and pancreatitis (e.g., pentamidine,
      valproic acid, co-trimoxazole) due to a possible increased toxicity risk.
      Since ddC is eliminated largely by the kidneys, concomitant admin-
      istration with nephrotoxic agents (e.g., amphotericin B, foscarnet,
      aminoglycosides, pentamidine) may decrease ddC clearance and
      potentially increase the risk of toxicity. Magnesium and aluminum-
      containing antacids may decrease the bioavailability of ddC, and
      probenecid appears to increase the bioavailability of ddC.
   d. **Dose and administration.** ddC is available in 0.375 and 0.75 mg
      tablets. The recommended **adult** dose of ddC is 0.75 mg every 8 hours.
      The dose should be reduced to 0.75 mg every 12 hours and 0.75 mg
      every 24 hours in patients with creatinine clearance of 10 to 40 mL
      per minute and <10 mL per minute, respectively. The safety and effi-
      cacy of ddC in **pediatric** patients < age 13 has not been determined;
      however, a dose of 0.04 mg per kg every 6 hours has been given with
      only mild adverse effects after 8 weeks. The effects of hemodialysis,
      peritoneal dialysis, and hepatic failure on the pharmacokinetics and
      dosing of ddC have not been fully determined.
   e. **Patient information.** ddC should be taken on an empty stomach.
      Patients should be instructed to report any new or unusual symptoms,
      particularly symptoms of peripheral neuropathy, to their physician.
   f. **Resistance.** Although clinical resistance does occur, and certain
      mutations can be selected *in vitro* by ddC, *in vivo* resistance muta-
      tions are rare.
4. **Stavudine (d4T)**
   a. **Pharmacokinetics.** The oral bioavailability of d4T is 80% to 86%
      and is not significantly affected by food. d4T is not appreciably
      bound to plasma proteins and has a volume of distribution of 0.9 to
      1 L per kg. Approximately 40% of the drug is excreted unchanged by
      the kidneys. A small amount of the drug is metabolized to thymine
      and unidentified polar compounds; however, the full metabolic dis-
      position of d4T has not yet been determined. The serum half-life of
      d4T is 1.2 hours, but the intracellular half-life of the active moiety,
      dideoxydidehydrothymidine triphosphate, is about 3.5 hours.
   b. **Adverse effects.** The major therapy-limiting adverse effect of d4T
      is dose-related peripheral neuropathy which may occur in up to 20%
      of patients taking d4T. d4T may also cause anemia, neutropenia, ele-
      vated hepatic transaminases, pancreatitis (particularly if adminis-
      tered concomitantly with didanosine), headache, gastrointestinal dis-
      turbances. Lactic acidosis with or without hepatomegaly and steatosis
      may also occur.
   c. **Drug interactions.** d4T should be used cautiously in combination
      with other agents that can cause peripheral neuropathy (e.g., iso-
      niazid, metronidazole, vincristine) due to a possible increased tox-
      icity risk.
   d. **Dose and administration.** d4T is available in 15, 20, 30, and 40 mg
      capsules. The usual **adult** dosage is 40 mg every 12 hours for patients
      ≥60 kg and 30 mg every hours for patients <60 kg. The **pediatric**
      dose appears to be 0.125 to 2 mg per kg every 12 hours. The dose
      of d4T should be reduced to 20 mg every 12 hours and 20 mg every
      24 hours in patients weighing ≥60 kg with creatinine clearance of
      26 to 50 mL per minute and 10 to 25 mL per minute, respectively. For
      patients weighing under 60 kg, the doses are 15 mg every 12 hours
      and 15 mg every 24 hours for patients with creatinine clearance of
      26 to 50 mL per minute and 10 to 25 mL per minute, respectively.
      The effects of creatinine clearance <10 mL/min, dialysis, or hepatic
      impairment on the pharmacokinetics and dosing of d4T have not
      been fully determined.

e. **Patient information.** d4T may be taken without regard to meals. Patients should be instructed to report any new and/or unusual symptoms, particularly symptoms of peripheral neuropathy (tingling, numbness, burning, pain in the extremities), to their physician.

f. **Resistance.** Although patients treated with d4T monotherapy demonstrate a gradual loss of response to d4T over time, the virologic basis for d4T failure has not been well characterized. No specific mutations in the RT gene have been identified. Recent information suggests mutations similar to those produced with ZDV therapy appear after prolonged d4T treatment.

5. **Lamivudine (3TC)**

a. **Pharmacokinetics.** The oral bioavailability of 3TC is about 86% and is not significantly affected by food. The drug is 36% plasma protein bound with a volume of distribution of about 1.3 L per kg. The majority of 3TC is eliminated unchanged by the kidneys, and the drug is only minimally metabolized by the liver. The serum half-life is 5 to 7 hours, but the intracellular half-life of the active moiety, lamivudine triphosphate, is 11 to 16 hours.

b. **Adverse effects.** 3TC is generally well tolerated. Possible uncommon adverse effects of 3TC include headache, fatigue, nausea, abdominal pain, diarrhea, peripheral neuropathy, neutropenia, thrombocytopenia, and elevated hepatic enzymes and bilirubin. Pancreatitis may occur rarely in adult patients, but is seen more commonly in pediatric patients (15%). Therefore, 3TC should be used cautiously in pediatric patients with either a history of pancreatitis or other risk factors for pancreatitis. Lactic acidosis, with or without hepatomegaly and steatosis, may also occur.

c. **Drug interactions.** 3TC increases peak serum levels of ZDV. Cotrimoxazole increases 3TC bioavailability.

d. **Dose and administration.** 3TC is available in 150 mg tablets and as a 10 mg per mL oral solution. The usual **adult** dose is 150 mg twice daily for patients weighing ≥50 kg and 2 mg per kg twice daily for adults weighing <50 kg. The **pediatric** dose for patients 3 months to 12 years of age is 4 mg per kg twice daily up to a maximum of 150 mg twice daily. Patients with creatinine clearances of 30 to 49, 15 to 29, 5 to 15, and 5 mL per minute should receive 150 mg once daily; 150 mg × 1 then 100 mg daily; 150 mg × 1 then 50 mg daily; and 50 mg × 1 then 25 mg daily, respectively. The effects of dialysis and hepatic impairment on the dosing of 3TC have not been fully determined.

e. **Patient information.** 3TC may be taken without regard to meals. Patients should be instructed to report any new or unusual symptoms while taking 3TC. Parents of pediatric patients receiving 3TC should be informed of the risk of pancreatitis and its associated symptoms.

f. **Resistance.** Resistance to lamivudine (3TC) is conferred by point mutations at RT codon 184. This appears rapidly (within weeks) if the patient is treated with 3TC in a regimen that does not completely suppress viral replication. Co-administration of ZDV and 3TC results in delayed emergence of resistance to ZDV, possibly because mutations at 184 restore susceptibility to ZDV even in viruses that have mutations at codons 41 and 215. 3TC resistant viruses appear to retain susceptibility to ddI.

6. **Abacavir**

a. **Pharmacokinetics.** Absolute bioavailability is 83% and absorption is unaffected by food. The drug distributed widely, with a volume of distribution of 0.86 L per kg, and is about 50% plasma protein bound. The drug is not significantly metabolized by cytochrome p450 enzymes, but is metabolized by alcohol dehydrogenase and glucuronyl transferase to inactive metabolites. Only 1% of the drug is excreted in the urine as unchanged drug. The half-life is 1.5 hours.

b. **Adverse effects.** The primary therapy-limiting side effect is a **hypersensitivity syndrome,** which may be fatal. Clinical manifestations of abacavir-induced hypersensitivity typically are fever, rash, fatigue, gastrointestinal disturbances, lymphadenopathy, elevated liver function tests, elevated creatinine phosphokinase or creatinine, and lymphopenia, but may also include myalgia, arthralgia, edema, shortness of breath, and paresthesias. The reaction usually occurs within the first 6 weeks of therapy, worsens with continued therapy, but is generally reversible following therapy discontinuation. **Patients who develop a hypersensitivity reaction must not resume abacavir therapy as fatal reactions have been described.** As with other nucleoside reverse transcriptase inhibitors, abacavir may cause lactic acidosis and hepatomegaly with steatosis, which may be fatal.

c. **Drug interactions.** Abacavir appears to be devoid of cytochrome p450-mediated drug interactions. Ethanol increases the abacavir area under the curve by 41% and half-life by 26%.

d. **Dose and administration.** The recommended adult oral dose is 300 mg p.o. b.i.d. The recommended dose for pediatric patients aged 3 month to 16 years is 8 mg per/kg (up to 300 mg) b.i.d. The drug has not been adequately studied in patients with renal or hepatic dysfunction to allow dosing modification recommendations to be made in these populations.

e. **Patient information.** Abacavir may be taken without regard to meals. Patients experiencing symptoms of hypersensitivity reactions, such as fever, rash, fatigue, or gastrointestinal disturbances should discontinue abacavir and consult with their physician immediately. Patients experiencing a hypersensitivity reaction should never again receive abacavir. It may be prudent for patients to avoid ingestion of ethanol while receiving abacavir, since ethanol increases exposure to abacavir and may put the patient at increased risk for adverse effects.

f. **Resistance.** *In vitro,* abacavir selects for mutations at codons 65, 74, and 184, similar to those observed with ddC, ddI, and 3TC, respectively. It seems that abacavir failure results in cross-resistance to 3TC, but it is less clear that cross-resistance to ddI or ddC develop. The presence of the M184V mutation does not seem to affect the virologic response to abacavir. However, the virologic response to abacavir is affected by ZDV resistance, and isolates that are dually resistant to ZDV and 3TC seem resistant to abacavir.

7. **Emtricitabine; FTC** (Investigational as of July 2000)

a. **Pharmacokinetics.** The oral bioavailability of emtricitabine in rats is about 90%. Food does not appear to affect the extent of absorption in humans. The volume of distribution in rats is 1.5 L per kg. The drug is 70% to 87% eliminated by the kidneys as unchanged drug. The half-life is approximately 7 to 8 hours.

b. **Adverse effects.** Potential adverse effects of emtricitabine are headache and nausea and hepatitis.

c. **Dose and administration.** The recommended dose appears to be in the range of 200 mg p.o. qd.

d. **Resistance.** The resistance profile of FTC seems identical to 3TC.

B. **Non-nucleoside reverse transcriptase inhibitors (NNRTIs).** Non-nucleoside RTIs are structurally dissimilar to the nucleoside RTIs and bind at distinct sites on the RT enzyme as compared to the nucleoside RTIs. These agents are potent inhibitors of RT and have activity against nucleoside reverse transcriptase inhibitor-resistant HIV strains. However, when NNRTIs are used as monotherapy, resistance rapidly develops. Broad cross-resistance occurs with this class of agents. Viruses resistant to one are typically resistant to all currently available NNRTIs. NNRTI resistance mutations occur in two clusters in the RT gene at codons 100 to 108 and at codons 179 to 190. The most common changes involve a K103N mutation [selected by efavirenz, delavirdine (DLV), and nevirapine (NVP)] and a Y181C mutation (selected by DLV and NVP).

1. **Nevirapine**
   a. **Pharmacokinetics.** The oral bioavailability of nevirapine is about 90% and does not appear to be significantly affected by food. The drug is about 60% plasma protein bound and has a volume of distribution of 1.4 L per kg. Nevirapine is primarily eliminated by hepatic metabolism via oxidative mechanisms. Nevirapine metabolites do not appear to be clinically active. Less than 3% is eliminated unchanged by the kidneys. The serum half-life is 40 to 45 hours, but decreases to about 25 to 30 hours after an initial 2 week dosing period due to autoinduction of hepatic enzymes.
   b. **Adverse effects.** The most common adverse effects of nevirapine are rash, headache, and depression. Fatigue, diarrhea, nausea, vomiting, fever, mylagias, arthralgias, elevated γ-glutamyl transferase and other liver function tests, and elevated mean corpuscular volume may also occur. **Rash** occurs in 7% to15% of patients and may be more common or more severe in women. The rash is usually self-limited and can be tolerated with antihistamines. In most cases, nevirapine can be continued; however, in a small percentage of patients (1% to 2%), a more severe rash with systemic involvement (e.g., hepatitis) and/or Stevens–Johnson syndrome have been reported. More severe rashes require discontinuation of nevirapine. In most cases, other NNRTIs can be substituted safely in patients with a nevirapine rash.
   c. **Drug interactions.** Nevirapine induces liver enzymes and may decrease levels of drugs metabolized through similar cytochrome p450 systems (e.g., protease inhibitors, phenytoin, methadone). Rifampin, rifabutin, and St. John's wort accelerate the metabolism of nevirapine and should not be administered concomitantly with nevirapine. Concomitant use of clavulanic acid-containing products (e.g., Augmentin, Timentin) within the first 4 weeks of nevirapine may increase the incidence of rash. Nevirapine may decrease the effectiveness of oral contraceptives when given concurrently.
   d. **Dose and administration.** The recommended adult dose is 200 mg p.o. qd for the first 14 days (to minimize the frequency of skin rash), followed by 200 mg p.o. b.i.d. thereafter. If the patient experiences a rash during the initial 14-day low-dose course, dose escalation to 200 mg p.o. b.i.d. should not be attempted until the rash has subsided. The pediatric dose for children aged 2 months to 15 years is 4 mg per kg (maximum 400 mg) qd for the first 14 days, followed by 7 mg per kg (maximum 400 mg) q12 hours or 4 mg per kg (maximum 400 mg) q12 hours for children aged 2 months to 8 years and >8 years of age, respectively. The effects of renal or hepatic failure and dialysis procedures on nevirapine dosing have not been established. Patients experiencing moderate to severe liver function abnormalities while on nevirapine should have nevirapine held until baseline hepatic function is achieved. Subsequently, the dose may be restarted at 200 mg p.o. qd; however, nevirapine should be permanently discontinued if liver function abnormalities reappear.
   e. **Patient information.** Patients should be instructed to report any new or unusual symptoms, particularly rash, while receiving nevirapine and consult with their physician or pharmacist prior to taking any new medications. Patients should be advised that if they experience a rash during the first 14 days of treatment with nevirapine, they should not advance to full dosing (200 mg b.i.d.) until the rash disappears. Nevirapine may be taken without regard to meals. Patients receiving oral contraceptives should be advised to

pursue additional nonhormonal contraceptive methods while receiving nevirapine.

2. Delavirdine

a. Pharmacokinetics. The oral bioavailability of delavirdine in humans is 85%. The absorption is not significantly affected by food, but is substantially decreased in the absence of adequate gastric acidity. The drug is 98% plasma protein bound and is primarily metabolized in the liver by cytochrome p450 3A enzymes and possibly also be CYP2D6. The drug is minimally excreted unchanged by the kidneys. Delaviridine exhibits nonlinear pharmacokinetics, with peak and trough levels and bioavailability increasing disproportionately with dose. The half-life of delavirdine is about 6 hours, but can range from 2 to 11 hours.

b. Adverse effects. The most common adverse effects of delavirdine are rash, mild headache, fatigue, and gastrointestinal disturbances. The rash is generally maculopapular and occurs usually between the first and second weeks of therapy. Transient, reversible elevations in liver function tests, insomnia, myalgia, anemia, neutropenia, thrombocytopenia, and elevations in uric acid may also occur.

c. Drug interactions. As delavirdine is dependent on gastric acid for absorption, drugs that decrease gastric acidity (e.g., antacids, H2 antagonists, omeprazole, lansoprazole) are expected to cause a significant decrease in delavirdine absorption. Concomitant administration with ddI also appears to decrease delavirdine bioavailability due to its buffering agent. As delavirdine is a cytochrome p450 3A inhibitor, it should not administered concomitantly with terfenadine, astemizole, cisapride, simvastatin, lovastatin, midazolam, triazolam, or ergot derivatives. Delavirdine may also increase plasma concentrations of other drugs metabolized by cytochrome p450 enzymes, including protease inhibitors. Rifampin, rifabutin, and St. John's wort significantly decrease delavirdine levels and should not be used concomitantly with delavirdine. Phenytoin, carbamazepine, and phenobarbital may also induce delavirdine metabolism and should be avoided. Ketoconazole, itraconazole, and erythromycin may inhibit metabolism of delavirdine and increase levels.

d. Dose and administration. The recommended dose is 400 mg (4 × 100 mg tablets), 3 times daily. The tablets may be dispersed uniformly in 3 oz. of water and ingested.

e. Patient information. Delavirdine should be taken with an acidic beverage such as orange or cranberry juice and staggered by at least 1 hour with any antacid or ddI doses. Delavirdine may be taken at the same time as ddI if resulting in improved compliance with antiretroviral therapy. The drug may be taken without regard to meals. Patients should be instructed to consult with their physician or pharmacist prior to taking any new medications or if they develop any new symptoms. Skin rashes, when they occur, typically are noted within the first few weeks of therapy and tend to resolve in 3 to 4 days despite continuation of therapy. Skin rashes should be brought to the attention of the physician.

3. Efavirenz (Sustiva)

a. Pharmacokinetics. The oral bioavailability of efavirenz is currently unknown. The drug may be taken without regard to meals of normal composition, but bioavailability increases by 50% when ingested with a high-fat meal. Efavirenz is 99.5% to 99.75% plasma protein bound and is eliminated primarily by hepatic metabolism via cytochrome p450 isozymes CYP3A4 and CYP2B6. The drug has a half-life of 40 to 55 hours and only minimal amounts are excreted unchanged in the urine.

b. **Adverse effects.** The most common adverse effects of efavirenz are rash, which typically occurs within the first 2 weeks and resolves within 1 month, and CNS disturbances, including dizziness, impaired concentration, abnormal thinking, somnolence, insomnia, and abnormal dreams. These CNS effects typically begin within the first couple days of therapy and usually resolve within 2 to 4 weeks. Delusions, behavioral disturbances, severe depression, and elevations in liver enzymes may also occur. Efavirenz may also cause total cholesterol elevations of 10% to 20% in some patients.

c. **Drug interactions.** Efavirenz is an inducer and inhibitor of CYP3A4 and should not be administered concomitantly with astemizole, midazolam, triazolam, cisapride, and ergot derivatives. Efavirenz decreases levels of protease inhibitors, clarithromycin, rifabutin, rifampin, and possibly warfarin, and increases levels of ethinyl estradiol and possibly warfarin. When used in combination with indinavir, the indinavir dose should be increased to 1000 mg p.o. q8 hours. Saquinavir should not be used as a sole protease inhibitor in combination with efavirenz due to the pronounced effect of efavirenz in accelerating saquinavir metabolism. Rifampin increases clearance of efavirenz and lowers serum levels, although no dosage adjustments of either drug are recommended. St. John's wort can decrease levels and should be avoided.

d. **Dose and administration.** The recommended dose is 600 mg p.o. qd, delivered as three-200 mg capsules. The drug should be taken at bedtime for the first few weeks to minimize the effect of CNS disturbances. As the drug is only minimally excreted unchanged in the urine, dosage adjustment in patients with renal insufficiency is not expected to be needed. It is unknown if dosage adjustment is needed in patients with hepatic impairment, although caution is recommended given the drug's extensive metabolism.

e. **Patient information.** Patients should be informed that the CNS disturbances, when they occur, usually begin very soon after therapy is started, but tend to resolve within a few weeks. Patients should be instructed to take their daily dose of efavirenz at bedtime to minimize the impact of possible CNS effects. If patients experience CNS symptoms, they should be cautioned against performing potentially dangerous activities, including driving. Patients should also be advised that although most rashes that occur resolve despite continuation of treatment, they should contact their physician if a rash is noted, as some may be serious. Patients should avoid eating a high-fat meal with efavirenz to potentially decrease the likelihood of side effects associated with increased efavirenz absorption. Additionally, patients should consult with their physician or pharmacist prior to taking any new medications due to the extensive drug interaction potential of efavirenz.

C. **Nucleotide analogs** inhibit HIV reverse transciptase without reliance on the initial intracellular phosphorylation step, which is a required step for intracellular activation of nucleoside analogs. The nucleotide analogs may possess broader activity than nucleosides against both resting and activated cells. Generally, there is no cross-resistance between nucleotides and nucleosides. Development of adefovir dipivoxil, a nucleotide agent being studied in clinical trials and clinically used under an expanded access program, was recently halted.

1. **Tenofovir disoproxil fumarate (PMPA prodrug)** (Investigational as of July 2000)

a. **Pharmacokinetics.** The oral bioavailability of tenofovir is 27% to 41% and is increased when taken with food. Tenofovir is negligibly protein bound. The primary route of elimination is renal excretion of unchanged drug. The estimated serum half-life is ≥17 hours. The half-lives in resting and stimulated peripheral blood mononuclear cells are about 50 and 10 hours, respectively.

  b. **Adverse effects.** Potential adverse effects of tenofovir include reversible elevations in creatine kinase, elevated hepatic transaminases, triglyceride elevations, neutropenia, exacerbation of peripheral neuropathy, fatigue, and headache.

  c. **Drug interactions.** Hydroxyurea appears to enhance the antiretroviral activity of tenofovir.

  d. **Dose and administration.** The recommended dose is probably 300 mg p.o. qd.

II. **Protease inhibitors** inhibit HIV protease, an enzyme required for the cleavage of viral polyprotein precursors and subsequent generation of functional HIV proteins. Inhibition of HIV protease does not allow HIV to produce infectious virions. Each of the protease inhibitors is associated with a fairly typical resistance pathway that initially involves unique mutations in the protease gene. Thus, at least initially, there is not complete cross-resistance among the members of this class of agents, and sequencing of protease inhibitors is possible (see Chapter 6). However, as the virus accumulate mutations in the protease gene, broader cross-resistance occurs and sequential use of these agents may not be possible. Although each of the protease inhibitors has individual side effects, some of the toxicity appears class-specific, notably the metabolic side effects on lipid, glucose and bone metabolism. These are discussed in detail in Chapter 17.

  A. **Saquinavir soft gel capsules (Fortovase)**

    1. **Pharmacokinetics.** The oral bioavailability of saquinavir soft gel capsules has not been firmly established, but appears to be at least 3-fold higher than the 4% bioavailability of the older hard gel capsule formulation when taken with a full meal. The drug is 97% plasma protein bound with a volume of distribution of 700 L. Saquinavir undergoes extensive hepatic metabolism, primarily by the cytochrome p450-mediated enzyme, CYP3A4. Only small amounts of the drug are excreted by the kidneys. The terminal elimination half-life is about 12 hours.

    2. **Adverse effects.** The most common adverse effects of saquinavir are gastrointestinal disturbances, including nausea, diarrhea, and abdominal discomfort. Other potential effects include elevated liver function tests, jaundice, confusion, seizures, headache, rash, paresthesias, and asthenia.

    3. **Drug interactions.** Rifampin, rifabutin, nevirapine, and St. John's wort significantly reduce levels of saquinavir. Other agents that induce CYP3A4, such as phenobarbital, phenytoin, carbamazepine, and dexamethasone, may also reduce saquinavir bioavailability. As saquinavir has CYP3A4 inhibitory activity, it should NOT be used concurrently with terfenadine, astemizole, cisapride, simvastatin, lovastatin, triazolam, midazolam, or ergot derivatives. Saquinavir may also increase levels of calcium channel blockers, quinidine, dapsone, clindamycin, triazolam, and sildenafil. Ketoconazole, clarithromycin, and other protease inhibitors substantially increase levels of saquinavir.

    4. **Dose and administration.** Saquinavir is available in 200 mg capsules. The usual **adult** dose is 1200 mg (6 × 200 mg capsules) 3 times daily within 2 hours after a full meal. When used in **combination with ritonavir** in a dual protease inhibitor-containing combination regimen, the dose is 400 mg b.i.d.. The safety and effectiveness in **pediatric** patients has not been established. The effects of hepatic or renal insufficiency and dialysis procedures on the pharmacokinetics and dosing of saquinavir have not been established; however, saquinavir should be administered cautiously in these settings, particularly in patients with hepatic insufficiency.

    5. **Patient information.** Patients should be instructed to take saquinavir within 2 hours of a full meal and that each dose (1,200 mg) should be

comprised of six-200 mg capsules. Patients should be clearly informed about the drug interaction potential of saquinavir and instructed to consult with their physician or pharmacist prior to taking any new medications or if they experience any new symptoms. The drug should ideally be refrigerated, but is stable at room temperature for up to 3 months.

6. **Resistance.** Resistance to saquinavir (SQV) is associated with acquisition of the G48V and L90M mutations in HIV-1 protease.

B. **Ritonavir**
   1. **Pharmacokinetics.** The bioavailability of ritonavir appears to be high and increased in the presence of food. Ritonavir is 99% plasma protein bound and is eliminated primarily via hepatic metabolism and biliary excretion. Only minimal amounts of the drug are excreted by the kidneys. The half-life of ritonavir is 3 to 5 hours.
   2. **Adverse effects.** The most common side effects of ritonavir are nausea, diarrhea, headache, dizziness, circumoral paresthesias, vasodilatation, pharyngitis, altered taste, elevated hepatic enzymes, elevated cholesterol. Ritonavir does not appear to be significantly myelosuppressive.
   3. **Drug interactions.** As ritonavir is a CYP3A4 substrate and inhibitor, it is associated with numerous documented and potential drug interactions. In addition, ritonavir has an affinity for several other cytochrome P450 isoforms, including CYP2D6, CYP2C9, CYP2C19, CYP2A6, CYP1A2, and CYP2E1. Specific drug interactions are below.
      a. Agents that decrease ritonavir levels. phenobarbital, dexamethasone, phenytoin, carbamazepine, rifampin, rifabutin, St. John's wort.
      b. Ritonavir increases levels of the following (contraindicated agents): amiodarone, astemizole, bepridil, buproprion, cisapride, clozapine, dihydroergotamine, encainide, ergotamine, flecainide, meperidine, pimozide, piroxicam, propafenone, propoxyphene, quinidine, rifabutin, simvastatin, lovastatin, terfenadine, clorazepate, diazepam, estazolam, flurazepam, midazolam, triazolam, and zolpidem.
      c. Ritonavir increases levels of the following (not strictly to the point of contraindication): clarithromycin (dose decrease recommended for patients with impaired renal function: 50% dose for ClCr 30 to 60, 25% dose for ClCr < 30), desipramine (dose reduction), and various narcotic analgesics, antiarrhythmics, antiinfectives, anticoagulants, antidepressants, antiemetics, antihypertensive agents, betablockers, calcium channel blockers, cancer chemotherapeutic agents, corticosteroids, hypoglycemics, hypolipidemics, immunosuppressants, neuroleptics, and stimulants that are metabolized by CYP3A4, CYP2D6, CYP2C9, or CYP2C19 (refer to product labeling for specific agents). Ritonavir also increases levels of sildenafil.
      d. Ritonavir decreases levels of the following: oral contraceptives (dose increase or alternative contraception recommended), theophylline (possible increased dose required).
      e. Disulfiram reaction. As ritonavir preparations contain alcohol, concomitant administration of ritonavir with disulfiram or metronidazole may result in the disulfiram reaction.
   4. **Dose and administration.** Ritonavir is available in 100 mg capsules and as an 80 mg per mL oral solution. The recommended **adult dose** of ritonavir is 600 mg p.o. b.i.d. with meals. When used in combination with saquinavir soft gel capsules, the dose is 400 mg b.i.d. Lower-dose regimens (100 to 200 mg b.i.d.) in combination with indinavir and saquinavir have also been studied. Safety and efficacy have not been completely determined in children. The oral solution may be mixed with chocolate milk, Ensure, or Advera to improve palatability. Gastrointestinal tolerance may be improved by titration to full dose over 4 days as follows (300 mg b.i.d. × 1 day, 400 mg b.i.d. × 2 days, 500 mg b.i.d. × 1 day, and 600 mg b.i.d. thereafter). Ritonavir pharmacokinetics have not been determined in patients with renal failure, but since the drug

is primarily metabolized by the liver, it is expected that its pharmacokinetics would not be altered in this setting. Because ritonavir is extensively metabolized by the liver, caution should be exercised when using the drug in patients with hepatic insufficiency.

5. **Patient information.** Patients should be instructed to report any new or unusual symptoms while taking ritonavir and should consult with their physician or pharmacist prior to taking any new prescription or nonprescription medications. Ritonavir should be taken with food and the dose slowly increased to the full 600 mg twice daily dose over the first 4 days of therapy and maintained at that full dose unless otherwise recommended. Patients should be informed that each 600 mg dose of ritonavir is six 100 mg capsules or 7.5 mL of liquid. Ritonavir capsules and solution should be refrigerated. If patients need to travel while receiving ritonavir, the capsules should be transported at refrigerated temperatures.

6. **Resistance.** Development of high-level resistance to ritonavir (RTV) involves the stepwise accumulation of multiple mutations. The first mutation generally appears at codon 82. Additional mutations at codons 36, 54, and 71 result in higher levels of resistance.

C. **Indinavir**

1. **Pharmacokinetics.** The bioavailability of indinavir is approximately 65% and is decreased in the presence of food. Plasma protein binding is 60% in humans and the volume of distribution is 1.5 to 2 L per kg in various animal species. Indinavir is eliminated < 20% as unchanged drug by the kidneys. Indinavir is metabolized in the liver by cytochrome P450 enzymes, primarily CYP3A4. Indinavir metabolites do not appear to provide any clinically meaningful antiretroviral activity. The half-life is 1.8 hours.

2. **Adverse effects.** Commonly reported adverse effects of indinavir are asymptomatic indirect hyperbilirubinemia and nephrolithiasis possibly associated with flank pain and hematuria. The nephrolithiasis generally resolves with hydration and/or a 1 to 3 day interruption of therapy. Hyperbilirubinemia and nephrolithiasis occur more frequently at doses greater than the recommended 2.4 gram per day dose. Nausea, vomiting, thrombocytopenia, headache, diarrhea, abdominal pain, aphthous stomatitis, insomnia, rash, and elevated hepatic transaminases may also occur.

3. **Drug interactions.** Ketoconazole increases the bioavailability of indinavir by approximately 40%; consideration should be given to indinavir dose reduction to 600 mg every 8 hours in this setting. Indinavir significantly increases rifabutin levels, and 50% rifabutin dose reduction is necessary. Conversely, rifabutin increases the metabolism of indinavir, necessitating an indinavir dose increase to 100 mg p.o. q8 hours. Rifampin and the herbal product St. John's wort significantly decrease indinavir levels, and concomitant use of these two medications is not recommended. Indinavir and didanosine should be staggered by at least 1 hour and administered on an empty stomach. Indinavir should not be administered concomitantly with terfenadine, astemizole, cisapride, triazolam, midazolam, simvastatin, lovastatin, ergot derivatives, and perhaps many other cytochrome P450 substrates. Other inhibitors (e.g., fluconazole, itraconazole, erythromycin, clarithromycin) and inducers (e.g., rifabutin, phenytoin, phenobarbital) of cytochrome P450 enzymes (CYP3A4, CYP2D6) have the potential to interact with indinavir. Indinavir increases levels of sildenafil.

4. **Dose and administration.** Indinavir is available in 200 mg and 400 mg capsules. The recommended dose of indinavir in adults is 800 mg **every 8 hours** (i.e., not t.i.d.) taken with water 1 hour before or 2 hours after a meal. Concomitant use of ritonavir improves the pharmacologic profile of indinavir such that it can be used twice daily and can be taken with food if necessary. Combination regimens that appear to be effective include

indinavir 800 mg p.o. b.i.d. with ritonavir 200 mg p.o. b.i.d., and indinavir, 400mg p.o. b.i.d. with ritonavir 400 mg p.o. b.i.d. Safety and efficacy in pediatrics has not been completely determined. Indinavir pharmacokinetics have not been determined in patients with renal failure, but since the drug is primarily metabolized by the liver, it is expected that the pharmacokinetics of the drug would not be altered in this setting. The dose of indinavir should be reduced to 600 mg every 8 hours in patients with cirrhosis-induced mild to moderate hepatic insufficiency.

5. **Patient information.** Patients should be instructed to drink at least six 8-ounce glasses of water daily in an attempt to minimize the possibility of nephrolithiasis. The drug should be taken on empty stomach, if not combined with ritonavir. Patients should be instructed to report any new or unusual symptoms, including symptoms of hyperbilirubinemia or nephrolithiasis, and should consult with their physician or pharmacist prior to taking any new prescription or nonprescription medications. When used as the sole protease inhibitor, the dose should remain at 800 mg every 8 hours (two 400 mg capsules per dose) unless otherwise directed. Patients should be informed about the importance of maintaining strict every 8-hour dosing as opposed to simply 3 times-daily dosing. Indinavir capsules are moisture-sensitive and should remain in the original container with a dessicant at room temperature.

6. **Resistance.** Indinavir resistance is very similar to ritonavir and isolates resistant to one are usually cross-resistant to the other. Indinavir resistance is also usually a result of multiple step-wise mutations, but the pattern is much more varied than that which occurs with ritonavir.

D. **Nelfinavir**

1. **Pharmacokinetics.** The bioavailability of nelfinavir is approximately 70% and is increased in the presence of food. Plasma protein binding is 98% and the drug is distributed widely with a volume of distribution of 2 to 7 L per kg. Nelfinavir is eliminated 1% to 2% unchanged by the kidneys. The drug is extensively metabolized in the liver by cytochrome p450 enzymes, primarily CYP3A. The half-life is 3.5 to 5 hours.

2. **Adverse effects.** The most commonly reported side effect of nelfinavir is diarrhea, which occurs in up to 20% of patients. It is typically controllable with antidiarrheals and not associated with weight loss, although it can be more severe. Asthenia, nausea, vomiting, depression, mild fatigue, rash, and elevations in liver function tests may also occur rarely.

3. **Drug interactions.** Nelfinavir is an inhibitor of CYP3A and should not be administered concomitantly with CYP3A substrates capable of causing toxicity, including terfenadine, astemizole, cisapride, midazolam, triazolam, simvastatin, lovastatin, or ergot derivatives. Rifampin and St. John's wort accelerate the metabolism of nelfinavir and should not be used concomitantly. No dosage adjustment of nelfinavir is necessary when it is administered with rifabutin or with inhibitors of cytochrome p450 enzymes such as ketoconazole, and presumably other azole antifungals and macrolide antibiotics. However, nelfinavir significantly increases rifabutin levels, and the dose of rifabutin should be halved when administered concomitantly with nelfinavir. Nelfinavir reduces ethinylstradiol levels, necessitating a dosage increase of ethinylstradiol and consideration of alternative contraception. Nelfinavir also increases levels of other protease inhibitors, and may increase levels of sildenafil.

4. **Dose and administration.** The recommended dose is 750 mg p.o. t.i.d. or 1,250 mg p.o. b.i.d. with food. Because nelfinavir is minimally eliminated by the kidneys, it is expected that no dosage adjustments are required in this setting. Consideration should be given to dosage adjustment in the presence of hepatic insufficiency.

5. **Patient information.** Nelfinavir should be taken with food to increase oral absorption. Patients should be instructed to report any new or unusual symptoms to their physician and informed that diarrhea occurs

in a significant percentage of patients, but rarely necessitates discontinuation of therapy and typically responds to antidiarrheals. The dose of nelfinavir should remain at 750 mg p.o. t.i.d. or 1250 mg p.o. b.i.d. unless otherwise directed. Patients should be instructed to consult with their physician or pharmacist prior to taking any new prescription or nonprescription medications.

6. **Resistance.** A mutation at codon 30 (D30N) is relatively specific for nelfinavir and usually appears first to emerge in isolates from patients failing nelfinavir. However, continued treatment with nelfinavir selects for the accumulation of additional resistance mutations, many of which are common to other protease inhibitors.

E. **Amprenavir**

1. **Pharmacokinetics.** The absolute oral bioavailability of amprenavir is unknown. The liquid formulation is 14% less bioavailable than the capsules; therefore the 2 dosage forms are not directly interchangeable on a milligram basis. The drug may be taken without regard to meals of a normal composition, but should not be taken with a high-fat meal due to potential for decreased absorption of the drug. The volume of distribution is 430 L and plasma protein binding is 90%. Amprenavir is metabolized in the liver by CYP3A4. Only minimal amounts of drug are excreted in the urine and feces. The half-life is 7.1 to 10.6 hours.

2. **Adverse effects.** The most common adverse effects of amprenavir are gastrointestinal disturbances, rash (amprenavir is a sulfonamide), and paresthesias.

3. **Drug interactions.** Amprenavir should not be administered concomitantly with astemizole, bepridil, cisapride, dihydroergotamine, ergotamine, midazolam, triazolam, simvastatin and lovastatin. Amprenavir may increase concentrations of pravastatin, cerivastatin, atorvastatin, diltiazem, nicardipine, nifedipine, nimodipine, dapsone, erythromycin, clorazepate, diazepam, flurazepam, clozapine, carbamazepine, loratadine, and pimozide. Serum levels and/or careful monitoring of possible adverse effects from amiodarone, lidocaine, quinidine, warfarin, sildenafil and tricyclic antidepressants should be performed as amprenavir may elevate levels of these agents. Rifampin or St. John's wort should not be used concomitantly with amprenavir. The dose of rifabutin should be halved if taken with amprenavir. Phenobarbital, phenytoin, and carbamazepine may decrease amprenavir concentrations. Delavirdine may increase and nevirapine and efavirenz decrease levels of amprenavir. Amprenavir may interact with oral contraceptives and additional nonhormonal contraception is recommended. As amprenavir contains significant amounts of vitamin E (daily capsule dose: 1744 IU; daily liquid dose: up to 8587 IU) that exceed the Reference Daily intake, supplemental vitamin E should not be taken. Amprenavir should be staggered by at least 1 hour with didanosine.

4. **Dose and administration.** The recommended dose of amprenavir is 1,200 mg p.o. b.i.d., delivered as 8×150 mg capsules. Ritonavir significantly improves the pharmacokinetic profile of amprenavir; if combined with ritonavir, 200 mg p.o. b.i.d., a dose of amprenavir, 600 mg b.i.d. can be used. Combination with ritonavir is essential if amprenavir is used with efavirenz, as the latter significantly decreases amprenavir serum levels. The pediatric capsule dose is 20 mg per kg b.i.d. or 15 mg per kg tid. The pediatric liquid dose is 22.5 mg per kg (1.5 mL per kg) b.i.d. or 17 mg per kg (1.1 mL per kg) t.i.d. The dosage of amprenavir should be reduced to 300 to 450 mg p.o. b.i.d. in patients with significant hepatic dysfunction. The need for dosage adjustment in patients with renal failure is unlikely.

5. **Patient information.** As amprenavir is a sulfonamide, patients should be questioned about a history of sulfa allergy prior to starting the drug. Patients should be advised to contact their physician if a rash develops.

The drug may be taken without regard to normal meals, but should not be taken with a high-fat meal. Each dose consists of eight capsules that should be taken in the morning and at night. Patients should consult with their physician or pharmacist prior to taking any new medications, and should be advised to pursue additional nonhormonal contraceptive methods. Patients should also be instructed to discontinue taking vitamin E supplements. The drug should be stored at room temperature and not refrigerated.

    6. Resistance. Use of amprenavir selects for mutations at codons 46, 47, and 50. The I50V mutation is unique to APV and does not appear to confer cross-resistance to other protease inhibitors.

F. Lopinavir, ABT-378/r (investigational as of July 2000)

    1. Pharmacokinetics. Plasma concentrations of lopinavir are low when it is administered alone. As a result, the drug is co-formulated with ritonavir 100 mg in an effort to capitalize on ritonavir's metabolic inhibitory properties and boost lopinavir concentrations to therapeutic levels. Lopinavir is the primary antiretroviral component of this combination product. Ritonavir concentrations achieved with this product (each capsule contains 133.3 mg lopinavir and 33.3 mg ritonavir) provide <10% of the area under the curve (AUC) of ritonavir given at the full 600 mg b.i.d. dose. The product appears to well-absorbed and food enhances bioavailability. The product is 98% to 99% protein bound, is extensively and rapidly metabolized by CYP3A4, and has a half-life of 5 to 6 hours.

    2. Adverse effects. Potential adverse effects of lopinavir include diarrhea, abnormal stools, nausea, asthenia, headache, rash, and vomiting. Elevations in triglycerides, cholesterol, hepatic enzymes, amylase, and glucose may also occur.

    3. Drug interactions. The CYP3A inhibitory capacity of lopinavir is approximately 6-fold less than that observed with standard dose ritonavir. However, lopinavir is expected to have the potential for drug interactions associated with cytochrome p-450 inhibition characteristic of other protease inhibitors (i.e., increase concentrations of astemizole, bepridil, cisapride, dihydroergotamine, ergotamine, midazolam, triazolam, pimozide). Rifampin accelerates metabolism of lopinavir and should not be used concomitantly. The rifabutin should be halved if administered concomitantly with lopinavir.

    4. Dose and administration. The recommended dose appears to be 400/100 mg (3 capsules) b.i.d. of lopinavir and ritonavir, respectively.

6. ANTIRETROVIRAL THERAPY

Effective antitretroviral therapy has been associated with dramatic improvements in mortality and morbidity from HIV infection and concomitantly with a fall in death rates from AIDS in the United States and other developed countries. Several issues have become clear over the last few years. Effective, durable therapy requires suppression of viral replication to very low levels because continuing viral replication in the presence of drugs only increases the risk of the emergence of resistant virus. Drug regimen failure almost inevitably is associated with resistance. Potent regimens usually require a combination of three or more drugs for durable effect. However, multiple drug combinations lead to increased complexity, increased risk of toxicity, and ultimately less adherence, which in turn leads to failure of the regimen. Consequently, antiretroviral therapy should be initiated with care, preferably by physicians with expertise in the use of these drugs, and with a view not only to short term virologic consequences, but also to long term benefit and safety.

I. **Surrogate marker testing in therapeutic decision making** (see Chapter 4). Both measurement of the amount of virus in the plasma, and measurement of the degree of immunologic impairment give vital information as to the stage of the patient. In general, the higher the viral load the greater the risk of progression to AIDS, and conversely the greater the degree of immune damage, the greater the risk of progression to AIDS or death. Thus both parameters, either individually or together, can be used to determine the urgency of treatment.
   A. **Viral markers**
      1. Direct measurement of the amount of virus present in the blood can predict the risk of disease progression. Increasing evidence suggests that direct measurement of viral load in body compartments is superior to CD4 count in determining the therapeutic efficacy of antiviral agents.
      2. Several **molecular techniques** are available that quantitate the amount of virion-associated plasma RNA (see Chapter 4). These techniques include reverse transcription followed by polymerase chain reaction (**RT-PCR**; Amplicor HIV Monitor Test, Roche Molecular Systems), branched DNA assay (**bDNA**; Chiron Corporation), and nucleic acid sequence-based amplification (**NAS-BA**; Organon Technika). Although the relative utility of these tests is unknown, one or more of them is increasingly used for patient management.
         a. Patients with **higher levels of plasma RNA** are at greater risk of progressing to AIDS than are those with lower copy numbers and that long-term nonprogressors in general have low levels of plasma RNA. There is no absolute threshold; the risk appears to increase steadily with increasing levels of plasma HIV RNA.
         b. **Short-term changes in viral load** (e.g., at 8 weeks after initiation or change in antiretroviral therapy) in individual patients have been shown to be predictive of disease progression. In general, patients with more than a log decrease in plasma viral load after treatment have a lower risk of progression to AIDS or death than do similar patients without such a virologic response. Patients whose plasma HIV RNA levels become undetectable with therapy have the lowest risk of progression; indeed many of these patients experience significant improvement in immune function.
         c. Viral load also adds information to the CD4 count. In general, patients with higher viral loads have a greater risk of disease progression despite the same CD4 count.
      3. Measurement of **p24,** one of the core antigens of HIV and the first virologic marker to be studied, has not proven useful as a marker of risk of disease progression or drug effect and has been largely abandoned in

routine clinical care. It is, however, still a useful test in the diagnosis of acute seroconversion (see Chapter 2).

4. **Quantitative culture of plasma for HIV**, and measurement of **syncytium-inducing phenotype** have been used largely in research to assess risk of disease progression and drug efficacy.

5. Measurement of **viral resistance** are increasingly being incorporated into clinical practice. Two measures of assaying for resistance are available (Hirsch MS, et al. *JAMA* 1998; 279:1984).

   a. **Genotypic testing.** Genotypic assays for drug resistance determine the nucleotide sequence of the reverse transciptase (RT) and protease (PR) genes. Such assays amplify HIV-1 PR and RT genes from viral RNA in plasma and then use automated DNA sequencing of the entire PR and RT genes. More limited assays such as the LiPA, selective PCR, or point mutation provide data limited only to specific codons that have already been implicated in drug resistance. These assays are relatively easy to perform and are fairly rapid (1 to 2 weeks).

   b. **Phenotypic testing.** In resistance testing the phenotype refers to the susceptibility of HIV-1 to inhibition by a particular drug. Drug susceptibility is defined as the amount of drug required to inhibit virus production *in vitro* by 50%, 90%, or 95% (IC_{50}, IC_{90}, or IC_{95}, respectively). The IC_{50} is usually measured. In general, IC_{50}s that are >4-fold higher than control isolates, suggest resistance to the drug in question. They have an advantage over genotypic assays in that cross-resistance is more easily determined.

   c. **Limitations of resistance assays**
      (1) Genotypic assays require **prior knowledge of the mutations** associated with resistance. Furthermore mutations **do not always predict phenotype** and cannot predict the effect of mutations on susceptibility to other drugs. This is particularly important with regard to the level of resistance to non-nucleoside reverse transcriptase inhibitors (NRTIs) such as ZDV. Not all mutations are associated with high-level resistance that would mean the drug will not be effective.
      (2) Phenotypic assays are slower to perform and **more expensive**.
      (3) Both assays are **relatively insensitive** to minor variants. Resistant variants may not be detected by most genotypic and phenotypic assays if they represent <20% of the circulating quasispecies. This is particularly important if the patient is not currently receiving the drug of interest. In general, if a drug is stopped, strains resistant to that drug disappear from the circulating plasma viral pool in 6 to 12 weeks and may not be detectable by resistance assays. However, this represents a **false negative** test as such resistant strains remain present in the body and can rapidly reappear if the drug is reintroduced.
      (4) Reliable results are difficult to obtain when the plasma HIV-1 RNA level is **<1000 copies/mL**.
      (5) Currently resistance assays **predict that a drug will not work**. They are less useful in predicting whether a drug will be effective as therapeutic success is more complicated than just assaying *in vitro* susceptibility.

B. **Immunologic markers**
   1. **CD4 cell count determination** has been the most frequently used marker of both disease progression and response to therapy. Measurement of the absolute number of CD4 cells is an excellent predictor of risk of disease progression, and periodic measurement of this value has become a cornerstone of patient management. However, changes in $CD4^+$ cell number do not appear to be optimal markers to assess the efficacy of antiviral therapy.

   2. b_2-Microglobulin and neopterin, additional surrogate markers of immunologic function, appear to offer only a modest increase in predicting risk of
   disease progression when done in conjunction with CD4 determination,
   are not of value in monitoring therapeutic response, and are now seldom
   used in routine practice.

C. Use of markers to initiate therapy. Most decisions regarding the initiation of antiviral therapy are based on viral load and CD4 cell determination.
In addition, the clinical status of the patient (presence of symptoms, AIDS
illness) can help decide if treatment is needed.

   1. All patients with advanced HIV disease (CD4 cell count < 200 cells/mm^3,
   prior AIDS-defining illness) should be treated.

   2. Many experts would initiate treatment at a CD4 cell count < 350 cells/mm^3
   regardless of symptoms and viral load. Many would initiate treatment at
   a CD4 cell count < 500 cells/mm^3.

   3. Most experts would initiate treatment at a plasma viral load of
   >30,000 copies/mL regardless of CD4 cell count because such levels are
   associated with a high risk of disease progression in the next 5 years.

   4. Most experts would not treat patients whose CD4 cell counts were
   > 500 cells/mm^3 and whose viral load was <5,000 copies/mL because such
   patients have a relatively low risk of disease progression in the next 3 to
   5 years. Such patients should be monitored closely for changes in CD4
   cell counts and plasma HIV RNA so that disease progression can be diagnosed early.

   5. No definitive recommendations can be made for patients with intermediate viral load levels and CD4 counts between 350 and 500 cells/mm^3.

   6. With increasing awareness of the long-term implications of antiretroviral therapy, experienced physicians are **individualizing the decision** to initiate treatment based not only on CD4 count and plasma HIV
   RNA, but also on the patient's acceptance of treatment and willingness
   to adhere to complex regimens.

D. Use of markers to monitor drug effect. The plasma HIV RNA, and to a
more limited extent the CD4 cell count, should be used to determine the effectiveness of an antiviral regimen.

   **1. The goal of treatment is in general to achieve plasma HIV RNA
   levels below the limit of detection.** This should always be the goal
   with the first regimen, and usually with a second treatment regimen.
   With more resistant virus, using salvage regimens, complete suppression
   of viral replication, while a goal, is often not possible and more limited
   virologic, immunologic or clinical goals may be established.

   2. Current approved tests have a **lower limit of detection** of ~400
   copies/mL (standard assays) or <50 copies/mL (ultrasensitive assays).
   Viral loads between 50 and 400 copies/mL usually indicate a greater risk
   of failure of a regimen. However, there is no consensus as to whether
   patients whose viral loads remain in this range should have their therapy altered.

   3. Generally a **1- to 2-log decrease** in viral load is taken as an indication
   of positive drug effect. At a minimum, a decrease of >0.5 logs (threefold
   change) is needed to overcome the variability of the test.

   4. Measurement at baseline and then 6 to 8 weeks after initiation
   is generally done, with subsequent periodic determinations every few
   months. If viral load fails to decrease at 8 weeks, in spite of the use of a
   potent regimen, then nonadherence to that regimen should be carefully
   considered. Patients who are nonadherent to one regimen are likely to
   be nonadherent to other regimens and may rapidly develop a multidrug
   resistant virus. Thus the reasons for nonadherence must be addressed
   before multiple successive therapies are used.

   5. Failure of a regimen is usually defined as the failure of the plasma
   HIV RNA to become undetectable, reappearance of detectable virus after
   a period of undetectability, or, in the case of salvage regimens where

undetectability cannot be achieved, the later return to baseline levels or higher. In these circumstances, most experts change therapy even in patients who are clinically stable. Changes in therapy are best guided by a combination of a history of prior antiretroviral drugs and resistance testing.

   6. Although decreases in viral load are usually accompanied by increases in CD4 number, cases have been described in which there is a lack of correlation in the direction of these changes. No data exists to determine which marker should be used in this situation to assess response; however, the majority of experts favor using viral load. When resistance develops, viral load appears to rebound before CD4 levels decrease.

   7. Data on laboratory variation and quality control are limited. In general, the intrapatient and intralaboratory variability suggest that a change that is <0.5 log (threefold) is within the normal variation of testing and should not be considered significant.

 II. **Approach to the initiation of therapy in the asymptomatic patient.** The decision to initiate therapy in asymptomatic patients is a complex one and ideally should be made after a full discussion of the benefits and risks between physician and patient. Early treatment is often accompanied by immediate side effects, which can diminish quality of life and in any event lead to a "medicalization" of a patient's life. In addition, the long-term toxicities of most available agents are only starting to emerge (see Chapter 17), and resistance to drugs may develop with early use, preventing a benefit of their use later in the disease. The need for more frequent monitoring may add a financial burden and interfere with the patient's work or other life activities.

   A. **The goals of treatment** must be determined and clearly discussed with the patient before initiation of therapy. From a virological perspective, it is generally agreed that **an important goal is to attempt to make the plasma viral load undetectable,** based on evidence that maximal inhibition of viral replication is associated with slower progression and prevent the development of resistance. This is a very rational approach to treatment, but important considerations must be discussed with and understood by patients before starting therapy.

      1. It is difficult, if not impossible, to achieve total inhibition of replication without the use of three-drug **combinations**, which increases the risk of drug intolerance and side effects.

      2. **Strict adherence to regimens is essential.** This approach is not suitable for noncompliant patients because intermittent or suboptimal therapy will considerably increase the probability of viral resistance. Thus it is vital that therapy be initiated **"when the patient is ready."** Given that there are very few instances where treatment needs to be initiated immediately, taking time to ensure patients' education and readiness can be very valuable in long-term success of antiretroviral therapy.

      3. The **long-term benefit** of early initiation of antiretroviral therapy is not known; specifically the durability of the viral response and the long-term tolerability and delayed toxicities of these regimens are still being evaluated.

         a. There are several theoretical **advantages of initiating therapy relatively earlier in the disease process**.

            (1) Earlier initiation of therapy is associated with a higher likelihood of suppressing viral replication.

            (2) More complete immune recovery may occur if treatment is started earlier.

            (3) Viral diversity increases over time and may be more limited if treatment is started earlier.

            (4) Transmission may be reduced if a higher proportion of infected individuals were treated and had very low viral loads.

            (5) If treatment is delayed, some patients may experience rapid progression and develop clinical illness in spite of appropriate monitoring.

b. There are also **considerations in delaying initiation of therapy.**
   (1) Toxicity of treatment is avoided or delayed.
   (2) Many patients will not completely respond to treatment. Earlier treatment will increase the population of patients with resistant HIV and increase the possibility of transmission of such virus.
   (3) Most patients treated with potent therapy have clinically relevant immune recovery even when they have very low CD4 cell counts.
4. Therapy is not curative. Current antiretroviral regimens do not eradicate HIV from latent, long-lasting cellular reservoirs.
5. Although complete suppression of viral replication in the plasma can be achieved with most potent drug combinations, the plasma represents only 1% of total body viral burden. It is not known whether complete suppression of viral replication in the body in all reservoirs can be achieved in all circumstances and with all regimens.
6. It is very important to counsel patients that complete inhibition of viral replication in the plasma cannot be achieved in all patients, especially those with prior therapy and more resistant virus. Patients may become depressed as a result of this "failure," and more realistic goals (perhaps attempting to keep the viral load below a more achievable level, e.g., 5,000 copies/mL) may need to be established with some patients.

B. The potency of different antiretroviral regimens should be considered when choosing treatment. The most commonly used method of comparing therapies is to examine the ability of a regimen to suppress viral replication to levels below detection 24 to 48 weeks after starting treatment. Most potent combinations, in clinical trials of previously untreated patients, achieve durable suppression of viral replication in at least 60% of patients treated. Regimens that are not associated with such rates of response should be regarded as potentially less potent. Response rates are often lower in clinical practice, as well as in studies of patients who have received prior therapy.
   1. Monotherapy usually results in a 0.5 to 1.5-log reduction of plasma RNA; however, this is rarely sustained because of resistance and **is never recommended.**
   2. Nucleoside analog combinations are generally more potent than is monotherapy. However, the combination of two nucleosides rarely achieves durable suppression of viral replication below detection and is **not recommended.**
      a. Dual nucleoside combinations are the backbone of most potent regimens however. The combinations of ZDV and 3TC, d4T and ddI, d4T and 3TC, and ZDV and ddI seem equivalent when used such potent regimens. The combination of ZDV and d4T is not recommended, as this combination proved inferior to others in a recent clinical trial. The combination of ddI and ddC is generally avoided because of cumulative neurotoxicity.
      b. The three nucleoside combination of ZDV, 3TC and abacavir is potent in early clinical trials and may be an effective initial regimen. Long-term studies assessing the durability of viral suppression with this regimen and comparisons to other potent regimens will be necessary to completely assess its role as initial treatment. However, the availability of these three drugs as a single pill may make it attractive in terms of patient compliance.
   3. The combination of **two nucleosides and a protease inhibitor** has become the gold standard of therapy.
      a. There are few large comparative studies among the various protease inhibitors when combined with two nucleosides, and current data does not support choosing one over any other based on **antiviral potency.**
      b. The initial mutations seen with **nelfinavir** failure (D30N most commonly) are not associated with resistance to other protease inhibitors (PIs). This has led some to suggest that nelfinavir is an attractive ini-

tial PI since its failure could be "salvaged" with other PI-based therapies. Small studies have indeed suggested that patients who fail nelfinavir can re-achieve successful viral suppression using combinations of ritonavir-saquinavir and ritonavir-indinavir.

   c. **Tolerability and long-term toxicity** become important issues in determining PI choices. However, long-term data comparing the different PIs is not available. There is general consensus that hyperlipidemia is most commonly seen with ritonavir.

   d. Several of the protease inhibitors are limited by frequent dosing schedules. The addition of a **small dose of ritonavir** (200 mg) significantly improves the pharmacokinetics of indinavir (allowing it to be given b.i.d.), saquinavir, and amprenavir. In this setting, the ritonavir does not appear to act as an additional antiviral agent.

   4. The combination of **two nucleosides and efavirenz** is equivalent to two nucleosides and a protease inhibitor. Emerging data suggests that the combination of **two nucleosides and nevirapine** is also equivalent to two nucleosides and a protease inhibitor, although some uncertainty remains with regard to patients with very high viral loads. There is less information using delavirdine as initial therapy.

   5. Combination of **two protease inhibitors** and of a **protease inhibitor plus a non-nucleoside inhibitor** have been less extensively studied, but also appear to be potent.

C. **The asymptomatic patient with >500 CD4 cells/mm³** has not yet been shown to have a long-term survival benefit from antiviral therapy; however, trials completed used only ZDV monotherapy.

   1. Some patients in this CD4 range may be **long-term nonprogressors** who may do well for many years without any therapy. Based on available data, most experts would regard patients with viral loads <5,000 copies/mL as possible slow progressors and not start antiretroviral therapy immediately.

   2. On the other hand, with evidence that viral replication is ongoing through the natural history of HIV infection and that immunodeficiency is ongoing, some experts now advocate therapy as soon as the diagnosis of HIV infection is made, especially in those patients with **high viral load** (and certainly those with >30,000 copies/mL) (see D below).

   3. Balanced against this is the observation that even at higher viral loads, CD4 count can remain at a high level for several years.

   4. Patients in this range should be encouraged to consider enrolling in clinical trials evaluating long-term strategies of treatment.

D. **The asymptomatic patient with CD4 cells in the range of 200 to 500 cells/mm³.** Most experts would consider treatment of such patients, especially at higher viral loads (Carpenter C, et al. *JAMA* 2000;283:381). In some patients, particularly those with CD4 cell counts between 350 and 500 cells/mm³, careful monitoring of patients may delay initiation of treatment for several years, but it is likely that all such patients will need to be treated eventually.

   1. **Combination therapy** should be used in all patients; the initial goal of therapy should be to maximally suppress viral load. Possible regimens are listed in Table 1 and include

      a. **Two NRTIs and an NNRTI** (either efavirenz, 600 mg p.o.daily or nevirapine, 200 mg p.o. b.i.d.). This regimen has the advantage of combining potency with relative simplicity.

      b. **Two NRTIs** (from list of possibilities in Table 1) **and one or two protease inhibitors.** As noted previously, there is no proven differences among the proteases. However, many experts advocate using ritonavir, in low doses (100 to 200 mg twice daily), combined with other proteases, to take advantage of favorable pharmacokinetics and allow for less frequent dosing. (see Chapter 5 for discussion of dosing

Table 1. Guidelines for antiretroviral therapy[a]

Two effective nucleoside reverse transcriptase inhibitors (NRTIS)	Potent protease inhibitor or NNRTI
PREFERRED (STRONG EVIDENCE OF CLINICAL BENEFIT AND SUSTAINED HIV SUPPRESSION)	
Zidovudine (ZDV) + lamivudine (3TC)	Ritonavir
ZDV + didanosine (ddI)	Indinavir[b]
Stavudine (d4T) + 3TC	Nelfinavir
d4T + ddI	Saquinavir (soft gel)
ddI + 3TC	Amprenavir[b]
	Ritonavir + saquinavir
	Efavirenz
	Nevirapine
ALTERNATIVES (LESS EVIDENCE OF ABILITY TO SUSTAIN HIV SUPPRESSION)	
2 NRTIs + delavirdine	
Abacavir + ZDV + 3TC	
NOT GENERALLY RECOMMENDED:	
2 NRTIs	
CONTRAINDICATED:	
Monotherapy	
Certain NRTI combinations:	
D4T + ZDV	
ddC + ddI	
ddC + 3TC	
ddC + D4T	

[a] Adapted from Guidelines for the Use of Antiretroviral Agents in HIV-Infected Adults and Adolescents. [US Health & Human Services, http://www.hivatis.org]
[b] Low doses of ritonavir (200 mg bid) may be added to improve plasma levels.

of individual PIs). This is particularly true when using indinavir, saquinavir, and amprenavir.

  c. The combination of ZDV 300 mg p.o. b.i.d., 3TC 150 mg p.o. b.i.d. and abacavir, 300 mg b.i.d. This regimen will have the advantage of being available as a single pill that can be taken twice daily.

  2. **Choosing an initial regimen** for patients is a complex process and requires careful consideration of issues for that individual patient, as well as future consequences in the event of failure of the regimen.

  a. There is no information yet available from prospective clinical trials to indicate that any one potent regimen is associated with a better long-term clinical outcome.

  b. **Adherence** is an important predictor of success. Many studies have shown that nonadherent patients will fail therapy and develop viral resistance. Adherence has been linked to complexity of therapy and to the development of apparently minor side effects. It is important to discuss with the patient in advance whether certain side effects are likely to lead to stopping treatment.

  (1) Physicians are poor predictors of likely adherence. However, **substance abuse,** especially alcohol and uncontrolled drug use, are associated with a higher risk of nonadherence and should be addressed before starting treatment.

  (2) In some patients, a **practice period** (using placebos, candy) that mimics drug schedules can help assess likely adherence and educate patients.

(3) Regimens that are complex, especially those that involve dosing more than twice daily or that have complicated food requirements are likely to have more problems with adherence.

c. **Baseline viral load** has been shown in many studies to predict viral success. Many experts would recommend a more potent regimen, often using four drugs, in patients with very high viral loads (e.g., plasma HIV RNA > 100,000 copies/mL). However, this approach has not been shown in prospective clinical trials to be superior to more standard three-drug regimens.

d. **Baseline CD4 counts** also predict success of regimens. However, this has not been shown to be as important in determining success of regimens in patients in this CD4 count range, as it is in patients with more advanced disease.

3. Patients receiving therapy while asymptomatic may be less willing than patients in more advanced stages to tolerate **subjective drug side effects.** A more complete discussion of the side effects of individual drugs is provided in Chapter 5. However the following issues are common and should be included in assessing which drugs to choose as initial treatment.

a. Headache, insomnia, myalgias, and nausea are common in the first few weeks of **ZDV** therapy. These symptoms usually resolve by 6 to 8 weeks, and therapy need not be stopped for these symptoms alone. However, if severe and/or limiting, the patient's ability to adhere with the regimen, substitution of ZDV by D4T is usually successful.

b. **Gastrointestinal side effects** (nausea, abdominal pain, cramping and diarrhea) are common with DDI and the protease inhibitors, especially ritonavir. Diarrhea is especially common with nelfinavir.

c. **Rash** may occur in the first few weeks of treatment with nevirapine, amprenavir, and abacavir. It may also occur less frequently with efavirenz and delavirdine.

d. When using abacavir, patients must be educated about the possibility of **hypersensitivity** (see Chapter 5).

e. Patients with a history of and/or risk factors for **pancreatitis** should not receive ddI.

f. **Peripheral neuropathy** may occur with ddI, ddC, and d4T.

g. Most patients (at least 50% to 60%) taking **efavirenz** experience vivid dreams and/or nightmares in the first 2 to 4 weeks.

h. Nephrolithiasis has been reported in 5% of patients taking **indinavir**. Avoidance of this requires considerable fluid intake.

i. Patients may need considerable support to comply with therapy while asymptomatic. Fitting in appointments for monitoring, dealing with the psychological implications of being a patient, and guarding confidentiality can all be significant sources of stress and can lead to noncompliance.

4. **A strategic approach** is needed to plan antiretroviral therapy at this stage of disease. In addition to determining patient preference, tolerance of likely side effects and ability to adhere, it is important to **preserve future options for treatment** as much as possible, given that life-long therapy is required. Unfortunately, long-term clinical trials are not completed and it is necessary to try and extrapolate from relatively short-term data.

a. In an effort to have options for treating in the event of failure, most experts would **limit the number of classes of antiretrovirals** used in initial therapy to two. An exception may be patients with very high viral loads where some experts would favor more intensive treatment.

b. Because of concern about long-term metabolic side effects (see Chapter 19), many physicians use initial **protease-sparing regimens** (such as two NRTIs and an NNRTI or three NRTIs), in preference to regimens containing protease inhibitors. It should be emphasized that a causal relationship between the use of protease inhibitors and all of these later syndromes has not been completely established.

  c. There is a limited amount of data in **sequencing protease inhibitors**. In general, treating patients with PI-resistant virus is difficult. However, some success has been achieved using dual protease regimens (ritonavir-saquinavir or ritonavir-indinavir) in patients who have failed nelfinavir. One reason for this may be that initial mutations associated with resistance to drugs such as nelfinavir or amprenavir may be less likely to lead to cross-resistance to other PIs. Thus, it may be possible to start initial PI-based therapy with these agents, knowing that second-line therapy with other protease inhibitors is still feasible.

  d. **Maintenance** therapy (i.e., starting with a three-drug regimen and dropping one of the agents at a later time point) has not been successful in clinical trials and is not recommended.

  e. **Simplification** of the initial regimen (usually involving switching from a protease inhibitor to either an NNRTI or abacavir) has been successfully employed in a limited number of studies. Patients should have had complete suppression of viral replication for at least 6 months if such a strategy is considered and should be monitored closely after the switch. The long-term success of such an approach, compared with continuation of the original regimen, is unknown.

  f. Most patients who adhere to these regimens will achieve durable complete suppression of viral replication. However, some patients may not suppress viral replication as rapidly and may be at greater risk of ultimate failure. In such patients, the possibility of **intensification**, i.e., adding another agent before viral resistance has occurred, is being evaluated in clinical trials and may emerge as an alternate strategy.

  5. The overwhelming majority of patients in this stage will not progress to AIDS in the short term even in the absence of therapy.

  a. Thus some patients in this range may still choose to forego therapy at this stage.

  b. If treatment is not begun, frequent (every 3 months) testing of CD4 and viral load should be performed to assess laboratory evidence of disease progression.

  6. Many patients who readily accept antiviral therapy will also wish to use alternative approaches such as acupuncture, visualization, or herbal therapy.

  a. They should be encouraged to share this information with their primary provider to prevent and detect side effects from such therapies.

  b. A nonjudgmental, supportive approach should be taken.

E. **The asymptomatic patient who has not been treated with antiviral agents and has <200 CD4 cells**. Patients with newly diagnosed HIV infection and CD4 counts <200 cells/mm^3 or those who have been monitored without antiviral intervention whose CD4 counts are less than this level require potent combination therapy. The approach to choosing a regimen is identical to that given in D above. However, clinical trials have shown **a survival advantage in patients with advanced disease who receive the combination of a protease inhibitor plus two nucleosides**. It is likely that other potent regimens that also effectively suppress viral replication and restore immune function would also have a survival advantage.

III. **Approach to the patient who is failing antiviral therapy.** Current antiviral philosophy centers on monitoring viral load carefully in patients receiving therapy and changing treatment when the patient starts to exhibit evidence of "virologic failure."

  A. The **definition of failure** may vary depending on the clinical circumstance.

    1. For patients receiving their initial treatment, most experts would define failure as

    a. Less than a 10-fold decrease (one log) from baseline HIV RNA levels receiving potent treatment after 8 to 12 weeks of therapy.

    b. Detectable HIV RNA levels after 4 to 6 months of therapy (may be longer when ultrasensitive assay is used).

    c. Repeated detection of HIV RNA in patients who had undetectable levels following initiation of therapy.

  2. In **patients who have failed several regimens**, where good therapeutic options are limited, some degree of viral replication may be tolerated, especially if the patients remain clinically and immunologically stable. In such cases, a sustained decrease in HIV RNA copy number of 1.5 to 2.0 $\log_{10}$ from baseline may justify continuation of the therapeutic regimen if acceptable antiretroviral options are not available. In this situation, virologic failure may be defined if the patient's viral load increases 0.5 to 1.0 logs over the minimum achieved by treatment or if the patient's viral load returns to within 0.5 to 1.0 logs of their baseline. Even then, if there are no good options, therapy may be continued.

B. The **cause of failure** should be carefully assessed.

  1. Nonadherence is a common cause of failure. If the reasons for nonadherence are not addressed, then it is extremely likely that the patient will not adhere to new regimens and failure will recur. If the patient is completely nonadherent, then wild-type virus will remain and the possibility of long-term success remains if adherence can be corrected. However, if the patient is partially adherent, then viral resistance is very likely and this will create great difficulties for ultimately successful treatment.

  2. Patients may fail because of **subtherapeutic drug levels**. This may reflect poor absorption, increased metabolism or drug-drug interactions (see appendix). The latter are particularly important when using combinations of protease inhibitors and NNRTIs. Failure of PI-based regimens without immediate appearance of resistant mutations has been attributed to subtherapeutic levels in individual patients and has been described with indinavir, nelfinavir and amprenavir. The addition of ritonavir, even in low doses, generally prevents this problem of inadequate drug levels. Therapeutic drug level monitoring is not yet widely available but should be considered in individuals who are apparently compliant, but failing a potent regimen.

  3. Failure will occur if the regimen is not **potent** enough. This should be unusual when typical three-drug regimens are used, but may be more likely in patients with very high baseline viral loads or lower CD4 counts.

C. Resistance testing has been shown to be of value in choosing new regimens for patients. At least over the short term (24 weeks), therapeutic changes guided by the results of resistance testing are associated with a greater likelihood of success.

D. The **choice of new regimens** is not always clear. Most experts advocate **three new drugs** that the patient has not previously taken in an effort to minimize resistance. In addition, if possible, a **new class of antiretrovirals** should be used. In all studies of patients who have failed a PI-based regimen, there has been a greater likelihood of success if the patient had not previously received an NNRTI, which was then included in the salvage regimen. However, switching to three new drugs and a new class may be confounded by issues of cross-resistance and toxicity, and often therapeutic options are limited for many patients after only one or two switches of treatments. Consultation with experts in antiretroviral therapy is recommended.

  1. Best results are seen if the entire regimen is switched, i.e., if the patient can receive **two new nucleosides and a new class of antivirals**.

  2. Cross-resistance among the protease inhibitors is an important issue. HIV strains resistant to indinavir tend to be resistant to ritonavir and vice versa. Indeed, indinavir failure is difficult to rescue and recent studies suggest that two new protease inhibitors should be used. The degree of cross-resistance with other protease inhibitors is more variable. Patients who have received therapy only with **nelfinavir** have a higher rate of success when given a second protease inhibitor based regimen such as ritonavir-saquinavir or ritonavir-indinavir (Tebas P, et al. *AIDS* 1999;13:F23).

3. **Cross-resistance among the NRTIs** is more variable.
   a. Resistance to **3TC** appears rapidly in patients failing regimens containing this drug. A single point mutation at position 184 of the reverse transcriptase gene confers high-level resistance to this drug and also to FTC. However, the appearance of this mutation may restore ZDV sensitivity in ZDV-resistant strains.
   b. Resistance to **ZDV** is a gradual process and initially may not be at a high level. However, the appearance of multiple ZDV resistance mutations is usually associated with high-level resistance.
   c. Viruses with high-level resistance to both ZDV and 3TC are usually resistant to **abacavir**.
   d. There is little cross-resistance between **ddI, DDC**, and ZDV. Although mutations at codon 184 decrease ddI susceptibility, the clinical relevance is uncertain.
   e. It is difficult to demonstrate **D4T** resistance by available resistance tests, but it is known to occur *in vivo*. Viruses with high-level resistance to ZDV tend to be resistant to D4T, although this may be difficult to demonstrate using resistance testing.
   f. Several mutations have ben described that are associated with **broad resistance** across the nucleoside analogs. These include a mutation at codon 151 and an insertion mutation at codon 69.
4. There is almost **complete cross-resistance among available NNRTIs**.
5. **Toxicity** also limits drug choices. This is especially true for peripheral neuropathy, which is seen with ddI, ddC, d4T, and to a limited extent, with 3TC.

E. **The patient who is clinically stable, but has worsening viral markers.** There is increasing evidence that some patients who are experiencing virologic failure while on a PI-based regimen may have prolonged periods where the CD4 count remains stable and there is no clinical progression. The reason for this is not clear, although there is some evidence that initial mutations associated with resistance to PIs makes the virus "less fit." This period of clinical and immunologic stability can last for several years, but is not associated with viral quiescence. Additional secondary mutations accumulate that may make salvage therapy more difficult. In general, therefore, if it is possible to change the patient's therapeutic regimen it should be changed.

F. **Therapy in patients with limited options.** It is important to discuss goals with patients in whom it is unlikely that durable viral suppression can be accomplished.
   1. It is important to realize that in general **any degree of viral suppression is associated with clinical benefit**. Disease progression is very rare in patients whose viral load remains less than 5,000 copies/mL and is slowed if the viral replication remains below baseline levels. Thus, even in the presence of drug resistance, antiretroviral therapy should be continued as long as it is tolerated and if some antiviral effect can be shown.
   2. **Hydroxyurea** increases intracellular levels of ddI and has been used as part of salvage regimens. However, it is myelosuppressive and reduces CD4 cell counts, so it should be used with caution. In addition, the use of hydroxyurea with ddI may increase risk of pancreatitis.
   3. Some physicians have advocated **recycling drugs** used previously, often in 5 to 7 drug regimens. However, such approaches usually have only transient success and are often poorly tolerated.
   4. Some physicians have advocated brief periods of **drug holidays** for 8 to 10 weeks to allow wild-type virus to become the dominant quasispecies and thus allow recycling of drugs. Again, this is rarely associated with

long-term benefit and if done, should be carefully monitored as precipitous drops in CD4 cell counts can occur.

G. The patient with prolonged antiviral experience who now has end-stage AIDS (see Chapter 10). Patients, especially those with advanced disease, take a large number of medications and are at significant risk of reversible and irreversible side effects. Gastrointestinal disturbances and peripheral neuropathy may be especially common with antiviral medications. In some cases, a switch to another antiviral medication may be possible, and it is especially important that such patients have a trial of drugs that might reduce viral load. However, in many patients, it is not possible safely to administer all appropriate medications. In this case, medications that treat patient symptoms and provide prophylaxis against opportunistic infections are usually given precedence over antiviral therapy. If symptoms can be controlled, antiviral agents are reintroduced.

IV. Mechanisms available to provide unapproved antiviral medication and to assist patients in paying for antiviral medications. Most antiviral medications used in AIDS are made available before FDA approval, and once clinical trials are under way through several different mechanisms most commonly referred to as "compassionate release" programs or "expanded access" programs. In general, these programs require that the treating physician document that patients are unable to tolerate or have failed on licensed therapies and, in addition, meet criteria for clinical and laboratory parameters set by the sponsor (usually a pharmaceutical company). In general, drugs are provided at no cost, although the costs of physician visits and laboratory testing must be borne by the patient or third-party payors or both. In addition, many companies provide assistance to patients who cannot pay for approved drugs to find sources of coverage or obtain drug at reduced or no cost.

7. OVERVIEW OF PEDIATRIC INFECTION

The epidemic of pediatric human immunodeficiency virus (HIV) infection continues at an alarming pace worldwide. The vast majority of new pediatric HIV cases are due to perinatal transmission of the virus. Transmission may occur during gestation (in utero), during labor and delivery (intrapartum), and through breastfeeding. Perinatal transmission of HIV can be greatly reduced by effective antiretroviral therapy of the mother during pregnancy and by early treatment of the newborn (see Chapter 9). With the introduction of such an approach in the United States and in the developed world, perinatal transmission has been reduced dramatically and many fewer babies are born with HIV infection. Indeed, the main factor in HIV transmission to infants now in the United States is lack of access to adequate prenatal care. However, the situation is much more grim in the developing world and in populations with less resources. Although pediatric AIDS cases, defined as children <13 years old, compose <2% of total cases in the United States, and account for 15% to 20% of cases in developing countries, the majority in sub-Saharan Africa.

Despite the encouraging data about new infections, there is still a large population of HIV-infected children and adolescents requiring ongoing medical care. **Management** of the HIV-exposed/infected child is multifaceted and includes an understanding of the unique manifestations and progression of pediatric HIV disease, determination of infection and immunologic status, unique aspects of antiretroviral therapy in children, optimal nutrition, prophylaxis against *Pneumocystis carinii* pneumonia (PCP) and other infections, and routine pediatric care. In addition, psychosocial assistance is essential in that this disease often infects or affects several family members.

I. **Pediatric exposure categories.** Of pediatric AIDS cases, 90% result from vertical or mother-to-fetus/infant transmission. Because women are one of the fastest growing groups of newly infected individuals, the pediatric epidemic will continue to grow. The other categories account for a small proportion of cases: coagulation-disorder therapy, 3%; receipt of blood components or tissue, 5%; and other (includes sexual abuse) or undetermined risk, 2%.

II. **Adolescents.** Recently there has been a marked proportionate increase in HIV-infected adolescents. Adolescent **risk factors** vary by gender such that treatment for coagulation disorders and homosexual contact are major categories in teenage boys, whereas heterosexual contact and, to a lesser extent, intravenous drug use predominate in teenage girls. Other risks include receipt of HIV-infected blood products or tissue and sexual abuse. Most worrisome is that 15% to 20% of all U.S. AIDS cases are thought to have been acquired between ages 13 and 19.

III. **Diagnosis of HIV infection in children** younger than 18 months poses a greater challenge than that in older children and adults, in whom standard serologic assays are used to diagnose HIV infection.

A. For infants, transplacentally acquired maternal HIV antibodies can persist up to 18 months. Therefore the diagnosis of HIV infection is based on direct demonstration of virus by viral blood culture, polymerase chain reaction (PCR) or immune complex-dissociated p24 antigen (ICD p24). It is possible to determine if infection has been acquired in utero and intrapartum. Infection acquired in utero tends to have a more rapid course.

   1. An infant is considered to have **in utero infection** if virologic tests (HIV DNA or RNA PCR or culture) are positive within 48 hours of life.

   2. Infants are considered to have **intrapartum** HIV infection if diagnostic tests within the first 48 hours of life are negative, but further virologic testing after 1 week of life is positive.

B. **Virologic testing** of exposed infants is performed initially by age 1 month (preferably in first week) and repeated with at least one test obtained after age 4 months. A presumptive diagnosis of HIV infection is based on one positive test (viral culture, PCR, or p24 antigen) and confirmed with a second specimen. More than 95% of infected infants test positive between ages 3 and 6 months. For infants who have not tested positive by age 6 months and have no clinical features consistent with HIV disease, HIV antibody testing is recommended until age 2 years to document loss of maternal antibody and lack of infection.

C. **Screening for HIV** should be done in infants and children with HIV-infected or high-risk mothers, children with sexually transmitted diseases (STDs), or any child with the following signs or symptoms of unclear origin: failure to thrive (FTT), diffuse adenopathy, hepatosplenomegaly, chronic thrush, chronic/recurrent diarrhea, recurrent invasive bacterial disease, lymphoid interstitial pneumonitis (LIP), encephalopathy, acquired microcephaly, chronic parotitis, or atypical immune-mediated thrombocytopenia.

IV. **Disease progression.** In general, children progress more rapidly than adults in the development of immune dysfunction and resultant illnesses. The highest incidence of AIDS occurs in the first year of life; however a wide spectrum of disease is seen from asymptomatic for years to severe immunosuppression with rapid progression to death in <1 year. A bimodal pattern of disease onset and progression has been described.

A. **Rapid progressors** comprise 10% to 25% of pediatric AIDS cases and develop symptoms within months to a year of life, with rapid decline in CD4+ counts and development of AIDS-defining conditions, followed by death within 4 years.

B. **Slow progressors** account for 75% to 90% of cases and have a more indolent course, with symptoms developing within the first several years. Median age at AIDS diagnosis is 6 years, but some live to adolescence. The latter often have evidence of lymphoproliferation (LIP, adenopathy, hepatosplenomegaly, or parotid enlargement).

C. **Nonprogressors** have no symptoms for 8 to 10 years, but comprise <5% of cases.

D. **Rate of disease progression** appears to correlate with the severity of maternal disease at delivery, timing of infection (intrauterine, intrapartum, or later), host genotype and immune response, viral burden, and viral genotype and phenotype.

E. **Laboratory abnormalities** noted in HIV-infected children include anemia, leukopenia, low CD4+/CD8, low absolute CD4+ count, hypergammaglobulinemia or rarely hypogammaglobulinemia, thrombocytopenia, reduction in lymphocyte response to mitogens, and decrease in antibody responsiveness.

V. **Pediatric HIV classification system.** In 1994, a revised classification system for HIV-1 infection in children younger than 13 years was published to incorporate the current state of knowledge about disease progression and to redefine the categories to describe the stage of disease and prognosis more accurately. The categories are based on the child's infection status, along with clinical and immunologic status (*MMWR* 1994;43:RR-12), and help in determining candidates for antiviral therapy (Table 1). The clinical categories are divided into mild (A), which includes children with lymphadenopathy, hepatomegaly, splenomegaly, dermatitis, parotitis, and recurrent or persistent sinusitis or otitis media; moderate (B), including various organ-specific dysfunctions (persistent anemia, neutropenia, or thrombocytopenia, LIP, cardiomyopathy, recurrent/chronic diarrhea, hepatitis, nephropathy, or leiomyosarcoma) or infections (invasive bacterial infection, persistent candidiasis, congenital CMV or toxoplasmosis, systemic neonatal HSV disease, recurrent HSV or herpes zoster, disseminated varicella, nocardiosis, or persistent fever); and severe (C) includes conditions listed in the 1987 CDC definition for AIDS, except LIP (*MMWR* 1987;36:1S).

A. **Differences between pediatric and adult HIV disease.**

1. **Primary mode of acquisition** is vertical transmission.

2. **A shorter incubation period and more rapid rate of disease progression** are generally seen in children with HIV, compared with adults. Mean survival without treatment is 9.4 years (Barnhart HX, et al. *Pediatrics* 1996;97:710).

Table 1. Classification for pediatric HIV infection

Immunologic categories[a]	Clinical categories (signs and symptoms)			
	N: None	A: Mild	B: Moderate	C: Severe
1. No evidence of suppression	N1	A1	B1	C1
2. Moderate evidence of suppression	N2	A2	B2	C2
3. Severe suppression	N3	A3	B3	C3

[a] Immunologic status based on age-specific CD4 counts and percentages as follows: 1, CD4% ≥25% or CD4 ≥1,500 in younger than 12 mo, ≥1,000 in age 1 to 5 yr, and ≥500 in age 6 to 12 yr; 2, CD4% of 15% to 24% or CD4 750 to 1,499 in younger than 12 mo, 500 to 999 in age 1 to 5 yr, and 200 to 499 in age 6 to 12 yr; 3, CD4% <15% or CD4 <750 in younger than 12 mo, <500 in age 1 to 5 yr, and <200 in age 6 to 12 yr. (From *MMWR* 1994; 43(RR-12):1, with permission.)

   3. **Diagnosis** of HIV infection in children younger than 18 months is more problematic because of the presence of maternal antibodies.
   4. Normal **CD4+ lymphocyte counts** in children younger than 6 years are higher than in adults *(MMWR* 1991;40:RR-2), such that opportunistic infections (OIs) occur with much higher CD4+ counts.
   5. **Infections.** Children have an increased incidence of recurrent invasive bacterial infections. Also, OIs often represent primary disease with a more fulminant course, given lack of prior immunity (i.e., PCP and CMV), rather than reactivation of latent infection seen in adults.
   6. Certain **noninfectious manifestations** are relatively unique to pediatric HIV, such as LIP, chronic parotid enlargement, and early onset of neurologic deterioration. Some conditions are less common in children, such as tuberculosis and malignancies. Of AIDS-defining illnesses in children, ~2% are malignancies compared with 10% to 15% in adults. Kaposi's sarcoma is rare in children.
VI. **Management** of pediatric HIV-infected patients requires a **multidisciplinary team approach,** including pediatrician, nurse, social worker, nutritionist, and health educator, with the availability of infectious diseases, immunology, developmental, neurology, ophthalmology, dental, chaplain, and gynecology consultants, among others. To provide **family-centered care,** several pediatric centers hold a joint clinic with the internists so parent(s) and child are seen simultaneously.
   A. **Evaluation** should include a complete history and physical examination with emphasis on infections, other illnesses, dietary and developmental history, along with growth parameters, oral lesions, lymph nodes, organomegaly and neurologic evaluation. Baseline and laboratory data obtained when the diagnosis of HIV infection is made (see Diagnosis section) should include plasma HIV RNA, complete blood count (CBC), lymphocyte subpopulations, quantitative immunoglobulins, liver, renal, and pancreatic profiles, Mantoux skin testing, rapid plasma reagin (RPR), hepatitis B surface antigen, HSV, CMV, Epstein–Barr virus (EBV) and toxoplasmosis titers after 6 months of age, and postimmunization antibody titers. Some centers also obtain a baseline chest radiograph, neuroimaging study, and neurodevelopmental assessment.
   B. **Goals of therapy** are similar to those in adults. Decreasing viral replication should enhance immune function, and prevent infectious and noninfectious complications. It is important also to address the child's and family's psychosocial needs, and improve quality of life. In addition, one must address the availability of pediatric medical preparations, pediatric pharmacokinetics, costs, side effects, and the capability of the child's caregivers to administer the therapy.

C. Criteria for initiation of therapy. Treatment should be initiated in children with a definitive diagnosis of HIV infection.

    1. The Working Group on Antiretroviral Therapy and Medical Management of HIV Infected Children in 1999 (http://www.hivatis.org) recommended that **all HIV-infected children be treated as soon as possible.**

        a. An exception was made for **children older than 1 year of age** with normal immune status and a low risk of disease progression (low virus load). In these children an individualized decision should be made taking into consideration issues such as safety, adherence and concern for the duration of antiretroviral response. In these circumstance, then treatment might be deferred to a later date.

        b. If treatment is deferred, children should be **monitored closely** with regular clinical evaluations, CD4$^+$ cell counts, and plasma HIV RNA measurements. Antiretroviral therapy should be initiated promptly in the HIV-infected child in the following situations.

            (1) **HIV RNA levels are elevated or increasing** (>5-fold increase for children <2 years and >3-fold for those >2 years of age).

            (2) **CD4$^+$ absolute number or percentage is declining** rapidly to Immunologic category 2.

            (3) Development of **clinical symptoms**

            (4) All children with **HIV RNA levels > 100,000 copies/mL**

            (5) Children older than 30 months who have HIV RNA levels consistent with treatment recommendations for HIV-infected adults (see chapter 6)

    2. **Antiretroviral therapies** should be used in **combination** in the treatment of all HIV-infected children. The principles of therapy are exactly the same as in adults (see Chapter 6).

        a. The only occasion when **monotherapy** is still used is during the 6 week course of **postexposure prophylaxis** of infants born to HIV-infected women. These infants usually receive zidovudine, although alternatives should be considered if the mother is known to have ZDV-resistant virus. However, if infants are diagnosed as having HIV infection during this period, treatment should be changed to combination therapy.

        b. **The agents** used in pediatric infection are the same as those used for adults; the only major difference is that not all drugs are available as a pediatric suspension (Table 2). Thus, there are limitations as to choices available for small children who are unable to take adult size tablet or capsules.

Table 2. Antiretroviral agents available as pediatric suspensions

NUCLEOSIDE ANALOGS INHIBITING HIV-1 REVERSE TRANSCRIPTASE (NRTIS):
Zidovudine (ZDV)
Didanosine (ddI)
Lamivudine (3TC)
Stavudine (d4T)
Abacavir (ABC)

NON-NUCLEOSIDE ANALOGS INHIBITING HIV-1 RT (NNRTIS):
Nevirapine

INHIBITORS OF HIV-1 PROTEASE (PIS):
Ritonavir
Nelfinavir
Amprenavir

c. The usual first choice regimen for children includes **two NRTIs and one protease inhibitor**. This approach has proven successful in reducing levels of HIV RNA to undetectable children.

d. There is less data available for **protease sparing regimens** in children. Although it might be possible to initiate therapy with two NRTIs in combination with an NNRTI (nevirapine or efavirenz) or three NRTIs alone, these combinations have not yet been studied as extensively in children as initial treatment.

e. Because **adolescents** can be treated with all available drugs, the approach to antiretroviral therapy in adolescents is identical to that of adults (see Chapter 6).

3. **Treatment failure** in HIV-infected children is similar to that in adults in that it is primarily defined virologically. However, clinical progression can be more rapid in children and viral failure can lead to growth failure, development of new infections indicative of immunodeficiency, or development or worsening of neurologic HIV disease. In general, it would be hoped that regular monitoring of virologic status would prevent immunological or clinical failure by offering new therapies.

a. As with adults, failure may result from problems with **drug delivery and drug adherence**. Failure to take the drug in children is even more complex than in adults and can involve failure of the parent or caregiver to administer the medicine as well as problems in formulation or taste of the medication. Pharmacokinetics are complicated in children and attention must be paid to correct dosing.

b. Definitions of **virologic treatment failure** in children include:
   (1) **Less than a 10-fold decrease** (one log) from baseline HIV RNA levels in children receiving potent treatment after 8 to 12 weeks of therapy.
   (2) **Detectable HIV RNA levels** after 4 to 6 months of therapy (may be longer when ultrasensitive assay is used). Ideally the goal is to suppress viral replication completely, however, this might not be achievable for every patient. Therefore, this is not an absolute indication and a sustained decrease in HIV RNA copy number of 1.5 to 2.0 $\log_{10}$ from baseline (if RNA levels are low) may justify continuation of the therapeutic regimen, if acceptable antiretroviral options are not available.
   (3) **Repeated detection of HIV RNA** in children who had undetectable levels following initiation of therapy.
   (4) **Persistent increase in HIV RNA** levels after initiation of treatment > than 3-fold in children >2 years, and > than 5-fold in children under 2 years of age

c. Indications of **immunologic treatment failure** in children include
   (1) Change in immunologic classification
   (2) Rapid and significant decrease in absolute CD4+ cell number.

d. **Clinical evidence of treatment failure** in children can include:
   (1) Progressive **neurodevelopmental deterioration**.
   (2) **Growth failure** defined as persistent decline in weight-growth velocity despite adequate nutritional support and without other explanation.

4. As with adults, the key to **management** is the introduction of new drugs, and new classes of drugs where possible. Resistance testing should be used to guide therapy in experienced patients. There have been fewer studies of different combinations in children, but the principles of using available drugs applies. A study of efavirenz combined with nelfinavir and at least one new nucleoside in NRTI-experienced children was associated with a response rate of 60% to 70%; children as young as 3 years were evaluated (Starr SE, et al. *N Engl J Med*, 1999;341:1874).

D. **Immunizations.** A key aspect of pediatric care is the administration of all routine childhood immunizations [diphtheria-pertussis-tetanus (DTaP),

Haemophilus influenzae type b (HIB), hepatitis B, and measles-mumps-rubella (MMR)] except varicella vaccine, which is not presently recommended. Inactivated polio vaccine should replace oral polio vaccine, and influenza vaccine (after age 6 months), plus pneumococcal vaccine (after age 2 years) should be included in the immunization schedule. Yearly influenza immunization is recommended for children over 6 months of age and family members.

1. **Suboptimal responses** to immunizations have been demonstrated in several studies of HIV-infected children, especially those with evidence of immunosuppression. Postimmunization titers, booster immunizations, and administration of vaccines at a younger age when the immune system is more intact have been suggested to optimize vaccine-mediated immunity.

2. **Passive immunization** against varicella, measles, tetanus, and hepatitis B should be provided after known exposures.

E. **Optimal nutrition** is crucial to treatment of the HIV-infected child, as malnutrition itself impairs many facets of the immune system. A large proportion of HIV-infected children develop FTT at some stage in their disease. This results from decreased intake (oral and esophageal lesions, poor dentition, nausea, zinc deficiency, neurologic dysfunction, anorexia, depression, pain, and decreased availability of food because of socioeconomic factors), increased losses [vomiting, diarrhea, pancreatic insufficiency, lactose deficiency, malabsorption, or OIs of the gastrointestinal tract], and presumed increased requirements (febrile illnesses, altered metabolic requirements, or cytokine production). Children generally have more muscle than fat wasting, and linear growth can be most affected. Intake in children must be sufficient to sustain basal energy expenditure, physical activity, and growth.

1. **A nutritionist** is an integral part of the HIV care team and assists with initial and ongoing evaluations along with recommendations regarding appropriate supplementation (Nicholas SW, et al. *J Pediatr* 1991;119: S59). **An initial assessment** should be carried out at diagnosis. All should take a multivitamin daily. Some children simply require a well-balanced, nutritious diet. For those who have **growth failure**, a more extensive evaluation is indicated, and a high-protein, high-calorie diet encouraged.

2. **Supplementation.** Macronutrient supplementation is necessary in those who have ongoing growth failure. In **infants**, caloric density can be increased by using a 24- or 27-calorie per ounce formula, by adding polycose or medium-chain triglyceride oil; **older children** can use a variety of 30-kcal per oz supplements. Elemental formulas may be needed for malabsorptive states. In addition to macronutrient supplementation, HIV-infected children may require replacement of micronutrients, such as zinc, iron, pyridoxine, or folate. If supplementation does not result in adequate weight gain, then nighttime or intermittent daytime **nasogastric tube feedings** may be necessary. **Gastrostomy tube** placement should be discussed when long-term supplementation is anticipated (Miller TL, et al. *Pediatrics* 1995;96:696). Children rarely need **total parenteral nutrition** for extended times.

3. **Appetite stimulants**, such as megestrol acetate or dronabinol (Marinol), have been used in some children and adolescents, with variable results.

4. **Neuroendocrine dysfunction**, such as thyroid and growth hormone disorders, have been described in a minority of children and should be evaluated in children with consistent symptoms.

G. **Neurodevelopmental intervention.** A large percentage of HIV-infected children develop neurologic involvement with motor or cognitive defects or both. Careful attention should be paid to development, school performance, and the neurologic examination each visit. With any signs of plateau or regression of milestones, a more detailed evaluation is warranted. Physical, occupational, or speech therapy or other interventions should be requested as indicated. Routine neurodevelopmental assessments and baseline neuro-imaging are recommended.

H. Psychosocial support is crucial for the HIV-infected or HIV-affected child and his family members, several of whom also may be infected. Children are often cared for by parents who are ill themselves, extended family members, or foster/adoptive parents because of parental death or illness. A family-centered **social worker/case manager** is a key member of the pediatric HIV-care team, providing invaluable emotional and psychological support, along with access to financial assistance for the families. In addition, many programs offer support groups, permanency planning, legal aid, chaplaincy services, and access to peer counselors, which is especially important for adolescents. Child-life specialists function as the child's advocate and play therapist.

VII. Infectious complications of pediatric HIV disease. More detailed information regarding prophylaxis for many opportunistic pathogens is found elsewhere in this manual.

A. Bacterial infections

1. **Recurrent bacterial infections.** HIV-infected children are at increased risk for systemic bacterial infections, including sepsis, meningitis, osteomyelitis, septic arthritis, or abscesses. The pathogens are often *Streptococcus pneumoniae, Haemophilus influenzae*, and *Salmonella* spp. Intravenous immunoglobulin (400 mg per kg every 4 weeks) is indicated for children with recurrent severe bacterial infections, hypogammaglobulinemia, or poor antibody responses to immunizations (see Immunization section for preventive measures).

2. *Mycobacterium tuberculosis* remains relatively infrequent in children. PPD skin testing is recommended even though some are anergic.

3. *Mycobacterium avium complex*, when disseminated, is seen with fever, night sweats, weight loss, malaise, abdominal pain, diarrhea, hepatosplenomegaly, abnormal liver enzymes, and neutropenia. It occurs in 12% to 24% of children with advanced HIV disease. Prophylaxis with rifabutin is recommended for those with CD4+<75 or a comparable degree of immunosuppression in children younger than 6 years. Treatment generally includes a three- or four-drug regimen, such as clarithromycin, rifabutin, ethambutol, ciprofloxacin, or amikacin.

2. Fungal infections

1. *Pneumocystis carinii pneumonia (PCP)* remains a major cause of morbidity and mortality in HIV-infected pediatric patients with a peak incidence in 3- to 6-month-old infants. Primary infection with a rapidly progressive pneumonitis can be devastating. Close to 50% of cases occur in children not previously identified as at risk or infected, further emphasizing the need for HIV screening and early prophylaxis.

   a. **Prophylaxis.** In 1995 revised guidelines for PCP prophylaxis were published (Table 3). These guidelines recommend identification of HIV-infected pregnant women and their infants, diagnostic and immunologic monitoring of the infants, and prophylaxis in all HIV-exposed infants regardless of CD4+ count (*MMWR* 1995;44(RR-4):1). Prophylaxis should continue throughout infancy for those with possible or definitive HIV infection but may be discontinued in uninfected infants older than 4 months. Beyond 12 months of age, continue PCP prophylaxis if the patient has severe immunosuppression or a history of PCP. It is anticipated that improved efforts at early identification of HIV-exposed infants and routine PCP prophylaxis for those younger than 1 year will result in marked savings with respect to costs and, more important, lives.

      (1) **The regimen of choice** is trimethoprim/sulfamethoxazole (TMP, 150 mg/m^2, and SMX, 750 mg/m^2) divided b.i.d. and administered on 3 consecutive days each week. Alternative schedules include the same dose given once daily on 3 consecutive days

Table 3. Recommendations for PCP prophylaxis

Age	Recommendations
Birth to 4 to 6 weeks	No prophylaxis
4 to 6[a] weeks to 4 months	PCP prophylaxis
4 to 12 months	
HIV infected or indeterminate	PCP prophylaxis
HIV infection excluded	No prophylaxis
1 to 5 years, HIV infected	
CD4 < 500 or <15%	PCP prophylaxis

PCP, *Pneumocystis carinii* pneumonia; HIV, human immunodeficiency virus; ZDV, zidovudine.
[a] Start prophylaxis at 6 weeks after ZDV discontinued if on perinatal ZDV protocol. [From *MMWR* 1995;44(RR-4):1, with permission.]

    a week, given b.i.d. 3 alternate days a week, or given b.i.d. daily. Routine hematologic monitoring should be carried out.

    (2) Alternative regimens. If TMP/SMX is not tolerated, then dapsone (2 mg per kg per day), monthly aerosolized pentamidine in those older than 4 years, or intravenous pentamidine are other options (*MMWR* 1995;44(RR-4)1).

  b. Treatment of PCP in children involves supportive care, often in a critical-care setting, TMP/SMX (20 mg per kg per day of TMP component dosed every 6 hours) for 21 days, administered intravenously and then orally when improved. Intravenous pentamidine, 4 mg per kg per day, is the second-line agent. Other options have not been well studied in the pediatric age group but include TMP-dapsone, atovaquone, trimetrexate and leucovorin, or clindamycin and primaquine.

    (1) Corticosteroids given to adults with moderate to severe PCP decreased the risk of respiratory failure and death. Two trials in pediatric HIV-infected patients also demonstrated a survival benefit (Sleasman JW, et al. *Am J Dis Child* 1993;147:30; McLaughlin GE, et al. *J Pediatr* 1995;126:821). Therefore in pediatric patients with PaO_2 <70 in room air, use of adjunctive corticosteroids is recommended.

  2. Candida causes thrush, esophagitis, and severe diaper rash in children. Nystatin is first-line therapy, but for persistent or recurrent disease or for esophagitis, the use of fluconazole, ketoconazole, frequent gentian violet applications (thrush), or amphotericin B may be necessary.

  3. Toxoplasmosis and cryptococcosis are uncommon in children with HIV disease.

C. Viral infections

  1. Varicella zoster virus infections, primary disease, recurrent zoster, or chronic infection, can be severe in children with HIV disease and usually require treatment with intravenous acyclovir. Famciclovir or valacyclovir are now available, but there is less pediatric experience with these newer agents. Although use of varicella vaccine is under study in HIV-infected children, it is not recommended; therefore any HIV-infected susceptible child should receive varicella-zoster immune globulin (VZIG) when exposed to varicella.

  2. Herpes simplex virus commonly causes oropharyngeal disease, but can occasionally cause esophagitis, recurrent genital infections, severe necrotizing infections, or disseminated disease. Depending on disease severity, oral or intravenous acyclovir is recommended. Famciclovir or valacyclovir also can be used. Chronic suppressive antiviral therapy may be necessary in children with frequent or severe recurrences.

3. **Cytomegalovirus** (CMV) infection has been reported in ~60% of HIV-infected children. Symptomatic disease, including pneumonitis, chorioretinitis, colitis, hepatitis, esophagitis, meningoencephalitis, and polyradiculitis, should be treated with ganciclovir, 5 mg per kg every 12 hours for 14 to 21 days, followed by maintenance therapy, 5 mg per kg per day. Foscarnet may be used for treatment failure or ganciclovir intolerance.

4. **Measles** causes severe, sometimes fatal, and occasionally atypical disease in HIV-infected children; therefore routine immunization with MMR is recommended. After exposure, prophylaxis with intravenous immunoglobulin (IVIG) is recommended, regardless of prior immunization status. Anecdotal reports indicate that intravenous or aerosolized ribavirin may attenuate the disease.

5. **Respiratory viruses**, such as respiratory syncytial virus, parainfluenza, influenza, and adenovirus, may be seen as severe acute disease, recurrent disease, or chronic viral shedding.

VIII. **Noninfectious complications**

1. **Malignancies** occur in ~2% of HIV-infected children reported to the CDC. Epstein-Barr virus is thought to play a role in 30% to 50% of peripheral lymphoma, as compared with the majority of cases of CNS lymphoma. Kaposi's sarcoma is rare, whereas the incidence of smooth-muscle tumors, leiomyomas, and leiomyosarcoma, is markedly increased in pediatric HIV-infected patients (Chadwick EG, et al. *JAMA* 1990;263:3182; Mueller BU, et al. *Pediatrics* 1992;90:460).

B. **Lymphoproliferative syndromes**, such as LIP, cystic tumors of the thymus, and lymphoproliferative disease, which are all probably EBV associated, are seen in HIV-infected children. Patients with LIP can develop progressive symptoms and may benefit from steroid therapy in confirmed cases.

IX. **Prevention** (see also Chapter 9)

A. **Prevention of vertical transmission.** Vertical transmission of HIV occurs via three different routes: intrauterine, intrapartum, and postpartum by breastfeeding. Without intervention, the rate of vertical transmission in the United States is ~25%, whereas studies report rates as low as 12.9% in Europe and as high as 50% in some areas of Africa.

1. **Maternal, fetal, and viral factors** (see Chapter 9) play a role in vertical transmission, including maternal timing of infection, immune function, $CD4^+$ and CD8 counts, duration of rupture of membranes, breast-feeding, viral burden, symptomatic disease and neutralizing antibodies, fetal genetic predisposition, prematurity and mode of delivery, and viral genotype and phenotype. One of the most important and encouraging studies demonstrated a significant reduction in vertical transmission of HIV.

2. **Antiretroviral therapy during and after pregnancy.** In a pivotal study, ACTG 076, a randomized, placebo-controlled trial in HIV-infected pregnant women who received ZDV or placebo orally antepartum, intravenously intrapartum, and their offspring were treated for 6 weeks (2 mg per kg orally every 6 hours). HIV transmission was reduced by approximately two-thirds, from 25.5% to 8.3% (Connor EM, et al. *N Engl J Med* 1994;331:1173). This set the stage for current recommendations that **all pregnant women receive optimal antiretroviral therapy** that can maximally suppress viral replication (see Chapter 9). For women who present late in pregnancy without prior antiretroviral care, intrapartum antiretroviral therapy (ZDV) still should be given. A single dose of nevirapine (200 mg) given once to the mother during labor, and once to the infant after birth, has been shown to reduce transmission. All infants born to HIV infected women should receive 6 weeks of zidovudine (2 mg per kg orally every 6 hours) after birth. Expert consultation should be sought if it is known that the mother had ZDV-resistant virus.

3. **Modification of obstetrical practices**, especially as mode of delivery, vaginal cleansing, and avoidance of invasive intrapartum procedures,

are also important in reducing risk of transmission (see Chapter 9). Elective caesarean section can reduce transmission risk from mothers who still have detectable viral loads at term.

4. **Other recommendations** to reduce vertical transmission include **avoidance of breastfeeding** in developed countries and intensive **HIV education** for women of childbearing age.

B. **Other modes of prevention**
   1. **Screening of blood products** has been under way since 1985, making acquisition by this mode very uncommon.
   2. **Adolescents.** Because 15% to 20% of all AIDS cases are thought to be acquired between ages 13 and 19 years, **HIV/STD education** is crucial in this age group. It remains to be seen whether the acquisition of knowledge will result in behavior change. Further studies on how to modify risk-taking behavior will be crucial to curbing this epidemic.

8. HIV DISEASE AND WOMEN

Women entered the human immunodeficiency virus (HIV) epidemic later than men, but now compose a significant proportion of new cases. Persons now at highest risk for HIV infection are women and adolescents, according to recent estimates. In addition, although African-American and Hispanic women compose 17% of the United States population, these minorities represent three-fourths of all reported cases of women with acquired immunodeficiency syndrome (AIDS). One of the most important issues regarding prevention and control of the HIV epidemic is development and implementation of culturally sensitive primary and secondary prevention strategies for women at risk. With respect to treatment of HIV disease, women need meticulous gynecologic and obstetric care, as well as recognition of the multifaceted social roles women have, especially in the family. In this chapter, gynecologic care, psychological needs, and social support of HIV-infected women and prevention strategies for women at risk for HIV infection will be emphasized. Refer to Chapter 9 for further information on obstetric HIV therapeutics.

I. **The epidemiology of HIV infection in women.** Women constituted 7% of AIDS cases in 1985, compared with 22% of newly diagnosed AIDS cases in 1997. In a large sampling of persons infected with HIV disease in 1996, women represented 26% of those infected in the United States (Bozzette SA, et al. *N Engl J Med* 1998;339:1897). Furthermore, the decline in mortality associated with more potent therapy was not as dramatic, at least initially, in women.

II. **Risk factors and risk reduction for HIV transmission in women.** Although injecting drug use (IDU) accounted for the majority of infection in women in the 1980s, by 1991 the primary mode of transmission to women and the current major source of new infection for women was acquisition from heterosexual activity. Given the continued increase in new HIV infections in minorities, women, and their children, risk-reduction strategies for these groups may require specific interventions.

A. **Heterosexual transmission** is clearly responsible for the continued increase in HIV infection in women in the United States, Asia, Africa, and India.

1. Bidirectional HIV transmission studies from discordant couples with one HIV-infected partner reveal 15% to 20% efficiency of HIV transmission from men to women, compared with variable rates of HIV transmission efficiency (1% to 20%) from women to men. This may be because of the greater volume of semen compared to cervical and vaginal secretions, and to the fact that HIV is found in greater concentrations in semen.

2. A number of risk factors have been demonstrated to increase risk of transmission to women.

a. The presence of any **sexually transmitted disease** in the seronegative partner increases transmission risk—this includes both ulcerative disease and nonulcerative disease, including trichomoniasis. Genital tract disease in the HIV-positive partner also increases risk as it appears to increase HIV viral load in the semen.

b. Certain **sexual practices**, e.g., sex during menses, bleeding during intercourse and receptive anal intercourse, increase the risk of transmission.

c. More **advanced HIV disease** in the seropositive partner—presumably because of higher seminal viral load.

d. **Uncircumcised** male partner.

e. **Cervical ectopy**—possibly because the cervical tissues become more friable.

3. **Risk-reduction** methods should emphasize skill building among healthcare workers (HCWs) on sexual history taking, followed by recommendations for limiting the number of sexual partners, discussing risks and

contraceptive use with potential partners, and implementing pregnancy and sexually transmitted diseases (STDs) protective measures (i.e., condoms). The male condom does reduce HIV transmission. The effectiveness of the female condom in the prevention of STDs, including HIV infection, has not been studied. Topical microbicides, such as nonoxynol-9, may also be effective in conjunction with condoms.

B. Substance abuse. IDU remains a dominant risk factor for HIV transmission among women in the certain parts of the United States and Europe. Risk-reduction measures include drug-maintenance programs, peer-support programs, educational programs, needle-exchange programs, and education regarding needle decontamination.

C. Homosexual transmission. Although unusual, isolated cases of female-to-female sexual transmission of HIV have been reported. In addition, bisexuality in women has been identified significantly more often in women with HIV compared with women without HIV attending an STD clinic in New York City (Bevier PJ, et al. *Am J Public Health* 1995;85:1366–1371). These data suggest that, as with other STDs, the frequency of female-to-female HIV transmission is low and that bisexuality may be a marker for engagement in other high-risk behaviors.

D. Intravaginal insemination. Although rare, transmission by this route has occurred. Because no procedures have been proven completely to remove HIV from semen, insemination with semen from HIV-infected men is not recommended. For risk reduction, all donors should undergo HIV-antibody testing. To ensure that semen is not collected from an infected donor who has no detectable HIV antibody, semen from donors should not be used until the donor has been tested again 6 months after semen donation.

III. Counseling and testing for HIV infection in women. In general, HIV should be considered when treating women with drug addiction, STDs, chronic vaginal candidiasis, cervical dysplasia, tuberculosis, and other serious infections. At health-care encounters for primary preventive, reproductive, and prenatal care, women need adequate counseling and testing for HIV infection. This is important not only for early detection of HIV in women, but also to limit vertical transmission.

IV. Initial assessment of nonpregnant HIV-infected women. The initial medical evaluation of nonpregnant women with HIV infection is similar to that of men (see Chapter 4).

A. Lack of access to care, attention to health care of children before self-care, and the large proportion of women who are economically and medically disenfranchised contribute to late detection of HIV and the sustained high frequency of *Pneumocystis carinii* pneumonia (PCP) and other acute opportunistic infections in women.

B. A careful medical history and physical examination should include evaluation for symptoms and signs of progressive immune dysfunction.

C. Serologic testing for syphilis, cytomegalovirus, hepatitis B, hepatitis C, and toxoplasmosis should be performed. These serologic results establish a baseline for potential clinical infections and future pregnancy. Women seronegative for toxoplasmosis should be carefully instructed regarding measures to avoid acquisition of this organism (see Chapter 4). **Skin testing** for tuberculosis should be performed and isoniazid prophylaxis given for those who test positive. Pneumovax immunization should be given at this visit, and additional vaccines, when warranted (see Chapter 4).

D. Assessment of **stage of HIV infection** should be obtained, including CD4+ cell count and HIV viral-load measurement (see Chapter 4 and Section V below).

E. Additional components of women's health care that should be evaluated when HIV is detected include

  1. Gynecologic evaluation. A thorough menstrual, sexual, obstetric, and contraceptive history should be elicited. Recurrent vaginal candidiasis is often a reason why HIV-infected women seek medical attention. However, women with HIV infection are no more likely than matched HIV-negative women to develop vaginal candidiasis.

2. **Physical examination.** Should include breast and pelvic examinations with good visual inspection of the lower genital tract.

3. **Laboratory examination.** Papanicolaou (Pap) smear is an adequate initial screen for cervical abnormalities and should be performed every 6 to 12 months. Cervical cultures or DNA probes for *Neisseria gonorrheae* (GC) and *Chlamydia trachomatis* should be performed periodically if the woman is sexually active, and a pregnancy test performed when indicated.

4. **Mammography.** The indication is every other year for women between 40 and 49 years and every year for women 50 years and older.

5. **Colposcopy** is not recommended initially unless there has been a prior diagnosis of atypical squamous cells of undetermined significance (ASCUS) or dysplasia. The procedure should be performed by an experienced physician.

V. **Evaluation of HIV in women.** Determination of HIV viral load and the effect of HIV on CD4⁺ and CD8 T lymphocytes is addressed in Chapters 2 through 4. Several studies have suggested that plasma HIV RNA levels in women might be lower (by 0.25 log) than those of men at similar stages of HIV progression, as determined by CD4⁺ count. However, the data are conflicting and the differences are small. Furthermore, there are inconclusive data as to whether men and women with the same viral load have different progression rates (some studies suggest a faster progression in women). At this point, there is no consensus that different therapeutic guidelines are needed for women compared to men.

VI. **Clinical manifestations of HIV infection in women.** HIV-associated opportunistic infections and malignancies and the respective therapeutic recommendations are not gender specific. PCP, wasting syndrome, and esophageal candidiasis are the most common AIDS-defining illnesses in women. Kaposi's sarcoma is the only AIDS-related syndrome that occurs with greater frequency in men and is seen in <2% of women. Rates of HHV-8 seropositivity among HIV-infected women are considerably lower than those seen in men. Clinical manifestations of HIV infection specific to women are predominantly gynecologic and obstetric.

A. **Gender-specific infections and malignancies**. These are, in general, less dependent on CD4⁺ cell counts than are the non-gender-specific clinical manifestations. Gynecologic conditions such as genital ulceration, vaginitis, cervicitis, salpingitis, genital warts, and dysplastic epithelial changes may be more frequent, more severe, and less responsive to treatment in HIV-infected women compared with women without HIV infection. The associations between these conditions and HIV infection are potentially confounded by sexual and drug-use behaviors that are independently predictive of both HIV infection and the occurrence of STDs. To date, breast cancer, lung cancer, and other malignancies are not increased in frequency in HIV-infected women compared with women without HIV infection. The American Cancer Society and CDC recommend annual Pap smears for HIV-infected women. Given the low false positive rate and high false negative rate (15% to 40%) of Pap smears and the prevalence of cervical dysplasia in HIV-infected women, many experts in HIV care suggest that HIV-infected women with CD4⁺ counts <500 cells/mm³ be seen at least twice a year for gynecologic examination and Pap smear.

1. **Menstrual problems**. HIV infection does not appear to increase the frequency of menstrual irregularities compared to matched controls. Ovarian failure in the form of **amenorrhea** is very common in advanced AIDS, particularly with severe wasting. Whether the origin is primary ovarian dysfunction, a functional disorder of the hypothalamus, or a combination of both remains undetermined.

2. **Vulvovaginal candidiasis.** Recurrent infections without a correctable potential cause (oral contraceptive or antibiotics) occurring >6 times per year may be an early warning sign of HIV infection. However, HIV

seropositivity per se is not an independent predictor of vaginal candida infection.

    a. Symptoms include vulvar pruritus, a thick white vaginal discharge, burning upon urination and dyspareunia. Examination can show local erythema, with typical thrush.

    b. Treatment. Initial episodes should be treated in a standard manner with a topical antifungal medication such as clotrimazole vaginal tablets, or miconazole cream or suppositories. **Recurrent or resistant vaginal candidiasis** can be treated orally with fluconazole, 100 mg daily for 14 days.

3. Genital herpes simplex virus (HSV). HSV may occur suddenly in an HIV-infected woman and become persistent, widespread, and more painful than HSV in women without HIV. In women with advanced HIV infection, HSV lesions may be difficult to treat (see Chapter 25).

    a. Treatment and prophylaxis. Acyclovir, 200 mg 5 times per day, or 400 mg, t.i.d., is usually effective. Additional measures include sitz baths and analgesic control.

4. HIV genital ulcer. Primary HIV ulcers test negative for HSV, chancroid, and syphilis. The lesions do not respond to empiric treatment of these pathogens.

    a. Treatment. Primary HIV ulcers may respond to antiretroviral therapy, topical or systemic corticosteroids, or thalidomide.

5. Human papillomavirus (HPV). Genital warts are caused by several types of HPV and are probably the most common STD in the United States. The prevalence of HPV infection in the United States is estimated at 40 million persons. Warts can occur anywhere on the external (condyloma acuminata) or internal genitalia or perianal area. HIV-infected women have a high prevalence of HPV and abnormal Pap smears. The correlation between these two strengthens as HIV disease progresses and cervical invasive neoplasia (CIN) appears. It remains uncertain whether the immunosuppression associated with HIV facilitates acquisition, reactivation, enhanced replication, or persistence of HPV infection in the genital tract with subsequent progression of HPV-induced cervical disease and possibly anal neoplasia. Certain HPV subtypes appear more oncogenic than do others, although documentation of HPV in asymptomatic women indicates that infection alone is insufficient to cause CIN. HIV-infected women are more likely to be infected with multiple HPV types, and are more likely to have HPV (particularly the more oncogenic subtypes) persist in the cervix.

    a. HPV, categorized by oncogenic potential risk.

        (1) Low oncogenic potential: HPV types 6, 11, and 42 through 44.

        (2) High oncogenic potential for high-grade CIN but rare invasive disease: HPV types 31, 33, 35, 39, 51, and 52.

        (3) High oncogenic potential for high-grade CIN and anogenital lesions: HPV types 16, 18, 45, and 56. HPV typing has not yet become standard clinical practice, partly because of the high prevalence of HPV found in women with normal cytologic characteristics.

    b. Treatment. Multiple regimens are used to treat HPV infection:

        (1) Cryoablation. Liquid nitrogen.

        (2) Topical ablation. Trichloroacetic acid or podophylline.

        (3) Surgical ablation. Laser therapy or cold-knife cone excision.

6. Pelvic inflammatory disease (PID). The etiologic agents of PID (GC, *C. trachomatis,* or aerobic and anaerobic organisms) in HIV-infected women are similar to those found in women without HIV. HIV-infected women with PID have less frequent leukocytosis and more frequent tuboovarian abscesses that require surgical intervention compared with women without HIV infection.

   a. Treatment. Inpatient regimens include cefoxitin, 2 g i.v. every 6 hours or cefotetan, 2 g every 12 hours i.v., and doxycycline, 100 mg every 12 hours i.v. or p.o. or clindamycin, 600 to 900 mg, every 8 hours i.v., and gentamicin, 5 mg per kg per day. Outpatient regimens include ceftriaxone, 250 mg single-dose i.m., and doxycycline, 100 mg b.i.d., p.o. for 14 days; ofloxacin, 300 mg b.i.d., p.o., and clindamycin, 300 to 450 mg q.i.d., p.o., or metronidazole, 500 mg b.i.d., p.o., for 14 days; or azithromycin, 1 g p.o. daily.

7. **Atypical squamous cells of undetermined significance (ASCUS).** Atypical squamous cells differ from truly dysplastic cells yet require close follow-up evaluation. Women with two consecutive Pap smears with ASCUS should be referred for colposcopy.

8. **Cervical invasive neoplasia (CIN).** Women with HIV are > 10 times as likely to develop CIN than are women without HIV infection. Although study designs and sample sizes have varied, it appears certain that CIN becomes clinically apparent as $CD4^+$ cell counts decline. As HIV-related HPV and CIN tend to be seen as multifocal and multisite disease, visual inspection of the lower genital tract, beyond the cervical transformation zone, is routinely recommended. Routine application of 5% acetic acid for better visualization of lesions and cervicography are not generally recommended. Detection of a lesion on colposcopy should be confirmed histopathologically and treated according to standard guidelines, including repeated cervical cytologic and colposcopic examinations every 3 months after therapy, until the patient has had three consecutive normal cytologic and colposcopic examinations. Subsequent examinations should occur every 6 months.

   a. Stages. CIN [also known as squamous intraepithelial lesions (SIL)] stages and the associated cytopathology are
      (1) CIN I: Low-grade SIL. Cellular changes associated with HPV and mild dysplasia.
      (2) CIN II: High-grade SIL. Moderate dysplasia.
      (3) CIN III: High-grade SIL. Severe dysplasia and carcinoma in situ.

   b. Ablation methods. The technologies in use for ablation of CIN are listed in order of increasing invasiveness.
      (1) Cryotherapy. This is the best tolerated procedure in an ambulatory-care setting. This method is probably adequate in patients with $CD4^+$ counts >350 cells/mm^3, depending on the severity of the lesion.
      (2) Laser therapy. This method is more aggressive than cryotherapy. For patients with $CD4^+$ counts <200 cells/mm^3, laser therapy should be combined with 5-fluorouracil and careful follow-up.
      (3) Loop electrosurgical excisional procedure (LEEP). This method has not been an effective intervention in HIV-infected women.
      (4) Cold-knife cone biopsy. Remains the gold standard in both diagnosis and treatment of CIN.

   c. It is as yet unknown whether **potent antiretroviral therapy** will change the natural history of HPV infection or SIL in HIV-infected women.

9. **Cervical cancer.** Squamous cell cancer (SCC) of the cervix results in ~7,000 deaths in the United States each year. Although the prevalence of HPV-associated CIN is significantly higher in HIV-infected women, the incidence of cervical cancer is not higher in HIV-infected women than in women without HIV infection. Possible explanations for this include effective Pap smear screening and follow-up, death from opportunistic infections before neoplastic transformation, and a relatively low percentage of HIV-infected women compared with uninfected women in

the United States. There is some data that suggests that HIV-infected women with invasive cervical cancer may present with more advanced disease, and have a poorer response to treatment (Maiman M, et al. *Cancer* 1993; 71:402).

10. **Anal cancer.** Engaging in receptive anal intercourse is a risk factor for HPV-associated anogenital cancer, especially in HIV-infected women. The anorectal junction shares many similarities with the transformation zone of the cervix, including a common embryologic origin and a confluence of squamous and columnar epithelia. Many of the risk factors for acquisition of HIV infection, such as multiple sexual partners, are the same as those for acquisition of anogenital HPV infection. For women with HPV disease who report anal-receptive intercourse, it is reasonable to screen for anal lesions with anoscopy followed by biopsy of any lesions. The time course over which anal intraepithelial neoplasia progresses to anal cancer has not been prospectively studied. The concern is that as HIV-infected individuals live longer with prophylaxis against opportunistic infections, the incidence of malignancies may increase.

VII. **Antiviral use in women.** (see Chapters 5 and 6). The recommendations for the use of antiretroviral regimens are the same for nonpregnant women as for men. Antiretrovirals have been prospectively studied in pregnant women and are strongly recommended to limit vertical transmission (see Chapter 9). Small case-series suggest that women may be at greater risk for side-effects from some antiretroviral therapy (e.g., rash with NNRTIs). Further evaluation of gender-specific issues with antiviral therapies is needed.

VIII. **Reproductive issues in HIV-infected women.**
A. **Contraception.** Definitive, effective contraception should be recommended to women with HIV infection who do not wish to become pregnant. These methods include tubal ligation, medroxyprogesterone (Depo-Provera), and levonorgestrel (Norplant). Clearly none of these protects from STDs or continued HIV exposure from HIV-infected semen. Condom use should be recommended concurrently (to prevent STDs) with any of these (see IIB). Other barrier methods such as the diaphragm and the sponge are generally not so effective as a contraceptive or as protection from HIV or other STDs.
B. **Pregnancy considerations**. Given the potential for reducing the risk of vertical transmission of HIV with ZDV, more HIV-infected women may contemplate pregnancy. Important issues in counseling HIV-infected women who are considering pregnancy include
1. Clinical stage of HIV infection,
2. Effect of pregnancy on HIV infection,
3. Effect of HIV infection on the pregnancy,
4. Sexual behaviors (unprotected sex, multiple sexual partners, and recurrent STDs during pregnancy),
5. Behaviors during pregnancy (substance abuse, tobacco use, and nutrition),
6. HIV disease in children, and
7. Permanency planning.

IX. **Psychological issues in the health care of HIV-infected women.** HIV infection may include a multitude of emotional traumas that may be faced immediately on diagnosis or with fluctuating frequency over the course of the disease. There seem to be some gender-specific psychological differences for HIV infection. Women are particularly concerned about financial difficulties, isolation, loneliness, disclosure, self-image, and sexual expression more than progression of illness or side effects of medication. Selected psychological issues for the treatment of HIV-infected women include
A. considerations for improving quality of life (symptom control),
B. considerations for medical treatment, including other family members,
C. issues in preventing ongoing risk behaviors by women who know they are infected with HIV,
D. mental health needs,
E. spiritual needs, and

F. recognition of the multiple roles of women.

X. Social issues in the health care of women infected with HIV. In general, health-care providers should recognize that the health of the family is often dependent on the health of the woman. The effect of AIDS on women involves women as individuals, as well as in their multiple roles in their families and communities. A case-management approach and peer-support groups can help address some of the identified social problems of women infected with HIV. Major sociocultural issues include

A. Access to care. Issues include limited providers of health care, health insurance, transportation, and child care.

B. Limitations to treatment. Issues include health insurance, fragmented and multireferral health-service delivery, ongoing financial support, supportive environment, and transportation.

C. Permanency planning. Issues include advance directives, durable power of attorney, and child care (fostering and adoption).

D. Terminal care needs. Most care provided to people with chronic illnesses is provided by female family members. For HIV-infected women, there may be no identifiable person to provide longitudinal terminal care.

XI. Establishment of a HIV service-delivery system for women. Programs that can enhance service-delivery systems for women infected with HIV include

A. One-stop comprehensive health care. Medical, psychological, gynecologic, obstetric, radiologic, laboratory, and social services at one site. Staff should have the necessary language skills and cultural competence to work with women infected with HIV.

B. On-site postpartum maternal and newborn care.

C. On-site child care.

D. User-led services for women. Provide knowledge, technical assistance, advice, and support to help focus on the way women prioritize their needs, and acknowledge the links between IDU and HIV and high-risk sexual practices and HIV.

E. Peer-support groups.

F. Case-management system. Provision of social workers to help maintain or retain self-control and order through the progression of HIV infection.

9. HIV IN PREGNANT WOMEN

I. **Overview of human immunodeficiency virus (HIV) in pregnant women**
   A. **The seroprevalence of HIV in childbearing women in the United States** based on studies of blood from newborn heel-sticks ranges from 0 to 8.9 per 1,000 with a mean of 1.7 per 1,000 live births (*MMWR* 1995;44 (RR-7):1–12).
   B. There are an estimated **12 to 15 million** HIV-infected women worldwide, the majority of whom are in their reproductive years.
   C. **All pregnant women** should receive counseling regarding the benefits and risks of HIV screening and be encouraged to undergo voluntary HIV serologic testing (*MMWR* 1995;44(RR-7):1–12). Screening pregnant women based only on reported risk factors will fail to detect at least half of the HIV-seropositive women.
   D. Issues to consider in caring for HIV-seropositive pregnant women:
      1. **Impact of pregnancy** on maternal HIV disease and therapy options
      2. **Perinatal transmission**: the risk and means of reduction
      3. **Impact of HIV** on pregnancy outcome and obstetric care
      4. **Infant** follow-up: early diagnosis and opportunistic infection prophylaxis

II. **Impact of pregnancy on maternal health and therapy of HIV**
   A. The **possibility of a shortened life expectancy** in the mother and the impact of maternal illness and potential death on long-term care of the child must be discussed with the mother and her family (see also Chapter 8).
   B. **Disease progression**
      1. In the United States and Europe, no clear acceleration of HIV disease by pregnancy (Hocke C, et al. *Obstet Gynecol* 1995;86:886–891) has been noted.
      2. In developing countries, the data are less clear about the potential impact of pregnancy on HIV disease.
   C. **Symptoms** of pregnancy and HIV may overlap. Fatigue, nausea and vomiting, dyspnea, and headaches are common among pregnant women regardless of HIV status. Skin lesions unique to pregnancy may mimic those of HIV and vice versa.
   D. **Drug therapy.** There have been few large prospective studies examining the effects of antiretroviral drugs and drugs used for opportunistic infection prophylaxis on pregnancy—specifically on maternal health. Given that, there is no evidence of adverse effects on the mother from treatment directed to HIV disease.
   E. **Physiologic changes in pregnancy**
      1. **Cardiovascular changes** (Brinkman CR III. Biologic adaptation to pregnancy. In: Creasy RK, Resnick R, eds. *Maternal-fetal medicine: principles and practice*. Philadelphia: WB Saunders, 1989:734–745). The **plasma volumes** increase by 45% over nonpregnant levels, whereas **red cell mass** increases by only 20% to 30%, leading to a normal dilutional drop in hematocrit to 33% to 36%. The iron requirement is ≥800 mg over the 9-month course of pregnancy. The total white blood cell (WBC) count increases to 10,000 to 12,000 cells/mm^3. During labor, the normal WBC count may be up to 15,000 cells/mm^3. The resting pulse increases ~10 beats per minute to 80 to 90 beats per minute. **Cardiac output** increases by 30% to 50% (6 to 8 L per minute), with most of the increase occurring early in pregnancy with a concomitant decrease in systemic vascular resistance (800 to 1,100 dyne/s/cm^5).
      2. **Pulmonary changes** (deSwiet M. Pulmonary disorders. In: Creasy RK, Resnick R, eds. *Maternal-fetal medicine: principles and practice*. Philadelphia: WB Saunders, 1989:875–879). **Increased pulmonary blood flow** leads to increased vascular markings on chest radiograph and potentially to increased systemic absorption of aerosolized medications. **Tidal volume** increases by 200 mL from 500 to 700 mL per breath in pregnancy.

Oxygen consumption increases 20%, which is more than compensated for by a 40% increase in resting ventilation because of increased tidal volume. **Respiratory rate** does not change with normal pregnancy. **Residual volume** is decreased by 20% in pregnancy. Arterial **pCO_2** decreases to 30 mm Hg in pregnancy. The **pH** is unchanged in pregnancy because plasma bicarbonate decreases to compensate for decreased pCO_2. **Dyspnea: >50% of healthy pregnant women will have symptoms of dyspnea because of the increased respiratory drive related to hormonal changes.**

3. **Gastrointestinal changes** (Key TC. Gastrointestinal diseases. In: Creasy RK, Resnick R, eds. *Maternal-fetal medicine: principles and practice.* Philadelphia: WB Saunders, 1989:1032–1037). Decreased tone in the **esophagus** may lead to acid reflux and esophagitis. **Stomach** acid secretion is unchanged, but emptying may be delayed, especially in labor, leading to poor absorption of oral medications in labor. **Pancreatitis** may be more frequent in pregnancy, although data are conflicting. The liver size, blood flow, and transaminase levels are unchanged in pregnancy. **Albumin** levels decrease 20% because of increased plasma volume, leading to decreased binding of many drugs. Serum bilirubin is slightly increased during pregnancy.

4. **Renal changes: The glomerular filtration rate** increases by 50%, leading to an increased creatinine clearance. Normal **creatinine clearance** for pregnancy is 130 to 170 mL per minute.

5. **Drug metabolism: The effects of pregnancy vary depending on method of drug administration and type of clearance. These effects can be predicted by changes described previously.**

III. **Perinatal transmission:** Transmission may occur in utero, during labor and delivery, or with breastfeeding.

A. **Rate:** The risk of perinatal transmission ranges from 9.1% to 55% in women not receiving antiretroviral therapy (Paz I, et al. *Obstet Gynecol Surv* 1994;49:577). The incidence in the United States and Europe ranges from 10% to 25%. In contrast, perinatal transmission of HIV-1 appears somewhat higher in Africa, with transmission rates of 40% to 50% noted in some studies. These geographic disparities may be related to a number of factors, e.g., breastfeeding, nutritional deficiencies and/or coexisting infections other than HIV-1, absence of adequate prenatal care, and increased rate of premature deliveries.

B. **Mechanisms of Transmission.** HIV may be transmitted from mother to infant in three ways:

1. Direct infection may occur **in utero**, via transplacental passage. 30% to 40% of transmission may occur by this means.

2. HIV may be transmitted to the infant **during the time of delivery**, by breaks in the skin and subsequent direct exposure to infected blood or secretions, or by ingestion of maternal blood or other fluids. It is estimated that at least 50% of mother-child transmission occurs during delivery.

3. HIV may be transmitted by **breastfeeding**. Breastfeeding is associated with a 5% to 32% increased risk of transmission above background antepartum/intrapartum risk and is not recommended when safe alternatives exist

C. **Factors associated with an increased risk** of transmission in women have been identified, particularly in women not receiving antiretroviral therapy. No test or group of tests can predict 100% lack of transmission.

1. **Maternal HIV viral load** has been shown in multiple studies to be very important in predicting risk of transmission to infants. Rates of transmission increase with increasing viral load, with very low rates in women (~5%) whose viral load is <1,000 copies/mL and increasingly higher rates as the viral load increases (Despina G, et al. *J Acq Immunodef Syndr* 1998;18:126). However, in women not receiving antiretroviral therapy, a

minimal threshold (i.e., a level below which transmission will not occur) has not been demonstrated.

2. **Antiretroviral therapy** of the mother during pregnancy and labor has been very effective in reducing the risk of transmission to the infant.

    a. Initial studies used **zidovudine** (ZDV) therapy. A randomized, placebo controlled trial (ACTG 076) showed that ZDV use in pregnancy and peripartum decreased transmission compared to placebo from 25% to 8% (Connor EM, et al. *N Engl J Med* 1995;331:1173). The regimen used in that trial was complicated. Women received ZDV, 100 mg 5 times per day (or 300 mg twice daily) after the 14th week of gestation. At the time of birth, intravenous ZDV was administered, at a dose of 2 mg per kg infused over 1 hour, and then 1 mg per kg hour by continuous infusion until delivery. Thereafter, the infants received oral ZDV syrup, at a dose of 2 mg per kg every 6 hours for 6 weeks. Subsequent studies have confirmed the success of this regimen in different patient populations and the true effectiveness in practice may be even greater.

    b. **Abbreviated courses of zidovudine** have been examined especially in situations where prenatal care is less available or where the financial issues of administering this intensive schedule of ZDV make it prohibitive. A trial performed in Thailand (Shaffer N, et al. *Lancet* 1999;353:773) studied the use of zidovudine beginning in the last month of pregnancy (week 36), 300 mg zidovudine orally every 12 hours (i.e, the first component of ACTG 076). A 51% decrease in perinatal HIV transmission occurred. Other observational studies (Wade NA, et al. *N Engl J Med* 1998;339:1409) suggest that shorter courses of zidovudine, even those beginning at the time of delivery, or during the first 48 hours of life, may be effective in decreasing the risk of HIV transmission to the newborn and that if no other recourse is available, **prophylaxis of the newborn in the immediate peripartum period** (labor and delivery and first 48 hours of life) is extremely important in reducing HIV vertical transmission.

    c. A recent trial in Uganda showed that a single oral dose of **nevirapine**, 200 mg p.o., given to the mother during delivery and to the infant (at a dose of 2 mg per kg) during the first 72 hours of birth, was capable of reducing the risk of vertical HIV transmission by half, when compared with short-course ZDV (Guay LA, et al. *Lancet* 1999;354:795).

3. **A lower CD4$^+$ count** confers an increased risk of transmission, with rates 2 to 3 times greater at lower CD4$^+$ counts. Whether this is independent of maternal viral load has not been completely clarified.

4. **Other maternal factors** have been associated in some epidemiologic studies with an increased transmission risk including cigarette smoking and older maternal age.

5. **Obstetric factors** are also important. **Premature rupture** of the amniotic membranes has been associated with higher risk of transmission, possibly related to increased duration of fetal exposure to infected cervicovaginal secretions. Membrane rupture over 4 hours is highly significant. **Chorioamnionitis** and placental membrane inflammation on histologic examination are also associated with an increased risk of transmission.

6. **Prematurity,** especially delivery at <34 weeks, is associated with an increased risk of infant infection.

7. **Mode of delivery** may be important in affecting risk of transmission as elective cesarean section may reduce perinatal transmission. Analysis of several studies conducted prior to the current era of potent antiretroviral therapy indicates that, even in women taking ZDV, elective cesarean section reduced the risk of transmission (The International Perinatal

HIV Group. *N Engl J Med* 1999;340:977). However, it is unknown whether there is an added benefit of an elective surgical delivery for women with very low to undetectable levels of virus. If attempting vaginal delivery, potential exposure of the infant to maternal blood by scalp leads, instrument delivery, and episiotomy should be limited as much as possible, and the duration of ruptured membranes should be as short as possible (Minkoff H, et al. *Am J Obstet Gynecol* 1995;173:585).

IV. Management of the pregnant HIV-positive patient (see Chapter 4 for routine care of HIV-positive patients). It should be emphasized that pregnancy, although important, represents a brief period in the life of an HIV-infected women. Consequently, therapy during pregnancy should be viewed in the context of the overall management of the infected women. In particular, antiretroviral therapy targeted to prevent transmission to the infant should not be given in a manner that might compromise future treatment of the mother.

  A. Antepartum
  1. Thorough **history and physical examination** including **funduscopic, neurologic, and pelvic** examinations should be performed.
  2. **Tuberculin skin testing** (*MMWR* 1995;44(RR-8):9–11). **All** newly diagnosed HIV-positive pregnant women or those not tested within the past year should be screened with intermediate strength (5-TU) purified protein derivative. **Evaluation and management** of pregnant women with positive TB skin tests is similar to those of nonpregnant women (see Chapter 23).
  3. Baseline **herpes simplex virus (HSV), cytomegalovirus (CMV), and *Toxoplasma gondii*** serologic studies should be performed if not already done, along with routine prenatal laboratory studies [complete blood count (CBC), blood type, Rh, and antibody screen; hepatitis B surface antigen, rubella antibody, and syphilis serology determinations; Pap smear and cervical *Chlamydia trachomatis* and *Neisseria gonorrhoeae* cultures].
  4. **Baseline laboratory studies** should include **CBC with platelets, differential, lymphocyte subsets, and liver function tests.**
  5. **Repeated lymphocyte subset testing** should be done every 3 months if CD4$^+$ count at baseline was <500 cells/ mm^3 to assess need for *Pneumocystis carinii* pneumonia (PCP) prophylaxis. The CD4$^+$ count decreases in pregnancy in all women, whether HIV positive or not (Biggar RJ, et al. *Am J Obstet Gynecol* 1989;161:1239–1244).
  6. **Antiretroviral therapy** should be strongly encouraged to reduce the risk of perinatal transmission. Women should be referred to a specialist knowledgeable about antiretroviral therapy and managed in conjunction with her obstetrician.
      a. HIV-1-infected pregnant women receive **standard clinical, immunologic, and virologic evaluation.** The initiation and choice of antiretroviral therapy should be based on the same parameters used for individuals who are not pregnant.
      b. Current guidelines in the United States (*MMWR* 1998;47:1) recommend the use of ZDV during pregnancy, based primarily on the extensive prior studies. However, **ZDV monotherapy should not be used.** Instead, a regimen designed to maximally suppress viral replication should be used (see Chapter 6). This is true even in women who do not plan to continue antiretroviral therapy after pregnancy, as suboptimal antiretroviral treatment of the mother will lead to the emergence of viral resistance, compromising the ability to treat her later.
      c. The **safety of antiretrovirals** taken in pregnancy for the fetus is not completely clear. Most of the reverse transcriptase inhibitors, with the exception of didanosine (ddI), are classified as FDA Pregnancy Category C, which means that safety in human pregnancy has not been determined, although animal studies are either positive for fetal risk or have not been conducted. Didanosine is categorized as a Cate-

gory B drug, which means that there is no evidence of risk in humans, though well-controlled studies not done and animal studies reveal no risk to the fetus. Most of the protease inhibitors are Class B agents, except indinavir. Although a class C agent, efavirenz should generally be avoided in pregnancy because fetal abnormalities have occurred in primate studies. Women who have not been taking antiretroviral therapy may want to consider delaying treatment until the end of the first trimester of pregnancy. For women who become pregnant while taking antiretroviral therapy, there are no clear guidelines. If they choose to temporarily discontinue therapy during the first trimester, all drugs should be discontinued, with re-institution of the full regimen again at week 14.

There remain some uncertainties as to long term side effects of drugs taken in pregnancy. It is therefore extremely important to monitor infants born to antiretroviral-exposed mothers. A registry for long-term follow-up of such infants has been established and physicians who care for such patients are asked to register patients by calling (800) 722-9292, extension 8465, in the US. For registrations from countries outside the US, physicians may call (919) 315-8465.

   d. For **women who present in labor** without prior antiretroviral treatment, the second and third parts of the recommended zidovudine protocol should be initiated, i.e., a 1-hour infusion of zidovudine at a dose of 2 mg per kg, followed by a continuous infusion of zidovudine at a dose of 1 mg per kg per hour throughout the duration of labor. Thereafter, the infant should be given zidovudine for the first 6 weeks of life. Consideration should also be made to the addition of a single dose of nevirapine to mother during delivery (200 mg p.o.) and infant (2 mg per kg). Infants born to mothers who received no antiretroviral therapy during pregnancy or delivery should still receive postpartum prophylaxis.

   e. Pregnancy in women who have previously received antiretroviral therapy may be complicated by the possibility of resistance. Thus, if the mother has a detectable viral load, resistance testing and use of optimal therapy guided by the results is recommended to suppress viral replication. Specialist consultation is advisable.

   f. There are no additional **toxicities** of the antiretroviral medications during pregnancy. Placebo controlled trials of zidovudine have not shown any additional adverse effects for mothers. However, it should be remembered that many antiretrovirals cause nausea and vomiting, which may exacerbate the nausea and emesis that occur with pregnancy, especially in the first trimester.

7. **PCP prophylaxis**. PCP prophylaxis is indicated for patients with $CD4^+$ lymphocyte count <200 cells/mm^3, unexplained fever (>100 °F) for >2 weeks or a history of oropharyngeal candidiasis; these indications are not different in pregnancy. The **first choice** for therapy in pregnancy is trimethoprim/sulfamethoxazole, one double-strength tablet daily. **Alternate** therapies in pregnancy include dapsone, 100 mg p.o. daily, or aerosolized pentamidine, 300 mg monthly via Respirgard II nebulizer. **Glucose-6-phosphatase deoxyhydrogenase** activity should be checked in patients at risk for deficiency before dapsone therapy. The **infant's pediatrician** should be notified of maternal sulfonamide therapy near delivery.

8. *Mycobacterium avium* complex (MAC). The usual indications for MAC prophylaxis apply ($CD4^+$ count <50 cells/mm^3; see Chapter 23). As in nonpregnant persons, azithromycin prophylaxis is the preferred therapy in pregnant women, with rifabutn or clarithromycin as alternates.

9. **Other opportunistic infections:** Optimal treatment or prophylaxis for other opportunistic infections during pregnancy must be determined on a case-by-case basis with the collaboration of an obstetrician and an

infectious disease specialist. For sight-threatening or life-threatening conditions, standard therapies should be used unless clearly contraindicated in pregnancy.

10. **Obstetric outcomes: No differences have been detected in birth-weight or prematurity rates in U.S. studies** (Alger LS, et al. *Obstet Gynecol* 1993;82:787; Johnstone FD, et al. *BMJ* 1988;296:467; Selwyn PA, et al. *JAMA* 1989;261:1289; Minkoff HL, et al. *Am J Obstet Gynecol* 1990;163:1598). **Increased rates of low birth weight and infant death** have been seen among pregnancies in HIV-infected women in developing countries (Temmerman M, et al. *Obstet Gynecol* 83:495, 1994; Braddick MR, et al. *AIDS* 1990;4:1001). **Maternal bacterial pneumonia and peripartum infection** rates appear to be increased even in developed countries. Peripartum infections (chorioamnionitis, postpartum endometritis, and episiotomy infections) are increased the most among women with low $CD4^+$ counts (Selwyn PA, et al. *JAMA* 1989;261:1289; Alger LS, et al. *Obstet Gynecol* 1993;82:787).

B. **Intrapartum**
   1. **Mode of delivery: Vaginal delivery** is generally indicated in women who have received effective antenatal antiretroviral therapy, unless there are obstetric indications for cesarean section. **Elective cesarean section** has recently been shown to reduce the risk of perinatal HIV-1 transmission to as low as 2% in pregnant women also taking zidovudine and should be considered in women whose viral load is detectable, even if on antiretroviral treatment.
   2. Every effort should be made to **minimize the duration of rupture of membranes** by avoiding artificial rupture of membranes and augmenting or inducing labor after rupture (Minkoff H, et al. *Am J Obstet Gynecol* 1995;173:585). Scalp leads, fetal scalp sampling, forceps, and vacuum extractor should all be avoided except in an emergency.
   3. **For HSV-seropositive women**, a careful vulvar and cervical examination for HSV lesions should be performed on admission for delivery, and vulvar and cervical HSV cultures should be considered, because HSV-2 seropositivity and genital reactivation are increased among HIV-positive women.
   4. **Body-substance isolation** is essential, including use of waterproof gowns, masks, and goggles for providers at delivery.
   5. **The infant** should be washed thoroughly before doing any blood draws or giving injections.
C. **Postpartum care**
   1. **Lactation** suppression is no longer used because of the potential for seizures and strokes with bromocriptine, which was of limited efficacy.
   2. **Contraception should always be addressed**.
      a. **Barrier methods** including foam and condoms are encouraged for all women.
      b. **Hormonal contraceptives** may be used unless contraindicated for medical reasons such as hypertension or because of interactions with other drugs patients may be receiving. With combination estrogen-progesterone oral contraceptives, the provider must consider potential effects of interactions with other therapies on efficacy (for example, rifampin) and toxicities of these medications.
      c. **Depomedroxyprogesterone acetate,** 150 mg i.m. every 3 months, may be used with less concern about potential drug interactions. The main side effects are irregular bleeding and weight gain.
      d. **Norplant** is implantable levonorgestrol in silastic capsules, effective for 5 years after insertion. Norplant is similar to depomedroxy-progesterone in terms of interactions and side effects.
      e. **The intrauterine device (IUD)** is not recommended for HIV-positive women because of a possible increased risk of pelvic infections.

3. **Psychosocial needs:** The provider must ensure adequate maternal **psychosocial support** during the postpartum period while awaiting determination of the infant's infection status. Normal postpartum hormonal fluctuations along with maternal anxiety and guilt over potential HIV infection in the infant lead to an increased risk for postpartum depression.

4. **Antiretroviral therapy.** The decision regarding continuing or changing maternal antiretroviral therapy depends on postpartum CD4$^+$ count and viral load, patient preference, and recommendations for therapy in nonpregnant individuals (see Chapter 6).

5. **Gynecologic medical follow-up.** See Chapter 8.

6. **Infant follow-up:** See Chapter 7.

10. MANAGEMENT OF THE TERMINALLY ILL AIDS PATIENT

John D. Stansell and William G. Powderly

Perhaps the most difficult decision an acquired immunodeficiency syndrome (AIDS) clinician faces is when to change from an aggressive, interventionalist treatment posture to a palliative mode of patient care. Despite recent advances in our understanding of the natural history of the human immunodeficiency virus (HIV) and the availability of potent agents to inhibit this virus, many patients with symptomatic HIV disease may face progressive debilitation and eventual death as a consequence of their infection and immunocompromise. This is particularly true for patients who develop multi-drug resistant virus (see Chapter 6) for whom effective antiretroviral therapy is no longer available. This chapter presents a clinical philosophy born from extensive clinical experience in the care and management of advanced HIV-related disease. Differing viewpoints, interpretations, and opinions are expected and appropriate. Every patient-care situation is unique, and the perspectives presented are not meant to be universally applicable. However, this chapter attempts broadly to define major issues facing persons ill with terminal HIV disease and to pose possible interventions. Care during dying is part of the continuity of care physicians should offer all patients who entrust them with their lives.

I. **Several general principles** should guide the astute clinician who ministers to a patient at the end of life.
   A. First and foremost, a clear understanding of the **patient's wishes for care** is paramount. This understanding should be achieved through discussion with the patient before the process of active dying. A new physician (e.g., a medical resident or intern) confronting decision making around end-of-life issues must turn to the primary care provider for guidance in the absence of clear-cut guidelines from the patient or his or her surrogates.
   B. **Symptoms that diminish quality of life are treatable** and should be approached aggressively. The approach of death does not indicate a need to forsake care, but simply to reorient thinking about what care is appropriate. Indeed this period of patient management may require the most intense and taxing physician involvement of any time during the course of AIDS.
II. **Recognition of the terminally ill AIDS patient.** Clinicians who manage large numbers of HIV-infected patients often see significant numbers of patients who have severely depressed CD4+ counts or high viral loads, but lead relatively asymptomatic lives. Similarly, prior diagnosis of AIDS-defining illnesses may not accurately reflect survival prognosis. Instead, the functional status of the AIDS patient most reliably predicts survival. The course of AIDS has been divided into four stages [*Canadian Report on Integrated Palliative Care for Persons with AIDS* (1989)]. The terminal stage of HIV disease discussed in this chapter combines the advanced and terminal stages proposed by the Canadian report.
   A. Persons with **early-stage** disease have a recent index diagnosis and good response to therapy. After treatment, these patients experience a full recovery of function and ability to resume normal activity and work.
   B. Persons with **progressive-stage** disease have episodic infections with shortening intervals. Weight loss and fatigue may emerge as significant problems. Mild neurologic or mental impairment may be present, and the person has a limited ability to perform work.
   C. Patients with **advanced-stage** disease have severe fatigue and debilitation. Significant neurologic or mental impairment such as dementia may be present. Response to therapy is poor, and infections are worsening and, perhaps,

The author acknowledges the contribution of John D. Stansell to the previous edition of this chapter.

constant. At the same time, emerging problems such as gastrointestinal (GI) disease, neuropathy, and renal failure, as well as drug allergies, narrow the spectrum of therapeutic options and increase the risk of these options. At this stage, the aim of medical care delivery should shift from an interventional, aggressive approach to palliation.

D. Terminal stage blurs with advanced stage. Death can be anticipated within days to a few months. It is important to recognize that most physicians generally overestimate life expectancy in late-stage HIV disease, but death can generally be anticipated within 6 months, based on the best clinical judgment and scientific data. At this stage, appropriate therapy is the provision of comfort care.

Although this classification is useful, it has important limitations. There is an important difference between patients who present in the advanced and terminal stages of AIDS without having received any prior treatment, and those who progress to these stages in spite of available treatment. Patients who present with advanced disease may still have a **reversible** course with aggressive and prompt antiretroviral therapy, and such patients should always be given the benefit of such treatment. However, patients who progress despite available treatment, often have virus that is very resistant to available drugs and a more palliative approach to such patients may be appropriate. Thus the **most critical decision** to make when assessing whether patients are at a terminal phase of the illness, is whether the patient has any realistic remaining antiretroviral options. This chapter largely deals with patients who do not have good alternatives for the treatment of HIV.

Caring for a Patient With Terminal-Stage HIV Disease

Four management areas should receive priority consideration: (a) diagnosis and treatment, (b) optimizing drug therapy,(c) symptom and pain control, and (d) preparation for a "good death."

I. Diagnosis and treatment. Patients with profound immunosuppression caused by HIV infection are at heightened risk for opportunistic infections and malignancy. Furthermore, these individuals risk end-organ disease from HIV itself (e.g., encephalopathy, enteropathy, and dermatopathic conditions). Unlike immunocompetent individuals or persons with lesser degrees of HIV-related immunodysfunction, multiple diseases often occur simultaneously. Moreover, infection with unusual organisms or unusual presentations with common pathogens are frequently seen.

   A. The role of **empiric treatment of complications** in HIV-infected patients and particularly in terminally ill AIDS patients is constantly debated. No single, simple, generalizable recommendation exists.

      1. Diagnosis and treatment in terminal AIDS patients must be a **patient-centered** decision. Empiric treatment may open the patient to unnecessary

      2. As much as possible, the patient needs to be completely apprised of the treatment options if a specific diagnosis is pursued and established. Certainly decisions will be altered based on the availability or unavailability of adequate treatment. If adequate therapy is available, however, the most effective form of palliation may be aggressive treatment.

   B. The frequency of **laboratory monitoring** and routine office visits requires individualization.

      1. Generally, patients with **stable signs and symptoms** are seen at intervals of 4 to 8 weeks. These visits should include time to review the laboratory work done in the interval, nutritional status, functional limitations, and adequacy of care delivery.

         a. In the absence of new signs or symptoms, routine blood work or cultures are unlikely to beneficially to affect the patient's course or quality of life.

  b. These visits are an excellent opportunity to review the patient's own sense about the course of events and his or her advance directives.

  c. The efficacy or advisability of continuing drug therapy should be assessed.

  d. These visits should be used to address social issues. Many people with HIV infection will be attempting to continue to work or have family and child-care responsibilities. There needs to be periodic review of the individual's support system and access to social-support services.

  2. New problems or complaints need more-focused visits, and generally involve more diagnostic testing and interpretation. It is appropriate to review the prior discussions regarding the **advance directive** and the possible problems that may be developing. There are often reasons to make a diagnosis even when the treatment options are limited, so that future discussions of prognosis and course of events can be more directed. However, as mentioned previously, the health-care provider must help the patient to anticipate future treatment choices before encouraging the patient to go through extensive invasive testing. Some patients, having seen friends or family go through a variety of HIV-related problems before death, have well-established limits for what they will endure.

II. Optimizing drug therapy. The advances in survival achieved in the treatment of HIV disease have been the development of potent antiretrovirals (see Chapter 6) and prophylaxis against commonly encountered opportunistic pathogens.

  A. However, the delivery of drug therapy to HIV-infected persons with very advanced disease is a double-edged sword. On the one hand, the medications may prevent diseases and their progression or sequelae, while on the other, they may provoke adverse drug reactions or interactions.

  1. Patients with more advanced HIV disease are increasingly prone to **drug allergy**, intolerance, toxicity, or interaction.

  2. Secondary complications of drug therapy, such as central-line sepsis, may complicate the course of late-stage patients.

  3. In some cases, **public health considerations** may enter into the decision as in patients receiving therapy for pulmonary tuberculosis.

  4. However, for the most part, the choice of drugs to offer or continue in late-stage patients must take into account the **desire of the patient** for aggressive therapy, the appropriateness of aggressive therapy versus palliation, and the impact drug therapy or its delivery will have on quality of life. In general, "the fewer, the better."

  B. Antiretrovirals

  1. Patients who have **never been treated** who present with very advanced HIV infection should **always** be offered potent combination antiretroviral therapy. Dramatic improvements in clinical well-being and immunologic function may occur when viral replication is controlled, and improved chance of survival can occur.

  2. Persons with terminal HIV disease who have **previously been treated** with all available classes may derive some benefit from continuation or resumption of these agents. In some patients, a moderate preservation of immune function occurs in spite of continued viral replication, and this immune benefit may last for several years. However, continuation or change to more drugs should be balanced with the patient's needs and quality of life.

  3. The status of treatment with **new drugs** is unclear, but it seems unlikely that patients with terminal-stage disease will have a protracted response to new drugs unless they can be given in combinations that use 2 or 3 new agents. Even in this case, resistance across classes is common and virological responses, if they occur, tend to be transient. Indeed, patients with very advanced HIV disease have decreased response to therapeutic interventions in general and to antiretroviral therapy in particular. Nevertheless, given the clinical improvements that clearly follow control of viral replication, if reasonably tolerable antiretroviral options become available, they should be offered to patients.

4. Antiretroviral therapy may complicate the delivery of **other medications** to prevent or treat opportunistic infections, malignancy, or to ease symptoms.

5. Clinicians should have a **low threshold for discontinuing antiretroviral therapy** in patients with clearly limited life expectancy. These patients receive little "bang for their buck" from antiretroviral therapy. **The exception to this recommendation** would be the patient who adamantly wishes to continue aggressive therapy despite terminal disease. The withdrawal of antiretroviral therapy may be seen as "cutting the lifeline" by these patients. Inasmuch as we should never strip a patient of hope, continuation of antiretrovirals, preferably those with the least side effects, for these terminally ill patients may be appropriate.

C. **Prophylaxis of opportunistic infections.** Patients with terminal disease are clearly at risk for the entire spectrum of opportunistic pathogens causing disease in AIDS patients. However, provision of prophylaxis must weigh the risk of disease from all these pathogens versus the impact of prophylaxis on patients' quality of life and life expectancy.

1. In general, even prophylaxis should be severely **limited** in the terminally ill patient.

2. Continued administration of systemic therapy to prevent *Pneumocystis carinii* **pneumonia** and *Toxoplasma gondii* **meningoencephalitis** is likely appropriate while a patient can continue to receive oral medications (see Chapters 4 and 22).

3. Similarly, those patients in whom superficial fungal infections or recurrent oral or esophageal candidal infections compromise quality of life are candidates for continuing **antifungal prophylaxis** with fluconazole, 100 to 200 mg p.o. daily.

4. Patients with **recurrent herpetic outbreaks are** likely to receive palliative benefit from continuing oral acyclovir.

5. However, the role of macrolide therapy to prevent *Mycobacterium avium* infection or ganciclovir to prevent cytomegalovirus (CMV) disease is less clear in patients with very advanced disease. It seems unlikely that terminally ill patients receive much palliative benefit from these latter prophylaxis strategies.

III. **Symptom and pain control.** Palliation of symptomatic complaints should be the major therapeutic intervention offered to the terminally ill AIDS patient. Prevention and relief of suffering in a person with limited life expectancy maximizes the opportunity for quality of life before death. As previously stated, symptoms are treatable and should be approached aggressively.

A. **Fever.** Not uncommonly, fever and accompanying night sweats complicate terminal-stage HIV disease.

1. Often these symptoms foreshadow **infectious or neoplastic diseases**. In such cases, treatment of the disease process is the most effective means of palliation.

2. However, occasionally no clear cause can be determined. In these patients, drug fever or adrenal insufficiency must be considered.

3. In the rare case in which a full workup, including drug discontinuation, adrenocortical axis testing, routine, fungal and acid-fast bacillus blood cultures, gallium scan, imaging studies of the chest and abdomen, and bone marrow biopsy have failed to document an origin, around-the-clock antipyretics are appropriate.

4. Although most AIDS clinicians are skeptical of "HIV fevers," changing or resuming antiretroviral therapy may very occasionally be of benefit and offer improved quality of life.

B. **Nausea/vomiting.** The list of causes of nausea and vomiting in the late-stage AIDS patient is legion (see Chapter 14).

1. **Diagnosis.** Although CMV disease, AIDS cholangiopathy, lymphoma, and central nervous system (CNS) lesions are causes of nausea/vomiting in AIDS patients, the leading cause is iatrogenic—medications. The most effective palliative intervention available is a reexamination and paring of the medication list of the terminal patient with GI complications. No drug therapy should be immune from reconsideration or elimination. The goal of therapy is patient comfort.

2. **Control of nausea and vomiting** may require all the pharmacologic acumen and ingenuity of the AIDS physician. Nausea may arise from stimulation of peripheral afferents, direct effects on the chemoreceptor trigger zone, or cortical stimulation. Insight into the mechanism of emesis is essential to the provision of effective therapy.

    a. The **benzamides** with or without phenothiazines are effective antiemetics in situations in which direct stimulation of GI afferents is the cause of nausea.

    b. Similarly, the **phenothiazines** or **butyrophenones** may provide relief of nausea caused by direct stimulation of the chemoreceptor trigger zone. Care must be exercised, however, as dystonic reactions are common.

    c. The judicious use of **benzodiazepines** or **butyrophenones** may aid in the control of anticipatory nausea.

    d. Frequently **combinations** of antiemetics, much like those used in cancer chemotherapy, are required to control nausea and emesis.

    e. **Dexamethasone** can be effective, especially in persons with CNS processes.

    f. The **cannabinoids** or inhaled marijuana can provide antiemesis and appetite stimulation. Unfortunately, many patients have significant dysphoria at the doses required to control nausea.

    g. The **selective serotonin receptor blockers** are highly effective at controlling emesis. However, the high cost of these drugs precludes their routine use in most AIDS patients.

C. **Diarrhea** with attendant dehydration and electrolyte imbalance is common and often life threatening in the late-stage AIDS patient. Causes of diarrhea include drugs, infections, and neoplasms (see Chapter 14). Control of diarrhea should always focus on diagnosis and treatment in treatable disease. However, many cases are idiopathic or caused by untreatable organisms. In these patients, **control of symptoms** is the goal of therapy.

    1. Initial therapy in **mild cases** may be diet modification or the use of bulk products (e.g., psyllium).

    2. More severe cases usually require regular administration of diphenoxylate or loperamide. If these agents fail to control diarrhea when used singly, they should be used sequentially or in combination. Upper limits of dosing have little meaning for the dying patient in whom the objective is to achieve symptom control.

    3. If these drugs fail to control diarrhea, **opiate antispasmodics** are appropriate. Deodorized tincture of opium or oral sustained-release morphine may be titrated to control diarrhea against unwanted sedation. In those persons in whom sedation becomes problematic, the use of stimulants such as methylphenidate or dextroamphetamine may preserve the level of consciousness while permitting adequate treatment of the diarrhea. In all these cases, the object of therapy is palliation and, clearly, the benefit of therapy must be measured against the discomfort of untoward side effects.

    4. The somatostatin analog **octreotide** is expensive, must be given by injection, and only partially controls diarrhea caused by infectious pathogens.

D. **Anorexia and weight loss.** Uncontrolled, unintended anorexia and weight loss often complicate late-stage AIDS (see also Chapter 17).

    1. Chronic disseminated infection, diarrhea with malabsorption, and GI complications of drug therapy frequently lead to wasting. The easiest

treatment is **control of the underlying infection or withdrawal of the offending medications.**

  a. The most frequent cause of weight loss is **inadequate caloric intake** rather than hypermetabolism. Most patients with wasting fail to meet minimal calorie consumption to support their metabolism. The goal is to increase calories.

    (1) Nutritional supplements are useful if they are truly supplements. Often, however, they are substitutes, and little is gained.

    (2) Appetite stimulants are rarely useful in terminally ill patients.

    (3) Total parenteral nutrition (TPN) can be initiated in patients with severe malabsorption in whom no treatable GI disease can be identified and other interventions have failed. This expensive treatment modality should not be initiated in an open-ended manner. A reevaluation of the indications for therapy and an assessment of the success or failure of TPN and its impact on quality of life should be undertaken at regular intervals.

E. Insomnia. The inability to sleep comfortably is a vexing problem for terminally ill patients.

F. Depression and anxiety (see also Chapter 13). Progressive physical impairment with loss of body image, loss of family and friends to AIDS, and impoverishment resulting from illness, all combine to produce severe depression in some terminally ill patients. Furthermore, depression can complicate the treatment of all other symptom complexes in the late-stage patient. Surprisingly, not all patients have depression. However, those that do should be aggressively treated. Psychiatric consultation should play a large role in any HIV practice. Individual psychotherapy can be extremely useful in some patients, and pharmacotherapy, especially with the serotonin-reuptake inhibitors, may achieve a remarkable reversal of vegetative symptoms.

G. Pain. Pain complicates the management of more than half of late-stage AIDS patients. AIDS patients admitted to hospice services most frequently cite the pain of peripheral neuropathy, chronic abdominal pain, and the discomfort associated with skin lesions or immobilization. Generally pain can be expected to increase as HIV disease advances, and in terminal stages, it is comparable to cancer pain. Perhaps nothing is more important in the management of the terminally ill AIDS patient than the effective control of pain. Unfortunately, physicians poorly manage pain. Inculcated, irrational fears of habituation often stand in the way of effective palliative pain therapy in terminally ill patients. Nothing could be more inappropriate. Clinicians need to be constantly aware of the goals of therapy and not allow misplaced apprehension to impede effective therapy. No patient should yearn for death because of our reluctance to offer adequate analgesia.

  1. A good **general rule to guide therapy** is that it takes much less analgesia to prevent pain than to treat it. Thus, patients with chronic pain should be offered analgesia on an around-the-clock, regularly timed basis. They should not be required to ask for pain relief other than for breakthrough discomfort. To administer adequate analgesia to an AIDS patient with chronic pain, it is invaluable for that individual to be followed up by a single, involved health-care provider. Fractionation of care among several providers leads to misunderstanding and, often, prejudice against the legitimate analgesia needs of the late-stage AIDS patient. This is particularly a problem when dealing with patients who are frequently undertreated for the pain of AIDS or cancer—women, the less educated, injection-drug users, or persons with more severe pain syndromes.

  2. The character as well as the intensity of the pain can guide therapy.

    a. Mild pain, particularly pain that results from an inflammatory process, may well respond best to a nonsteroidal antiinflammatory agent (NSAID) like ibuprofen or naproxen. Usually classified as mild analgesics, NSAIDs may be much more effective at relieving pain from inflammatory sources than are opiates. These drugs have the added benefit of not developing a pattern of tolerance or psychologic dependence. However, there is a ceiling effect to the analgesia offered by the NSAIDs. Dosing above this level, although it may improve the antiinflammatory effects, yields no further improvement in analgesia. In moving to more powerful analgesics, however, clinicians should always bear in mind that the NSAIDs offer significant benefit as adjunctive therapy. Additional analgesics, usually the weak opiates, should be added, not substituted.

b. In **escalating analgesia**, the clinician should scale a ladder from the weak to the stronger analgesics.

  (1) When NSAID therapy alone is insufficient, most clinicians turn to the **weak opiates** (e.g., codeine). These medications are usually oral and require 20 to 60 minutes for onset of analgesia.

  (2) If this drug proves inadequate, **oxycodone or hydrocodone** may be used.

  (3) If more careful titration of analgesia is required, **oral morphine suspension** may be tried. It must be kept in mind, however, that oral morphine is only a fraction as effective as intramuscular or intravenous morphine. The mixed agonist–antagonist drugs, butorphanol and pentazocine, may precipitate withdrawal in narcotic-dependent persons and generally should be avoided in the management of chronic pain.

  (4) If **further analgesia** is required, parenteral morphine, hydromorphone, or fentanyl may be used. The **fentanyl patch** is a particularly attractive form of pain management for AIDS patients. It requires no parenteral access and avoids the concentration peaks and valleys of repeated dosing. Several facts must be kept in mind when using the patches, however. The patch requires 12 to 24 hours to become effective, as a depot of drug must accumulate in the skin and subdermal tissues. Similarly, drug continues to enter the bloodstream for significant periods (half-life, 17 hours) after the patch is removed. Finally, drug delivery can be affected by fever; absorption can dramatically increase in the face of significant temperature elevations.

c. **Adjunctive nonopiate drugs** can be added to the pain regimen of late-stage AIDS patients and yield greater pain control at lower opiate doses.

  (1) The **tricyclic antidepressants** and serotonin-reuptake inhibitors can significantly improve pain control, possibly by treating neuropathic pain or depression.

  (2) Similarly, neuropathic pain management can be improved with the use of the **anticonvulsants,** phenytoin or carbamazepine. These drugs, however, have a narrow therapeutic window and require frequent drug-level monitoring.

  (3) The **glucocorticoids** can be particularly useful in terminally ill patients with pain caused by CNS lesions.

  (4) The addition of small doses of **amphetamine or methylphenidate** in patients with refractory pain or untoward sedation can yield significant improvement in quality of life.

  (5) The judicious use of the **benzodiazapine anxiolytics** can improve pain control for some late-stage patients.

  (6) **Dronabinol or marijuana** can provide anxiolytic and euphoric effects palliative to some patients with chronic pain.

d. All the opiates share a common pattern of **untoward side effects**.

  (1) **Constipation** is a formidable problem in the patients with chronic pain. AIDS patients begun on chronic opiate therapy should be begun on a regular bowel regimen.

(2) **Nausea** caused by direct stimulation of the chemoreceptor trigger zone can require dose reduction, alteration in opiate, or use of antiemetic agents.

(3) **Sedation** invariably occurs with opiate administration, although to a smaller degree in patients with severe pain than in persons with mild pain.

(4) **Tolerance** is a predictable consequence of repeated opiate administration and is manifest by increasing opiate dose requirements to maintain the same level of analgesia. Tolerance usually begins to emerge several weeks into chronic pain management. Tolerance is also a major problem in treating chronic pain in active narcotic users or persons in methadone maintenance programs. To achieve adequate analgesia, sufficient drug must be given to overcome the tolerance to their usual level of narcotic. Thus, offering acetaminophen with codeine to an addict who injects upward of 0.3 to 0.5 g of street heroin per day has very little impact. Tolerance can be minimized by combining different analgesics or alternating opiates. It does not indicate addiction, and fear of narcotic habituation should never be the reason to withhold pain medication from a terminally ill AIDS patient.

e. **Neuropathic pain** requires a special approach to pain management. Opiates are generally ineffective.

(1) The **tricyclic antidepressants**, amitriptyline, nortriptyline, and desipramine, are the first-line drugs for managing neuropathic pain. Discernible effects usually occur within a few days, but these drugs can be escalated to doses effective for treating depression over a period of weeks to treat peripheral neuropathy. A second agent may be added in the face of incomplete, although diminished, pain. The serotonin-reuptake inhibitors, trazodone, and other antidepressants are not effective treatments for neural pain.

(2) If the tricyclics fail to control neuropathic pain, most literature suggests proceeding to the **anticonvulsants.**

(3) **Mexiletine,** the antiarrhythmic, can provide analgesia in patients for whom other therapy has failed. This drug requires thrice-daily dosing and has been associated with CNS side effects.

(4) **Capsaicin**, the substance P depletor extracted from peppers, should be reserved for the last resort and only for persons with limited painful areas. The substance causes severe pain when first applied, and patients should receive other forms of analgesia until the ointment has had the opportunity to deplete the cutaneous nerves of substance P. More important, both the clinician and the patient must know that the drug does not respect boundaries; care must be taken to limit the area to which the medication is applied to that which is painful.

IV. **Orchestrating the "good death."** Physicians have an obligation to their patients to aid in the process of dying. Effectively to fulfill this responsibility, physicians need to discuss frankly issues vital to facilitating a dignified death with their patients. These issues include(a) durable power of attorney for health care,(b) advance directives,(c) do-not-resuscitate orders (DNRs), (d) hospice care, and(e) aid in dying.

A. **Durable power of attorney for health care (DPOA).** Perhaps no directive is more important in the process of dying than the execution of a DPOA. By designating a person intimately familiar with the patient's own wishes for care at the end of life, the patient ensures that his or her desires are followed. In the absence of this document, the decision-making responsibility goes to the nearest relative, who may not share the patient's attitudes toward end-of-life care. The designation of a secondary agent is extremely important, especially if the primary agent is also HIV seropositive.

B. Advance directives. Although carrying less legal weight in most states compared with the DPOA, advance directives convey to caregivers and support systems the patient's desires for specific care at the end of life. This may be particularly important in dealing with withdrawal of life support or nutritional therapy or the patient's desire for the actual location of death.

C. DNRs. Discussions of heroic measures at the end of life are essential to the provision of a dignified death. In the absence of these discussions, primary-care HIV physicians and housestaff are left to flounder about trying to reconstruct the desire of the patient for aggressive therapy. It must be stated that no physician is required to provide futile therapy; however, a patient's desires generally should hold sway. Patients must understand the components of a DNR order. Chest compression, pressor therapy, cardioversion, intubation and ventilation, invasive lines, and intensive care are all procedures that should be explained when discussing DNR orders. Finally, patient desires need to be clearly and prominently reflected in the medical record.

D. Hospice care. Most patients do not have an adequate understanding of hospice care. Oftentimes, it is "just a place you go to die." The ability of hospice care to offer psychosocial support, as well as palliative therapy should be discussed with the terminally ill AIDS patient considering hospice admission. Moreover, attitudes toward continuing medication and the provision of nutrition or hydration should be thoroughly examined.

E. Aid-in-dying. It is not unreasonable to want some control over how one dies. Patients do not cede responsibility for themselves to others when diagnosed with a terminal illness. Unfortunately, we cannot always make death a tolerable process. Despite our best efforts, some incurably ill AIDS patients wish for deliverance from suffering and a quiet, pain-free death. However, public attitudes toward aid-in-dying are at odds with professional positions on the issue. This conflict recently has been increased with judicial rulings that will likely increase the availability of aid-in-dying.

    1. It is important to understand **why some patients request aid-in-dying.** First, it is a need to maintain control over their lives. Most patients who request aid-in-dying do not kill themselves! Second, it is often a fear of the process of dying—dementia, incontinence, immobility, etc. These people are not invariably depressed or psychiatrically disordered. The request is, however, a signal to the caregiver and family that the patient's needs and fears have not be adequately addressed. When confronted with a request for aid-in-dying the caregiver's first responsibility is to elicit these fears and needs and attempt to alleviate them.

    2. Aid-in-dying may be appropriate for some terminally ill AIDS patients, and ethics committees are struggling to offer guidelines for use. In the absence of institutional guidelines, some **general recommendations** are offered.

        a. The AIDS patient should have **advanced illness associated with severe, unrelieved suffering.**

        b. The **patient must be able to understand all therapeutic alternatives and initiate the request** for aid-in-dying. The decision to use aid-in-dying and when to implement the plan must reside solely with the dying patient. Adequate comfort measures, sometimes including psychiatric evaluation, should be exhausted. The decision should be made within the context of a long-term patient—physician relationship, and the best time to discuss aid-in-dying is early in the course of AIDS.

        c. All physicians must adhere to their **personal codes of ethics.** If an HIV caregiver believes aid-in-dying is morally incompatible with personal ethical standards, then the caregiver should refer the patient to another physician for aid-in-dying while continuing to offer supportive care to the patient.

    d. The **methods of deliverance** should be reliable and not add to the patient's suffering. Commonly, the combination of opiates, barbiturates, and alcohol is used.

    e. Provision of a lethal prescription does not end a **caregiver's responsibility for care.** There must be a clear understanding of the caregiver's role in aid-in-dying beyond the provision of medications. What is the physician's availability and involvement if the attempt is unsuccessful? What further measures should be used? Should the support group call an ambulance? Further, the physician must familiarize the patient support group with the process of death—gasping, incontinence, seizures, etc.

3. These are weighty issues and responsibilities, and those who question their involvement would do well to consult with **senior staff or ethics committees.**

11. PULMONARY ASPECTS

I. **Overview of pulmonary processes in human immunodeficiency virus (HIV) infection**
   A. **Changes in pulmonary immune function.** The lung is the most frequent site of opportunistic infection in acquired immunodeficiency syndrome (AIDS), because, along with the gastrointestinal tract, it serves as an interface with all of the available potential pathogens in the environment.
   B. **Pulmonary infection.** The epidemiology of pulmonary infection varies by time period, geography, and patient population. In the inner-city population in the United States (a population less likely to have had access to ongoing care), the lung is affected in 90% of patients and *Pneumocystis carinii pneumonia* (PCP), is the most common. In populations with better access to care, prophylaxis for PCP is more likely and other pulmonary processes are more common, especially bacterial pneumonia. In patients with CD4⁺ counts >250 cell/mm³, the most common respiratory problems are upper respiratory infection, acute bronchitis, acute sinusitis, and bacterial pneumonia. Only a small minority (<5%) are the result of PCP.
II. **Diagnostic approach to the HIV-infected patient with thoracic manifestations** (The general approach is outlined in Fig. 1).
   A. **History.** The history should emphasize both pulmonary and systemic symptoms. These include dyspnea on exertion, cough, and systemic symptoms such as fever, sweats, malaise, and weight loss. All are relatively nonspecific, but may point to the chest. Travel and residential history should be obtained, both domestic and foreign, as it may serve to expand or narrow the differential diagnosis. Similarly, exposures to other sick individuals, particularly those with mycobacterial disease or the patient's social history, or both, may suggest the diagnosis of tuberculosis (TB). A history of prior prophylaxis for PCP, *Mycobacterium avium* complex (MAC), cryptococcus, or toxoplasmosis may also be useful.
   B. **Physical examination.** The eyes should be carefully examined for signs of CMV, disseminated Pneumocystis, or Toxoplasma infection. The skin should be examined for cutaneous manifestations of Kaposi's sarcoma (KS) or disseminated fungal disease. Evidence of pulmonary consolidation strongly favors bacterial pneumonia, although it may occasionally be found in KS. Physical signs of pleural effusion strongly favor mycobacterial disease or KS. The presence of peripheral adenopathy suggests lymphoma, TB, and fungus, and is unusual in Pneumocystis infection. Hepatosplenomegaly can be seen in any disseminated fungal or mycobacterial infection, as well as lymphoma. When it is present, the underlying diagnosis is unlikely to be PCP or KS. In general, the chest radiograph should initiate the algorithm shown in Fig. 1.
   C. **Laboratory investigations.** The lactate dehydrogenase (LDH) is increased in PCP, but is not specific. A very high LDH suggests the diagnosis and provides prognostic information. If the complete blood count (CBC) is often not helpful, medication-induced neutropenia may suggest that the patient is at greater risk for bacterial or Aspergillus infections. The CD4⁺ count helps to determine which infections and tumors are likely. In particular, opportunistic infections are less likely at CD4⁺ counts >200, whereas TB and bacterial pneumonia are quite common in that situation. Blood culture may be useful for detecting bacteria, MAC, *Mycobacterium tuberculosis* (MTB), and histoplasmosis. A serum protein electrophoresis may reveal polyclonal hypergam-

The author acknowledges the contribution of Daniel M. Goodenberger to the previous edition of this chapter.

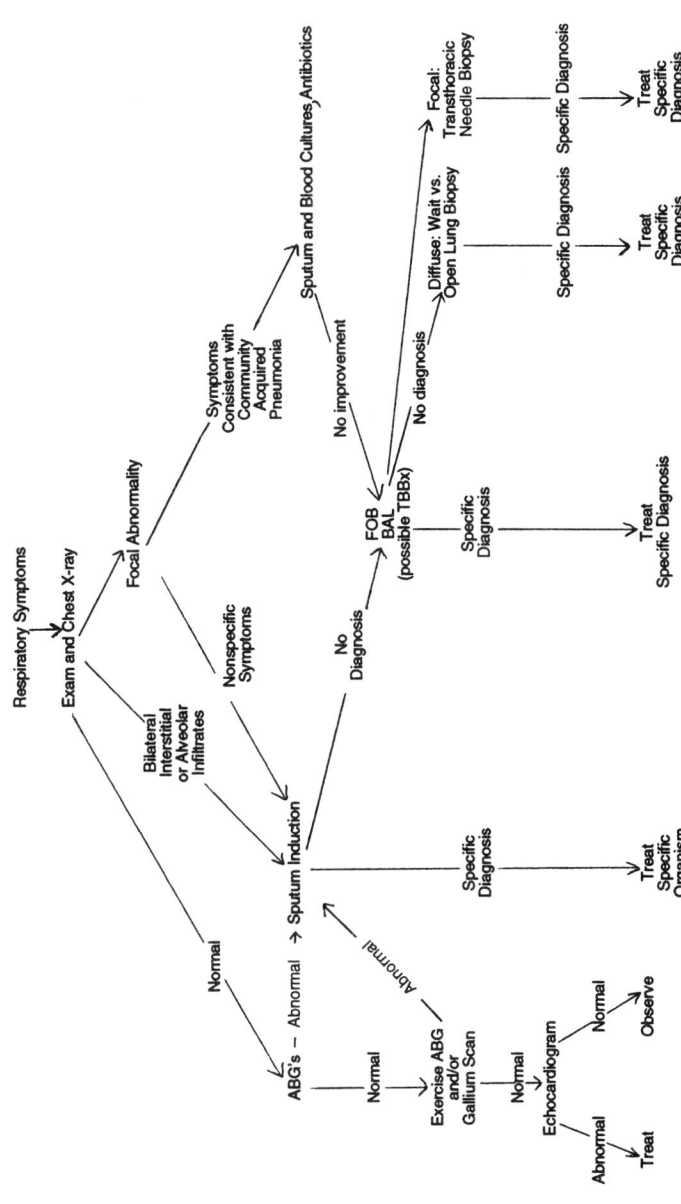

FIG. 1. Diagnostic algorithms for human immunodeficiency virus–infected patients.

maglobulinemia associated with lymphoid interstitial pneumonitis (LIP). Cryptococcal antigen in blood, cerebrospinal fluid (CSF), or a BAL is a very useful finding. Histoplasma antigen should be sought in urine, where it may also be diagnostic. Coccidioidal complement-fixation levels should be sought when the patient gives the appropriate history of residence or travel. If no diagnosis has been reached after this workup, including induced sputum, fiberoptic bronchoscopy with bronchoalveolar lavage (BAL), or transbronchial biopsy or both, the practitioner should consider biopsy of liver, marrow, or lymph nodes, guided by physical examination or laboratory abnormalities.

    D. Chest radiograph findings are not usually diagnostic alone, but the pattern of involvement may guide further investigation and empiric treatment (see Table 1).

III. Specific pulmonary processes (Table 2)

    A. Community-acquired bacterial pneumonia

        1. General

            a. Pathophysiology/natural history. Bacterial pneumonia is increased in HIV-infected individuals because of defects in $CD4^+$ T-cell–B-cell interactions, with resultant defective humoral immunity. Community-acquired bacterial pneumonia (CAP) is common. The most common organisms causing CAP are *Streptococcus pneumoniae* and *Haemophilus influenzae*. The risk of CAP is increased 4.3 to 6 times over that of the general immunocompetent population. Pneumococcal pneumonia in AIDS is more likely to be bacteremic (50% to 80%), with a mortality reported to be >4 times as high as that in the normal population (Caiaffa et al. *Am J Res Crit Care Med* 1994;150:1493–1498). Gram-negative organisms (especially *Pseudomonas aeruginosa*) are associated with pneumonia in patients with more advanced disease; typically nosocomial, they may also occur in the community setting.

            b. Risks. An increased risk for bacterial CAP is associated with intravenous drug use, low $CD4^+$ counts (greatest incidence with a count <200/mm^3), cigarette smoking, previous infection with PCP, and smoking of illicit drugs (cocaine, crack cocaine, and marijuana).

            c. Clinical presentation is usually similar to that for community-acquired pneumonia in normal hosts.

            d. Laboratory findings are nonspecific. The white blood count is generally increased, similar to that in HIV-negative individuals. The LDH may be modestly increased. Arterial blood gases typically reveal an increased A–a gradient.

            e. Radiographic imaging. The chest radiograph most often shows focal airspace disease, ranging from patchy bronchopneumonia to segmental or lobar consolidation with air bronchograms. However, the patient may have interstitial infiltrates difficult to distinguish from PCP pneumonia.

            f. Diagnosis. Diagnosis is suspected by presentation with the characteristic clinical syndrome, with an onset of illness substantially more rapid than that typically seen with PCP or other opportunistic pulmonary infections. Ultimately, specific diagnosis relies on positive cultures from sputum, blood, pleural fluid, or respiratory tract cultures. In a typical case, fiberoptic bronchoscopy may be deferred while the patient undergoes a trial of therapy.

            g. Therapy. For those HIV-infected individuals with an onset typical of encapsulated aerobic organisms, a second- or third-generation cephalosporin is a reasonable first choice (e.g., ceftriaxone, 1 g per 24 hours i.v., or cefuroxime, 1 g per 8 hours i.v.). If the patient fails to respond or worsens, trimethoprim/sulfamethoxazole, 5 mg per kg per 8 hours TMP i.v., should be added and investigations should proceed to fiberoptic bronchoscopy, assuming sputum examination is negative. If gram-negative pneumonia is suspected, an antibacterial

Table 1. Radiographic patterns of thoracic involvement in the HIV-infected patient

Chest Radiograph	CT Correlates
NORMAL	
Mycobacterium avium-intracellularae[a]	
Pneumocystis carinii[a]	
Mycobacterium tuberculosis[a]	
Histoplasma capsulatum[a]	
Coccidioides immitis	
Nonspecific interstitial pneumonitis	
Lymphoid interstitial pneumonitis	
DIFFUSE INTERSTITIAL INFILTRATES	
Pneumocystis carinii[a]	Thin-walled cysts, airspace ground-glass infiltrates
Disseminated *Mycobacterium tuberculosis*[a]	Low-attenuation adenopathy with sharply marginated rim of enhancement, miliary nodules that may grow quickly, frequent effusions
Disseminated *Histoplasma capsulatum*[a]	Miliary nodules
Disseminated *Cryptococcus neoformans*[a]	Miliary nodules
Disseminated *Coccidioides immitis*[a]	Miliary nodules
Disseminated *Blastomyces dermatiditis*	Miliary nodules
Mycobacterium avium-intracellulare	
Nonspecific interstitial pneumonitis[a]	
Lymphoid interstitial pneumonitis	Variable-sized nodules
Penicillium marneffei[a]	Cavitary upper-lobe infiltrates better seen on CT
Non-Hodgkin's lymphoma	
Extracerebral *Toxoplasma gondii*	
Hyperinfection with *Strongyloides stercoralis*	
FOCAL INFILTRATES AND CONSOLIDATION	
Bacterial pneumonia[a]	Segmental/lobar distribution; effusions common
Kaposi's sarcoma[a]	Peribronchovascular distribution with intralobular septal thickening; irregular, variable-sized nodules; effusions and adenopathy common
Mycobacterium tuberculosis[a]	Occult cavities; effusions
Cryptococcus neoformans[a]	
Coccidioides immitis	
Blastomyces dermatiditis	
Pneumocystis carinii	
NODULE(S)	
Lung cancer[a]	One-third have extensive pleural disease
Kaposi's sarcoma[a]	Numerous ill-defined nodules, 1 to 2 cm; linear opacities; effusions in 50%
Lymphoma[a]	Usually asymmetric adenopathy elsewhere

continued

Table 1. *Continued*

Chest Radiograph	CT Correlates
METASTATIC CANCER	
Cryptococcus neoformans[a]	
Coccidioides immitis[a]	May be occult cavities
Blastomyces dermatiditis[a]	
Mycobacterium tuberculosis	May be occult cavities
Pneumocystis carinii	
CAVITIES	
Pneumocystis carinii (especially upper lobe after inhaled pentamidine)[a]	Thin-walled cysts
Mycobacterium tuberculosis (CD4 >200 cells/mm^3)[a]	Associated adenopathy
Aspergillus fumigatus[a]	
Coccidioides immitis	
Rhodococcus equi[a]	
Septic pulmonary emboli	
Kaposi's sarcoma	
Lymphoma	
THORACIC ADENOPATHY	
Mycobacterium tuberculosis[a]	
Histoplasma capsulatum[a]	
Other fungal infections	
Mycobacterium avium-intracellulare[a]	
Kaposi's sarcoma[a]	
Lymphoma	
Lung cancer	
Pneumothorax	
Pneumocystis carinii[a]	

CT, computed tomography.
[a] Principal or important manifestation of this disease.

with activity against *P. aeruginosa* (e.g., cefepime or ciprofloxacin) should be used.

    h. Prevention. Trimethoprim/sulfamethoxazole prophylaxis, as described in the section on PCP, results in a 67% decrease in risk for bacterial CAP. All previously nonimmunized HIV-positive individuals should receive pneumococcal vaccine.

2. *Rhodococcus equi*

    a. Pathophysiology/natural history. The responsible organism is a gram-positive bacillus that is weakly acid fast (because of cell-wall mycolic acids). It multiplies and resides intracellularly in macrophages. It occurs naturally in the soil, and is a well-known veterinary pathogen. Of human infections, 83% to 88% are pneumonia.

    b. Clinical presentation. The onset is usually insidious, with fever, productive cough, and pleurisy in up to half. Chest radiographs typically show focal infiltrates, of which approximately three fourths cavitate. The cavities are often more apparent on computed tomog-

Table 2. Lung involvement in HIV infection

BACTERIA	VIRUSES
Streptococcus pneumoniae	*Cytomegalovirus*
Haemophilus influenzae	*Adenovirus*
Pseudomonas aeruginosa	*Herpes simplex*
Staphylococcus aureus	
Moraxella catarrhalis	PROTOZOA
Rhodococcus equi	*Toxoplasma gondii*
Nocardia asteroides	
	METAZOA
MYCOBACTERIA	*Strongyloides stercoralis*
Mycobacterium tuberculosis	
Mycobacterium	MALIGNANCIES
avium-intracellulare	Kaposi's sarcoma
	Non-Hodgkin's lymphoma
FUNGI	Lung carcinoma
Cryptococcus neoformans	
Histoplasma capsulatum	OTHER
Aspergillus fumigatus	Lymphoid interstitial pneumonitis
Coccidioides immitis	Nonspecific interstitial pneumonitis
Blastomyces dermatitidis	Pulmonary hypertension
Pneumocystis carinii	Emphysema
	Bronchiectasis

raphy (CT) scan. The parenchymal findings are often accompanied by effusions. Specific diagnosis depends on successful culture of the organism.

c. **Therapy.** The optimal therapy has not been defined. Erythromycin, 1 g per 6 hours i.v., and rifampin, 600 mg per day p.o., are given for 2 to 6 weeks, followed by oral continuation of both medications for 4 to 6 months. Alternatively, vancomycin, 1 g per 12 hours i.v., with dosage adjusted by serum levels, may be given.

3. **Nocardiosis**
   a. **Clinical presentation** is most often the result of pulmonary infection. Symptoms include cough, which is often productive, fever, weight loss, and malaise. Dyspnea and pleurisy also may occur. A substantial portion of patients have disseminated disease. Involvement of the brain is particularly common. Chest radiograph may reveal focal infiltrates or nodules of varying size. Cavitation is common, and pleural effusion may be present. The presence of a detectable brain abscess(es) in combination with the other clinical and radiologic findings makes *Nocardia* very likely. The other major AIDS-associated illness that may cause brain abscesses with cavitary pulmonary infiltrates is aspergillosis.
   b. **Diagnosis.** Gram stain of pulmonary secretions may reveal branching, beaded, gram-positive filaments that are weakly acid fast. Definitive diagnosis requires culture, which may take 2 to 4 weeks. When a pulmonary process is identified as a *Nocardia* infection, careful evaluation of the central nervous system and other organ systems should be done to rule out dissemination.
   c. **Therapy.** Sulfamethoxazole, 6 to 8 g daily in four divided doses, is the drug of choice. Sulfonamide blood levels should be measured and doses adjusted to keep serum levels between 100 and 150 µg per mL. An alternative therapy is TMP/SMX in a dosage of trimethoprim, 15 to 20 mg per kg per day, which should be given in two divided doses.

B. Viral pulmonary infections
   1. CMV rarely causes pneumonitis as a sole pathogen. CMV is usually discovered as a co-pathogen in the lung with another primary diagnosis, most often PCP. In the occasional patient with pulmonary infection caused only by CMV, the patient may have fever, malaise, fatigue, myalgias, tachypnea, and nonproductive cough.
      a. Diagnosis. The presence of CMV on cultured BAL fluid is not definitive. CMV should be considered to be the primary process only if cytopathic changes are found in a characteristic clinical setting with no other pathogen or other pulmonary process identified. Transbronchial biopsy may lend weight to the diagnosis.
      b. Therapy. If other pathogens, particularly PCP, are identified, treatment is given for the primary infection. In this circumstance, the presence or absence of CMV appears to have no adverse impact on either short- or long-term outcome. If CMV is the only pathogen identified, with a positive culture and cytopathic changes, the treatment of choice is ganciclovir, 5 mg per kg per 12 hours i.v. for 14 days, followed by 5 mg per kg per day i.v., indefinitely (see Chapter 25 for discussion of drugs used for CMV infection).
   2. Herpes simplex virus (HSV). Pneumonitis caused by HSV is very uncommon, and when it occurs may be a result of either extension of herpetic tracheobronchitis or hematogenous dissemination. Diagnosis requires the isolation of HSV from appropriate respiratory secretions in a compatible clinical setting. Acyclovir, 10 mg per kg per 8 hours i.v. for 10 to 14 days, with dosage adjusted for renal function, is the preferred therapy.
C. Mycobacterial pulmonary infections (see Chapter 23)
   1. MTB
      a. Pathophysiology/natural history. MTB is a widespread human pathogen causing disease in normal hosts. Because of its natural virulence, it causes disease early in HIV infection, with a median CD4+ count of 345 cells/mm^3. Among the common HIV-related pathogens, it is remarkable for person-to-person communicability as a respiratory aerosol. Because of the high prevalence of TB in much of the Third World, where HIV infection is increasing, it is becoming the most important lethal opportunistic infectious pathogen in the worldwide HIV pandemic. Moreover, TB accelerates the progression of onset of other opportunistic infections, shortens life, and causes an increased death rate (not caused directly by TB itself). The rate of reactivation in HIV-positive patients is greatly increased, approaching 10% per year.
      b. Risks. In the United States, the risk for TB in HIV infection is increased among intravenous-drug users, homeless persons using shelters, Haitians, prison inmates, and on open hospital wards in which patients with TB and HIV are cared for. Multidrug-resistant TB [defined as strains resistant to both isoniazid (INH) and rifampin], is increased in HIV-positive patients, particularly those hospitalized within three rooms of a patient with multidrug-resistant TB, having hospital stays of >10 days, and ambulating on wards with inadequately masked patients with TB.
      c. Clinical presentation. The presentation of TB in HIV-infected patients can be roughly separated into two kinds, depending on CD4+ count
         (1) Early (higher CD4+ counts). The patient has symptoms typical of pulmonary TB, with fever, cough, night sweats, malaise, and weight loss. In this group, the tuberculin skin test is positive in 40% to 80%. The chest radiograph more closely resembles that seen in TB in the immunocompetent patient (with infiltrates in the upper lobes, particularly the apical or poste-

rior segments, or the superior segment of the lower lobe). Cavitation is frequent. Histopathologic studies show granulomatous inflammation.

   (2) **Late.** In these patients, the CD4+ count is generally <200/mm³. Disease is usually disseminated, and the patient has constitutional symptoms. The tuberculin skin test is almost always negative, associated with general anergy. The chest radiograph is less typical of classic TB, and histopathologic studies show abundant organisms with few or no granulomata. It is more likely to reflect dissemination, with diffuse or lower lobe reticulonodular interstitial infiltrates or miliary-appearing lesions, mediastinal or hilar adenopathy, and pleural effusions. The chest radiograph also may be normal.

  d. Diagnosis
   (1) If a tuberculin skin test is positive and the patient's disease is consistent with TB, the patient should be treated as though active TB is present while awaiting definitive evidence.
   (2) The diagnosis of pulmonary disease can often be made by obtaining sputum for smears and cultures. Sputum should be induced by using 3% saline, but only in a setting that minimizes the chance of spread to others (a negative-pressure box or negative-pressure isolation room). In HIV infection, the sputum may be positive even in the absence of cavitary disease.
   (3) If the sputum is unrevealing, fiberoptic bronchoscopy should be undertaken; transbronchial biopsy provides a more rapid diagnosis than BAL with acid-fast stains and culture. Postbronchoscopy sputum should be obtained.
   (4) When extrapulmonary sites of disease are identified or suspected, biopsy of an involved organ may be very useful.
   (5) Mycobacterial blood cultures may also be positive in a surprisingly high number of patients.

  e. Therapy (see Chapter 23)
  f. Impact of potent antiretroviral therapy. Paradoxical reactions have been described in patients with tuberculosis treated with potent antiretroviral therapy. Such patients may develop increasing pleural effusion (often with many neutrophils), increased adenopathy and fever. This does not represent worsening of the tuberculosis and can respond to corticosteroid therapy (Narita et al. *Am J Respir Crit Care Med* 1998;158:157–161).

 2. MAC
  a. Pathophysiology/natural history. MAC is a recognized, but uncommon cause of pulmonary disease. The most common pattern of pulmonary involvement is a bilateral diffuse or lower lobe reticulonodular interstitial infiltrate. Treatment and prevention are discussed in detail in Chapter 23.

D. Fungal infections (see also Chapter 24)
 1. *Histoplasma capsulatum* is found in temperate river valleys throughout the world. In North America, it is endemic in the St. Lawrence, Ohio, and Mississippi River Valleys. It is also endemic in the Caribbean, notably Puerto Rico, and the river valleys of South America. In 20% to 30% of cases, chest radiographs are normal. The remainder shows a variety of abnormalities, with a diffuse interstitial infiltrate or miliary pattern most common. Occasionally there are focal infiltrates, and rarely, pleural effusions. Mild to moderate disease may be treated with itraconazole, 200 mg b.i.d. (see Chapter 24). Severe disseminated disease should be treated with intravenous amphotericin B 0.5 to 1 mg per kg per day to 500 to 1,000 mg total, if an adequate response is achieved. This is followed by chronic life-long maintenance with itraconazole, 200 mg/day.

2. ***Cryptococcus neoformans.*** Meningitis is the initial manifestation in AIDS in 70% to 85% of cases. Simultaneous pulmonary involvement occurs in ~30% to 40%, and primary pulmonary involvement is uncommon (only 5% to 10%). Pleurisy is relatively common (40%) in those with pulmonary infection. The serum cryptococcal antigen titer is positive in 75% to 90%. Even in the absence of central nervous system findings, positive serum antigen should prompt spinal tap and fluid analysis. The most common findings on chest radiograph are focal (patchy segmental) and diffuse interstitial infiltrates. Patients with isolated pulmonary disease can be treated with fluconazole, 400 mg daily. All other patients should be treated initially with amphotericin B, 0.7–1.0 mg per kg per day, with flucytosine, 100 mg per kg per day p.o. in four divided doses. Treatment of meningitis is discussed in Chapter 24.

3. **Coccidioidomycosis.** This dimorphic fungus is an uncommon cause of infection in HIV-infected patients in general, but in the American southwest, where the disease is endemic, up to 25% of HIV-infected patients will have the disease over a 3.5-year period. The CD4$^+$ count is usually <250/mm^3, and often <150/mm^3. Occasional primary infection occurs after dusty exposure, including archeologic excavation, construction work, and so on.

   a. **Presentation.** The most common symptoms are fever and dyspnea. Weight loss and cough are other common symptoms. Pulmonary disease is present in 70% of patients. The most common chest radiographic findings are a diffuse or reticulonodular infiltrate or both. Other radiographic findings include nodules, cavities, patchy infiltrates, and hilar adenopathy. The definitive diagnosis requires identification of coccidioidal spherules from sputum or BAL fluid, or a subsequent positive culture.

   b. **Therapy** (see Chapter 24)

4. **Aspergillosis** is an uncommon, but increasing cause of pulmonary disease in AIDS, in which it most often involves the lungs, but can disseminate. It most often involves the pulmonary parenchyma, but can involve the tracheobronchial tree. Tracheobronchial disease is associated with dyspnea and wheezing caused by obstruction of large airways. Therapy is discussed in detail in Chapter 24.

5. ***Penicillium marneffei*** is a dimorphic fungus that is endemic in Southeast Asia and is emerging as a pathogen for HIV-infected individuals who are native to the region or who have traveled there. The disease is usually disseminated at presentation. Symptoms include fever, weight loss, skin lesions, hepatomegaly, lymphadenopathy, and pulmonary infiltrates. Blood cultures are often positive, as is marrow examination and culture. Biopsies should be obtained of skin lesions, and cultures of these are often positive as well. Amphotericin-B, 0.5 to 1.0 mg per kg per day for 2 to 8 weeks followed by itraconazole, 200 mg b.i.d., is appropriate initial therapy (see Chapter 24).

E. **Protozoa** (see also Chapter 22)

1. ***Pneumocystis carinii.*** One of the first two illnesses associated with the AIDS epidemic, it remains common, and is currently the cause of death in 15% to 20% of HIV-positive individuals. The major risk is low CD4$^+$ count, with risk increasing sharply after CD4$^+$ count decreases to <200.

   a. **Clinical presentation.** The onset is typically subacute over 2 to 4 weeks, with prominent symptoms of fever, sweats, nonproductive cough, dyspnea, fatigue, weight loss, and on occasion retrosternal chest pain. Examination may reveal tachypnea, but there are seldom adventitious lung sounds of any sort.

   b. **Laboratory findings.** Arterial blood gas analysis may reveal hypoxia or an increased A–a gradient. The serum LDH is elevated in ~93%, representing the LDH-3 fraction. An LDH >450 IU/L is strongly predictive of PCP. A normal level suggests that an alternative diagnosis is more likely. When the diagnosis is PCP, the LDH is prognostic; in one study, survivors had a mean level of 394 IU/L, whereas those who died had a mean level of 717 IU/L.

c. **Radiographic imaging.** The chest radiograph is normal in from 6% to 23% of individuals with PCP. The most common radiographic pattern is bilateral diffuse interstitial infiltrates, which may progress to alveolar consolidation. Other patterns include localized infiltrates, cystic changes (most commonly in the upper lobes), cavitary nodules, and rarely, effusions. In the patient who has received inhaled pentamidine prophylaxis, there is a tendency toward apical infiltrates with cystic changes.

d. **Diagnosis** requires demonstration of the organism in secretions or tissue.

(1) **Sputum induced** with 3% saline has a sensitivity ranging from 55%, by using a silver stain, to as high as 81% to 92% when a direct fluorescent antibody against PCP is used. The sensitivity is diminished with prior pentamidine prophylaxis to ~64%. Fiberoptic bronchoscopy with BAL has a sensitivity of 80% to 98%. This is decreased to ~80% when the patient is receiving prophylaxis. The sensitivity of the procedure can be increased by performing BAL in both the right middle and the right upper lobe, to a level approaching 95% (Yung et al. *Am Rev Respir Dis* 1993;148:1563–1566).

(2) If induced sputum is negative for PCP, the patient should rapidly undergo **fiberoptic bronchoscopy** (FOB). The induced sputum can be obtained in the morning, with the results known by early afternoon. If negative, the patient can undergo BAL the same day. If the BAL is negative, PCP is very unlikely, and an alternative diagnosis is more likely. At that point, a decision will need to be made about whether to repeat bronchoscopy with transbronchial biopsy; the principal risk is pneumothorax, which occurs in ~8% of individuals with AIDS. In summary, we recommend that when a patient known to be HIV-infected has a compatible clinical history and diffuse interstitial infiltrates, systemic therapy for PCP should be begun. Sputum for PCP should be induced at the first opportunity; if positive, treatment should be continued. If sputum is negative, the patient should undergo FOB/BAL. If there is no diagnosis, and the patient fails to respond to anti-PCP therapy, further diagnostic procedures are indicated, including transbronchial lung biopsy. In the event that the patient continues to improve, despite a negative BAL, treatment can be continued under observation.

(3) If the chest radiograph is negative, but the patient has compatible clinical symptoms, a **gallium scan** may be obtained. If there is diffuse uptake consistent with PCP, sputum may be obtained; if negative, bronchoscopy should be performed with BAL and transbronchial biopsy.

e. **Therapy** (see Chapter 22)

2. *Toxoplasma gondii.* Pulmonary involvement in toxoplasmosis in HIV infection occurs in a small minority of patients. The major symptoms are nonspecific and include cough, dyspnea, and fever. Treatment is discussed in Chapter 22.

F. **Pulmonary malignancies**

1. **Kaposi's sarcoma** (see Chapter 29). The lungs are involved in 20% to 40%. Pulmonary KS is responsible for the respiratory symptoms in approximately one-third of those patients who have mucocutaneous KS (Meduri. *Am J Med* 1986;81:11–18). This may result in symptoms through a variety of mechanisms; the malignancy may obstruct the trachea or bronchi; it may cause pulmonary edema as a result of lymphatic

obstruction; it may cause large effusions; and it may cause lung consolidation and hemorrhage.

a. Clinical presentation. Mucocutaneous KS is present in most, but not all, patients with pulmonary KS. Nonspecific symptoms include dyspnea on exertion and cough. Symptoms specifically suggestive of KS include hemoptysis and stridor. Individuals with obvious KS outside the lungs frequently have respiratory symptoms leading to diagnostic difficulties. In this group, ~40% of respiratory symptoms have been caused by KS alone or in association with an opportunistic infection, and 60% are the result of other causes. It has proven to be nearly impossible to differentiate between those with pulmonary KS and those without on the basis of chest radiographs or clinical criteria or both.

b. Radiographic imaging. Nodular infiltrates, which may be accompanied by mediastinal adenopathy, are common. However, the tumor may have interstitial infiltrates difficult to differentiate from PCP.

c. Diagnosis. Assuming induced sputum is negative, FOB should be undertaken. In a substantial number of patients with pulmonary KS, there may be visible endobronchial disease, which is a red or purplish, spreading, slightly raised, stain-like area tending to occur at bronchial bifurcations. In addition, FOB may be helpful in diagnosing alternate or associated opportunistic infections.

d. Therapy. (see Chapter 30)

2. **Lymphoma.** Thoracic manifestations are rare, and thoracic adenopathy is uncommon.

3. **Lung carcinoma.** Tobacco exposure from cigarette smoking appears to be the major risk factor and is causative in nearly all individuals with HIV infection who develop lung carcinoma. However, the incidence of lung cancer appears to be increased in HIV infection, and to occur at a younger age, with an unusually high percentage of adenocarcinomas. Interestingly, the lung cancer often is seen before the diagnosis of AIDS (Grudon et al. *J Thorac Imaging* 1995;10:99–105) and is typically advanced at presentation. Therapy should be planned in consultation with an experienced oncologist.

G. **Idiopathic HIV-related diseases**

1. **Lymphocytic interstitial pneumonitis (LIP)**

   a. Pathophysiology/natural history. This illness is seen most commonly in children younger than 13 years, most of whom acquired HIV perinatally. Thirty percent to 50% of children infected by this route will develop LIP. The origin and pathophysiologic characteristics are unclear. It may be caused by simultaneous infection with Epstein–Barr virus (EBV) and HIV, as there is some evidence of HIV RNA expression in the affected tissue (Travis et al. *Hum Pathol* 1992;23:529–541). The most common chest radiographic finding is bilateral reticulonodular infiltrates. These may involve all the lung fields or may be predominantly in the lower lobes. BAL fluid reveals principally CD8+ lymphocytes. One can be reasonably confident of the diagnosis if there is a characteristic presentation, age, and risk factors, if the chest radiograph reveals reticulonodular interstitial infiltrates, and if the FOB is otherwise negative for opportunistic infection.

   b. Therapy. Prednisone, antiretroviral therapy, and intravenous immunoglobulin have all been tried without definite proof of efficacy.

2. **Nonspecific interstitial pneumonitis (NSIP)**

   a. Pathophysiology/natural history. The pathophysiology and origin are unclear. Some cases may be related directly to HIV infection with or without EBV infection. NSIP is much more common than LIP in adults (11:1). Histologic examination reveals a chronic round-cell interstitial infiltrate, consisting principally of CD8+ lymphocytes.

b. The most common **radiographic finding** is bilateral reticulonodular interstitial infiltrates. However, the chest radiograph may be normal in 14%.

c. Diagnosis. NIP is a diagnosis of exclusion. When the radiograph and syndrome are characteristic, and FOB, BAL, and ultimately transbronchial biopsy are histologically negative, with persistently negative cultures after prolonged incubation, the diagnosis may be seriously entertained. Under these circumstances, the patient may be observed, and the course will typically be stable.

d. Therapy. This is usually a stable entity, and therapy is rarely necessary.

3. **"Primary" pulmonary hypertension**
   a. There appears to be an increased risk of pulmonary hypertension associated with HIV disease. In one study, a rate of 0.5% was found, compared with an incidence of primary pulmonary hypertension of 0.0005% in the normal population (a 1,000-fold increase). Investigation of the pulmonary artery endothelium revealed no evidence of direct HIV infection, although HIV-induced mediator release has been proposed as a mechanism.

   b. The **clinical presentation** is nonspecific, with atypical chest pain, shortness of breath, and dyspnea on exertion. Physical examination may be consistent with pulmonary hypertension, revealing a right ventricular heave, prominent P_2, or murmur of pulmonary insufficiency, or a combination of these.

   c. The **chest radiograph** is typically normal or reveals signs of pulmonary hypertension.

   d. Echocardiography to measure pulmonary artery peak pressures noninvasively should be done when this diagnosis is suspected. An exercise study may reveal the characteristic increase in dead space to tidal volume ratio or increase in A–a gradient or both. Ultimately, right heart catheterization, with or without pulmonary arteriography to exclude chronic thromboembolic disease, may be necessary to confirm this diagnosis.

   e. Therapy. There is very little information regarding vasodilator therapy. However, the disease does appear to respond to epoprostenol in a way similar to that in non–HIV-infected patients with primary pulmonary hypertension.

4. **Pneumothorax**
   a. The predominant origin of pneumothorax in the HIV-infected individual is prior or current subpleural necrotizing pneumonitis and secondary bleb formation caused by **PCP**. Pneumothorax occurs spontaneously. It also occurs more easily than normal in patients undergoing FOB, brush biopsy, and transbronchial biopsy. It appears to occur somewhat more frequently in those receiving prophylaxis with aerosolized pentamidine. Other interstitial diseases may predispose to pneumothorax, and KS may cause apical disease with cavities.

   b. Presentation is similar to that with other individuals with pneumothorax, including chest pain and acute onset of shortness of breath. In severely affected individuals, or those with tension pneumothorax, there may be hypoxemia and hypotension. The pneumothoraces in HIV-infected individuals are bilateral with an unusual degree of frequency (34%) and are recurrent in a similar percentage.

   c. Radiographic imaging. Chest radiograph will show a pneumothorax, which may be bilateral. In all cases, both lung fields should be examined carefully. Blebs or bullae may be visible, particularly in the upper lobes, when the lung has collapsed away from the chest wall. There may be associated signs of infiltration or infection.

   d. Therapy
      (1) Standard therapy with a **chest tube and doxycycline or minocycline pleurodesis** has been noted to have a poor

success rate. This may be related in part to treatment with steroids or dapsone or both, both of which reduce the inflammatory response to tetracycline. Also, large apical bullae, particularly those associated with PCP, may lead to prolonged air leaks and incomplete expansion. It is impossible to sclerose the lung adequately when the pleural surfaces are not in close apposition. In one series, the standard thoracostomy and inflammatory therapy had only a 26% success rate and was associated with a 28% death rate. By comparison, video-assisted thoracoscopic surgery and talc pleurodesis resulted in 88% success rate with only a 4-day hospital stay. A similar success rate may be obtained with thoracotomy, partial pleurectomy, and bleb stapling, but the average length of stay approached 3 weeks.

(2) Based on this, the **following algorithm** is suggested.

(a) When there is a **very small unilateral pneumothorax**, a small chest tube should be placed for suction. If there is complete and prompt reexpansion of lung without a persistent air leak, pleurodesis with doxycycline or minocycline may be attempted.

(b) If, however, there is a **large or persistent air leak** or incomplete expansion, an additional chest tube should be placed if necessary for relief of symptoms or hypoxemia, and the patient should proceed to VATS-assisted talc pleurodesis (Wait and Dal Nogare. *Chest* 1994;106:693–696). In all instances, consultation should be sought from an experienced pulmonologist or thoracic surgeon.

IV. **Medical intensive care for the HIV-infected patient**

A. **Background.** This issue was muddied by early reports of mortality approaching 91% of mechanically ventilated HIV-positive patients with PCP (Schein et al. *Crit Care Med* 1986;14:1026–1027). However, by the late 1980s, survivals approaching 40% were being reported in this same situation (Wachter et al. *JAMA* 1995;273:230–235). Later studies suggest a decline in survival, in part because of exclusion of brief episodes of respiratory failure caused by bronchoscopy and perhaps because of inclusion of sicker patients undergoing mechanical ventilation, to an overall survival level of 18% to 24% (Staikowsky et al. *Chest* 1993;104:756–762; Wachter et al. *JAMA* 1995;273: 230–235). In general, these studies were not well stratified with physiology scores such as APACHE, but predictors of outcome were identified. In particular, those with short duration of treatment before mechanical ventilation for PCP (TMP/SMX and prednisone <5 days) had higher survival rates, approaching 50% (Staikowsky et al. *Chest* 1993;104:756–762).

B. **Outcomes.** Survival outcomes are as noted previously. Those surviving mechanical ventilation for PCP in general spend only ~5% of their remaining life in a hospital. Costs are high and approach $175,000 per year of life saved (Wachter et al. *JAMA* 1995;273:230–235). There are fewer data for intensive care of nonventilated HIV-positive patients. At the National Institutes of Health (NIH), at a time when survival for mechanically ventilated PCP was ~10%, the overall intensive care unit (ICU) survival was approximately twice as high (Rogers et al. *Crit Care Med* 1989;17:113–117). Additionally, the risk of HIV infection to health-care personnel in the ICU was low.

C. **Recommendations.** We recommend that plans for intensive care in various circumstances be discussed with HIV-infected individuals well before any need for such intervention. In particular, these discussions should be accompanied by information regarding realistic estimates of survival and allow time for input by both the patient and his or her family members.

12. DERMATOLOGIC MANIFESTATIONS

Human immunodeficiency virus (HIV) infection produces a panorama of cutaneous signs and symptoms. The initial infection by HIV may produce a transient macular roseola-like eruption. Progression results in infectious processes, neoplastic disease, and a variety of poorly characterized skin reactions. Patients may also have symptoms such as pruritus without visible skin lesions.

I. **Management of noninfectious cutaneous findings in HIV infection**. Patients with HIV infection may have one or more well-defined cutaneous lesions that have a significant association with HIV infection and acquired immunodeficiency syndrome (AIDS).

A. **Seborrheic dermatitis**. Perhaps the best known dermatosis associated with HIV infection, seborrheic dermatitis, has an incidence of ~80% in the context of HIV infection. Its presence correlates inversely with decreasing CD4$^+$ counts. Seborrheic dermatitis is a common benign dermatosis. A red, scaly eruption occurs most frequently in the malar areas, nasolabial folds, eyebrows, bearded area, and the retroauricular areas of the face. In severe cases, seborrheic dermatitis also can affect the hair-bearing areas of the axillae, chest, and groin. The origin of seborrheic dermatitis is poorly understood. In the context of HIV, seborrheic dermatitis may be chronic and recurrent. Management relies on applying antifungal or corticosteroid creams or both. There is a wide array of antifungal creams [miconazole cream, ketoconazole (Nizoral) cream, and so on] from which to select. These should be applied sparingly to affected areas 2 to 4 times daily for initial control, followed by intermittent application to suppress recurrence. A similar approach can be used with topical corticosteroids, either alone or in combination with antifungals. Low-potency corticosteroids (hydrocortisone cream, either 1% or 2.5%; aclometasone dipropionate cream, 0.05%), applied as needed up to 4 times daily, are effective in managing seborrheic dermatitis. Potent topical corticosteroids (class IV and above) should not be used on the face, where they may produce local side effects such as atropy.

B. **Pruritus** is a common symptom in HIV-infected persons.
1. Pruritus may be essential (no identifiable cause) or may be a consequence of an external agent such as crusted scabies, an internal metabolic abnormality, neoplasia, or reaction to medication. Pruritus leads to scratching and the production of secondary lesions. These lesions are generally nondescript macular, papular, and follicular. Severity of pruritus can be assessed by determining whether the symptom awakens the person at night and by the degree of excoriation.
2. Therapy for pruritus must be directed at the underlying cause, if identifiable.
a. For essential pruritus, therapies include application of antipruritic preparations containing ingredients such as menthol, camphor, phenol, and pramoxine. These ingredients are present in a variety of antipruritic agents and can be added extemporaneously to topical corticosteroid preparations if inflamed excoriations are present. Topical doxepin cream can be applied up to 4 times daily to individual itchy lesions. If the secondary lesions are inflamed, topical corticosteroid preparations can be applied. Finally, antihistamines can be given for generalized pruritus.

The author acknowledges the contribution of Neal S. Penneys to the previous edition of this chapter.

b. For unremitting pruritus, referral to a dermatologist for ultraviolet light B therapy is appropriate. Controlled administration of ultraviolet light has been shown to be effective therapy for widespread pruritus in HIV-infected individuals who do not respond to more limited forms of therapy.

C. Psoriasis may be aggravated by the coexistence of HIV infection. Therapies for psoriasis range across a spectrum, depending on the extent of the psoriatic flare.

    1. For limited disease, intermediate-strength topical corticosteroid preparations (triamcinolone acetonide cream or ointment, either 0.025% or 0.1%, or equivalent) applied from 1 to 4 times daily is the mainstay for control. If control is not obtainable with topical corticosteroids, then the patient should be referred to a dermatologist for other topical antipsoriatic agents such as calcipotriol, coal tar, and anthralin-containing preparations.

    2. The safest approach to widespread psoriasis is to use phototherapy, either ultraviolet light A (PUVA) or ultraviolet light B wavelengths. Systemic agents that have been used in the context of HIV-infection include retinoids such as etretinate at ~1 mg per kg per day; generally these agents are used in conjunction with ultraviolet therapy. Immunosuppressive therapies are usually avoided in psoriatics with HIV infection. Antiretroviral therapy has been reported as efficacious, in some cases.

D. Atopic dermatitis may have a slight increase in incidence and severity in HIV-infected persons. The extent of the rash can vary from localized disease of flexural areas to generalized dermatitis. Care of atopic dermatitis in HIV-infected individuals parallels that used in immunocompetent persons. The hallmarks of dermatologic care of atopic dermatitis include avoidance of irritants, hydration, the judicious use of intermediate-strength topical corticosteroid creams and ointments (see the agents used in management of psoriasis), and antihistamines. If the process is widespread, the patient should be referred for phototherapy applied in a manner similar to that in psoriasis.

II. Superficial cutaneous infections are a common feature of AIDS. Their causes represent a variety of agents of viral, fungal, and bacterial origin. Ectoparasites also produce cutaneous disease in immunosuppressed persons. Common skin infections can have atypical appearances. Furthermore, multiple pathogens may coexist and produce unusual and complex cutaneous infections.

A. Cutaneous human papillomavirus infection (HPV), a common viral infection with a variety of forms in immunocompetent hosts, has a wider spectrum of presentations in AIDS.

    1. HPV infection will respond to ablative therapies, such as cryotherapy with liquid nitrogen, superficial electrodesiccation, and curettage, but will frequently recur, particularly if immunosuppression is profound. Many topical anti-HPV agents can be applied, followed by debridement to debulk warty lesions.

    2. For extensive HPV infection, referral for sensitization therapy with dinitrochlorobenzene (DNCB) or other antigens can be effective as long as the patient can respond immunologically. However, as CD4+ counts decrease, HPV infections may become refractory to treatment.

    3. For treatment of **condyloma**, all of the ablative methods can be used. In addition, topical podophyllin may be applied, either by the physician or by the patient by using a commercially available preparation (Condylox).

B. Molluscum contagiosum, a pox virus, found commonly in children, has a venereal pattern of transmission in adults. Lesions are usually delled. In HIV, systemic fungal diseases such as histoplasmosis, cryptococcosis, and *Penicillium marnefii* can mimic molluscum contagiosum. If there is clinical doubt, or if the patient is acutely ill and has delled cutaneous papules, a skin biopsy should be obtained to confirm a diagnosis. Treatment of Molluscum contagiosum is by simple ablation of the lesion with a curette, cryotherapy with liquid nitrogen, or inducing vesiculation and sloughing of the lesion with cantharidin.

C. Herpes simplex (HS) and varicella-zoster viruses (VZV) produce an array of skin lesions in the immunocompromised person. Herpes zoster may be a reliable sign of the presence or progression of HIV infection in an otherwise asymptomatic young person. Both herpes simplex and VZV may produce disseminated skin lesions in HIV-infected individuals. With a diminishing immune response, herpetic infections that usually are self-limited become chronic and fail to heal. Further to confound the problem, chronic herpetic and VZV lesions may not have the characteristic structure of acute lesions in immunocompetent individuals.

1. The **diagnosis** of herpetic infections rests on the form of the clinical lesion, examination of a Tzanck preparation (Wright stain of a scraping taken from the base of a lesion), skin biopsy, viral culture, molecular diagnostic methods, or a combination of these.

2. For chronic or recurrent herpetic infection and for long-term suppression, either oral acyclovir or famciclovir therapy is the best approach. Low dosages (200 to 400 mg daily) can be used indefinitely as a suppressive; however, there is a risk of the development of resistant strains of both HS and VZV. Standard herpetic and VZV dosage can be used to suppress active disease. An advantage of famciclovir in the management of VZV is that dosing is only 3 times daily versus 5 times daily for acyclovir. In resistant cases, intravenous therapy with foscarnet is the most effective alternative (see Chapter 25).

D. Candidiasis is a mucocutaneous infection whose presence correlates directly with degree of immunosuppression. Mucosal candidiasis may be an early sign of immunosuppression. Severity of infection correlates inversely with declining CD4+ count.

1. Candidal infections produce lacy white plaques on the palate and buccal regions. An erythematous erosive lesion produced by *Candida* may be on the gingival margin and lips. Diagnosis is easily made on site. For confirmation, KOH preparations can be examined and cultures obtained. Candidal infection also can be present at other body sites including the genitalia and periungual areas.

2. Application of topical antifungals, or the use of systemic antifungals, or both are the mainstays of anticandidal treatment. For exposed areas, topical application of antifungal creams (ketoconazole cream or equivalent, 1 to 4 times daily) eradicates the process. On mucosal surfaces, clotrimazole oral troches, 10 mg dissolved slowly in the mouth 5 times daily, or equivalent, is an effective treatment (see also Chapter 24).

E. Dermatophytosis is a common problem in the immunosuppressed. Of patients with AIDS, ~40% have dermatophytosis. These infections may be widespread and have unusual morphologies. The most common forms of dermatophytosis include tinea pedis, tinea cruris, and onychomycosis. KOH preparations can be used to confirm the presence of hyphal forms. Limited cutaneous dermatophyte infections can be treated with antifungal creams (miconazole or equivalent, ~4 times daily). Extensive dermatophytosis can be treated with griseofulvin orally (500 mg twice daily or adjusted dosages for microsized or other forms). For onychomycosis, oral itraconazole (Sporonox) can be taken at a dose of 200 mg daily for 3 months with significant cure rates, although this agent has not been formally tested in HIV-seropositive patients.

F. Infestations by scabetic mites can be an unrecognized problem in HIV-infected persons. Crusted forms occur, associated with myriad mites. Failure to recognize this form of scabies can be associated with scabetic epidemics if patients are hospitalized before treatment. A KOH or oil preparation reveals mites, eggs, and feces. Treatment is with permethrin (Elemite) cream or its equivalent. Persons with extensive crusted lesions may require retreatment. Contacts also must be treated to prevent reinfection.

G. Oral hairy leukoplakia is a mixed floral infection of the mucosal epithelium, most often affecting the sides of the tongue. Oral hairy leukoplakia was initially observed in HIV infection, but has since been found in other venues.

If symptomatic, the most effective treatment is the application of 25% podophyllin resin solution (an alcoholic extract of Podophyllum peltatum) to the area. A cotton swab soaked in the solution is dabbed to the lesional area 2 or 3 times. Patients rinse their mouths thoroughly with water as soon as the application is completed (30 seconds to 1 minute contact time). Occasionally a second application is needed at a later time.

   H. **Bacterial infections** of the skin in HIV are approached in a manner similar to that in immunocompetent individuals. Cultures should be obtained from suspected lesions and antibiotics directed toward the identified pathogens.

III. **Systemic infectious processes** may produce a variety of cutaneous lesions. Generally these skin lesions are nondescript; however, systemic fungal diseases may produce skin lesions resembling molluscum contagiosum. Bacterial septic lesions span a range from purpuric macules to ulcers with eschars. Systemic therapies should be directed toward the appropriate pathogen. Treatment of cryptococcosis, histoplasmosis, pneumocystosis, and so on, are dealt with elsewhere in this text. However, three infectious processes with prominent cutaneous involvement are handled mainly through their cutaneous manifestations. These are Reiter's syndrome, bacillary angiomatosis, and syphilis (as well as other sexually transmitted diseases).

   A. **Reiter's disease** can be seen with the classic triad of keratosis blennorrhagica, conjunctivitis, and circinate balanitis. Antimetabolites such as methotrexate should not be used to treat Reiter's syndrome with HIV infection. Good clinical responses have been described by using the systemic retinoid, etretinate, alone or in combination with intermediate-strength topical corticosteroids. Referral for phototherapy is a useful adjunct.

   B. **Bacillary angiomatosis** is a systemic infection caused by *Bartonella quintana* and **B. henselae**. Skin lesions range from small flesh-colored papules, solitary lesions resembling Kaposi's sarcoma or hemangioma, to multiple angiomatous papules, nodules, and eschars. The infection has been reported in the lungs, liver, spleen, and bone, as well as the skin. The diagnosis is suspected clinically and supported by history and suggestive changes in a skin biopsy, which include a proliferation of small vessels, neutrophils between vessels, and clumps of basophilic material that represent bacteria. The infection responds to a number of antibiotics including erythromycin (500 mg, 4 times daily), doxycycline (100 mg, twice daily), tetracycline, minocycline, and azithromycin (see Chapter 26).

   C. **Syphilis** and other sexually transmitted diseases occur with HIV infection. Chlamydial infection, bacterial vaginosis, chancroid, and lymphogranuloma venereum have not been noted to behave in an atypical fashion in immunosuppressed persons. Their treatment continues to be as described for immunocompetent individuals.

     1. Syphilis can appear and behave in traditional ways in HIV-positive patients. However, atypical presentations are well documented. Patients need not have recognizable skin lesions; for example, keratoderma with chorioretinitis has been reported in secondary syphilis. Therefore physicians should be alert to unusual and potentially unique presentations of syphilis. Although serologic testing is reliable in most cases, the well-documented immune abnormalities in HIV patients may lead to serologic aberrations in some cases. Patients have been reported in whom serologic changes did not occur, but spirochetes were detected in tissue, so a skin biopsy may be indicated in some instances.

     2. The treatment for syphilis is described in Chapter 27.

IV. **Cutaneous malignancies in HIV** are common. Although all varieties of skin cancer have been described in HIV infection, there are three common groups: Kaposi's sarcoma, cutaneous lymphoma, and squamous cell carcinoma.

   A. **Kaposi's sarcoma** is an autochthonous, multicentric neoplasm of vascular origin that was one of the first lesions associated with the AIDS epidemic. Before the advent of HIV infection, Kaposi's sarcoma occurred primarily in elderly Italian or Ashkenazic Jewish men, in black equatorial Africans, and in patients with lymphoma or who were iatrogenically immunosuppressed. Kaposi's sarcoma with AIDS occurs more commonly in homosexual men.

  1. The pathogenesis of Kaposi's sarcoma is complex. However, there is now compelling evidence that a key factor is infection with human herpesvirus 8 (HHV-8) that otherwise tends to be aymptomatic. In most circumstances, HHV-8 infection is acquired sexually. As with other opportunistic complications, Kaposi's sarcoma has decreased in incidence since the introduction of more potent antiretroviral therapy.

  2. Kaposi's sarcoma can affect skin, mucous membranes, and internal organs, including the gastrointestinal tract and lungs. In the skin, lesions range in color from pink to violaceous and dark brown and can be macular, papular, or nodular. Lesions can expand rapidly or remain indolent. Diagnosis is easily made clinically and confirmed by skin biopsy.

  3. For the most part, cutaneous lesions of Kaposi's sarcoma can be ignored. If lesions are extensive or interfere with a bodily function such as ambulation, then referral for intralesional chemotherapy, local radiation, circumscribed surgery, or another limited modality such as laser ablation can be used to control symptoms. Treatment of Kaposi's sarcoma is discussed in Chapter 28.

B. Both T-cell and B-cell lymphomas are found in the skin in HIV-infected individuals.

  1. Although **B-cell lymphomas** are common at other body sites in HIV infection, cutaneous involvement is uncommon. Skin lesions are infiltrated nodules and plaques. The diagnosis is confirmed by skin biopsy. Involvement of the skin in B-cell lymphoma is usually an indicator of widespread disease. Therapies are discussed in Chapter 29 and are directed at the underlying process.

  2. **T-cell lymphomas** also have been reported in AIDS. Cutaneous T-cell lymphoma produces skin lesions in AIDS patients that are similar to those in noninfected persons, generally infiltrated plaques. A skin biopsy coupled with immunohistochemical studies is sufficient to confirm the diagnosis. The treatment of cutaneous T-cell lymphoma is highly variable. If there is no evidence of internal involvement, treatment may involve a progression of therapies including application of topical corticosteroids, phototherapy, the use of topical antimetabolites such as nitrogen mustard, and ultimately systemic antimetabolites.

C. Other cutaneous neoplasms have been described in the AIDS patient. Infection with carcinogenic forms of HPV can lead to bowenoid changes and ultimately to **invasive squamous cell carcinoma**, particularly in the anogenital regions. Sporadic cases of melanoma and basal cell carcinoma also have been noted. Whether there is an altered incidence of these cutaneous malignancies in AIDS is not clear. Treatment of cutaneous malignancy involves referral for surgical excision with margin control and, less often, irradiation.

V. Poorly classified skin eruptions are common in HIV infection.

A. **Eosinophilic folliculitis** is a clinicopathologic entity described in HIV patients. The clinical lesion is a papulopustule that coalesces with adjacent lesions to form irregular plaques. In some instances, the lesions are discrete, producing a purely follicular pattern. Skin biopsy reveals folliculitis with eosinophils frequently in follicular epithelium. This eruption may represent a point in a spectrum of nonspecific pruritic follicular eruptions that are described in HIV-seropositive patients. Successful treatment regimens have included applications of intermediate-strength topical corticosteroids, antipruritics, metronidazole (250 mg, 3 times daily, for 3 to 4 weeks), isotretinoin (40 to 80 mg daily for ~8 weeks), phototherapy as described for the management of psoriasis, and systemic antihistamines such as cetirizine, cromolyn sodium, and astemizole.

B. **Drug reactions** can produce a spectrum of reactions ranging from insignificant mild dermatitic processes to life-threatening syndromes (such as erythema multiforme and toxic epidermal necrolysis). All have been described in HIV infection. In general, reactions to medication resolve when the offending agent is discontinued. A nonchemically related alternative can be substituted if needed. Severe drug reactions should be referred. They may require considerable support, particularly if there is extensive denudation and risk of sepsis. Certain reactions are frequent in HIV-infected individuals because of the nature of the medications used

1. **Trimethoprim-sulfamethoxazole** produces a cutaneous reaction in a significant proportion of patients, perhaps up to 30%. In most cases it is a mild pruritic erythema, often with fever, but occasionally can be more severe and progressive. In many patients, the rash does not necessarily recur on rechallenge. Rechallenge should not be performed in patients who have had serious reactions such as erythema multiforme. The protease inhibitor, **amprenavir**, has structural similarity to the sulfonamides, and rash may also occur in patients who start it.

2. **Zidovudine** produces a curious nail pigmentation in many patients. Fingernails are affected more severely than toenails. Discoloration produced by ZDV is probably similar to nail pigmentation produced by other chemotherapeutic agents such as doxorubicin. Zidovudine also produces pigmentation of the oral mucosa.

3. Skin rash is common with the **non-nucleoside reverse transcriptase inhibitors (NNRTIs)**. It appears to be most frequent with nevirapine use, and more severe reactions (including erythema multiforme) have been described with nevirapine. In most circumstances, NNRTI-associated skin rash, which occurs in the first 2 to 3 weeks after starting treatment can be managed without drug interruption, using antihistamines for pruritus. Interestingly, there does not appear to be significant cross-reactivity among the drugs and it is often possible to substitute an alternative NNRTI in the event of skin reactions.

4. Rash (usually mild erythema) may be part of the **abacavir** hypersensitivity reaction, but is not a necessary feature of this syndrome (see Chapter 5).

5. **Foscarnet** produces penile ulcerations in a significant percentage of men receiving the drug. Ulcerations are more severe in uncircumcised men. The ulcerations resolve when foscarnet is discontinued.

C. **Photosensitivity** has been described in HIV-infected patients. Most likely, this process represents a form of drug hypersensitivity. Black patients are disproportionately affected. Treatment consists of discontinuation of suspected medication, the use of sunscreens, the application of intermediate-strength topical corticosteroids, and possibly referral for hardening by exposure to graded intensities of light.

D. **Porphyria cutanea tarda** has been described many times in HIV-infected persons. Many patients have independent risk factors associated with precipitation of porphyria cutanea tarda. Patients generally respond to traditional therapy with phlebotomy. One patient was described as responding solely to ZDV.

13. NEUROLOGIC AND PSYCHIATRIC COMPLICATIONS

I. **Spectrum of neurologic and psychiatric complications in human immunodeficiency virus (HIV)**
   A. **HIV-associated complications** are those most closely associated with the retroviral infection alone. **Aseptic meningitis**, characterized by fever, headache, nuchal rigidity, and a lymphocytic pleocytosis in the cerebrospinal fluid (CSF), is common during primary infection and may frequently recur during otherwise asymptomatic early years of infection. **Acquired immunodeficiency syndrome (AIDS) dementia complex** (also known as AIDS encephalopathy) is the most common HIV neurologic complication in advanced disease, occurring in roughly 20% of all cases of AIDS. A less severe manifestation of neurologic deterioration, which occurs frequently, has been termed **HIV-associated motor cognitive disorder**. The spinal cord may be affected **by vacuolar myelopathy**, resulting in progressive deterioration of lower extremity and bladder function. Peripheral nerve syndromes associated with HIV include **Guillain-Barré** syndrome (demyelinating motor neuropathy), which occurs more frequently in early stages of HIV infection and may be a presenting complication, and distal sensory **peripheral neuropathy**, a common source of foot pain in advanced HIV stages. Weakness may develop as a result of **polymyositis**. Thus, no part of the neuromuscular system is spared from direct HIV-associated consequences of HIV infection.
   B. **Psychiatric disease** is frequently encountered in HIV-infected subjects. These individuals must confront life-threatening complications of both the primary infection and opportunistic infections, the social scrutiny that accompanies this diagnosis, and the effects of the polypharmaceutic battle waged during illness. **Depression** is common and must be differentiated from early stages of AIDS dementia. **Substance abuse** is frequently associated with acquiring HIV and complicates medical management by special concerns regarding compliance and appropriate use of therapies prescribed. Financial pressures associated with progressing disability and costly therapy often compound patients' frustrations and prevent them from attaining optimal functional status. **Mania** also may complicate AIDS dementia, but requires specific psychiatric management.
   C. **Opportunistic neurologic complications** are important considerations in the evaluation of subjects with new neurologic symptoms and signs. The most common secondary neurologic complications include those that cause focal mass lesions [*Toxoplasma* **encephalitis and central nervous system (CNS) lymphoma**], those that result in multifocal demyelination (**progressive multifocal leukoencephalitis**), those causing meningitis (*Cryptococcus neoformans*), and those causing encephalitis [**cytomegalovirus** (CMV)]. In addition, **neurosyphilis** can appear in a variety of ways in HIV and requires particularly aggressive therapy. Increased incidence of tuberculosis also raises the concerns that **tuberculous meningitis** be retained as a special and highly lethal potential complication during HIV infection.
II. **AIDS dementia complex** (ADC) is diagnosed by recognizing its characteristic clinical manifestations and by excluding alternative diagnoses.
   A. The **clinical presentation of ADC in adults** includes progressive **cognitive deterioration, declining motor performance, and behavioral changes** (Navia et al. *Ann Neurol* 1986:19:517). Careful history will generally document a progressive course over several months. Abrupt onset

The author acknowledges the contribution of David B. Clifford to the previous edition of this chapter.

should raise the suspicion of alternate diagnoses. Subjects often characterize their cognitive problems as a slowing of thought with loss of interest in
prior activities and tendency to forget details. Motor deterioration is often
characterized by slowing of gait or unsteadiness, deterioration of handwrit-
ing, and loss of bladder control, resulting in urgency, frequency, and eventually incontinence. Behavioral problems are most commonly a withdrawal
from prior interests and activities consistent with depression, but often
devoid of overt affective complaints. Less commonly, psychotic behavior may
be quite florid. Seizures are a regular behavioral manifestation of this
encephalitis, occurring in ~10% of such patients.

B. **Pediatric HIV-associated progressive encephalopathy** is characterized
by a triad of clinical manifestations including impairment of brain growth,
resulting in acquired microcephaly or parenchymal volume loss or both on
neuroimaging studies, progressive motor dysfunction, and plateau or loss in
neurodevelopmental milestones (Mintz M. *Adv Neuroimmunol* 1994;4:207).
Pediatric HIV neurologic involvement is contrasted with the adult experience
in that opportunistic complications are less common, as is the development of
peripheral neuropathy. Diagnostic and therapeutic objectives are the same as
in the adult encephalopathy.

C. **Diagnosis** of ADC requires the presence of an appropriate clinical syndrome, almost always in advanced HIV, characterized by CD4$^+$ counts
<200 cells/mm^3.

1. **Magnetic resonance (MR) or computed tomography (CT) brain
scan** should be obtained to rule out opportunistic mass lesions. MR is
more sensitive for several of the opportunistic complications of HIV and
is preferred if available. The MR (or CT) may be normal in the presence
of ADC, but generally cerebral atrophy is present. White matter is often
affected either in a diffuse manner or with several multifocal areas. Contrast enhancement is not characteristic of HIV encephalitis associated
with ADC. Quantitative evaluation of groups of AIDS dementia scans
demonstrate preferential atrophy of the deep gray matter (Dal Pan et al.
Neurology 1992;42:2125), but this may not be obvious in isolated cases.
MR spectroscopy shows promise in its ability to detect changes associated with AIDS dementia, but it is not useful as a clinical tool.

2. **Lumbar puncture** (LP) should be performed primarily to exclude
alternate diagnoses, including cryptococcal meningitis, CMV encephalitis, progressive multifocal leukoencephalitis, and neurosyphilis.

   a. The Cerebrospinal fluid **(CSF) formula** typically seen in ADC may
   be normal, but modest elevations in protein (50 to 80 mg per dl) and
   a few lymphocytes (0 to 20) are frequently present.

   b. In advanced ADC, the HIV core antigen (p24 antigen) becomes
   measurable in the CSF, increasing with severity of ADC (Brew et al.
   J Neurol Neurosurg Psychiatry 1994;57:784). Sensitivity of CSF p24
   antigen is low, making it an unsatisfactory diagnostic test for ADC.

   c. The role of quantitative HIV RNA measurement is under investigation. HIV may be recovered at any stage of infection from the CSF,
   so presence of virus is not helpful.

   d. Cytokines b$_2$-microglobulin and neopterin also increase in the CSF
   with progression of ADC, but are nonspecific, being increased with
   other opportunistic CNS processes as well.

3. **Blood tests** that should be ordered in evaluating a patient for ADC
include measurement of thyroid function, serum serologic testing for
syphilis, and B$_{12}$ levels. Absence of CMV viremia reduces the chance
that CMV encephalitis is the cause of dementia, but CMV PCR on CSF
should be negative to rule out CMV encephalitis.

4. **Neuropsychologic testing** provides a more accurate way to follow
neurologic function, most appropriate to the research setting. A systematic mental-status examination is an important part of the examination and should be repeated at intervals. If there is uncertainty about

the degree or presence of declining neurologic function, quantitative neuropsychologic tests may be obtained and followed up subsequently. Most clinicians use a battery of tests weighted to timed motor tasks, which routinely show the deterioration of function typical of ADC.

D. The **differential diagnosis** for ADC includes the full spectrum of diseases causing declining cognitive and motor function. In addition to alternate opportunistic neurologic processes considered in the previous evaluation, the physician also must consider **toxic causes,** including the consequences of polypharmacy typical of this population or use or abuse of other substances by the subject. Excessive sedative-hypnotic drugs, medications taken for gastrointestinal (GI) complaints, and pain medications may easily mimic ADC. **Metabolic** derangements also may impair neurologic performance. When several metabolic parameters are out of normal range, they may produce surprisingly severe impairment. **Behavioral changes** associated with marked anxiety and depression also may mimic ADC and are eminently treatable.

E. **Therapy** for ADC is based on the understanding that the virus itself is necessary to the development of the disease, but considerations for development of improved therapy recognize the likely interplay between the virus, the neural substrate, and the immunologic response to this infection.

   1. At present, it appears that a **rational approach** to therapy for AIDS dementia would be to **optimize HIV therapy** according to the latest studies based on virologic parameters (see Chapter 6). We must be mindful that some of the newly developed drugs may not effectively cross the blood–brain barrier and might thus be substantially inferior to other antiretroviral therapy for dementia. It must also be recognized that resistance to antiretrovirals develops with extended use. Consequently, a change in therapeutic agents is likely necessary if dementia develops while taking a regimen.

F. **Adjunctive therapies** for AIDS dementia are under development, based on the observation that there is often a poor correlation of direct viral load in the brain with the degree of dementia seen clinically, thus implicating indirect mechanisms for neurologic dysfunction. **Cytokines,** such as tumor necrosis factor, have been associated with advancing dementia in AIDS patients and represent a potential therapeutic target, which is under investigation. Neurotoxic cascades set in motion by portions of the virus, such as the envelope glycoprotein **gp120,** probably involve excitatory amino acids, platelet activating factor (PAF), arachidonic acid, and calcium-mediated toxicity have been demonstrated in experimental paradigms (Lipton et al. *N Engl J Med* 1995; 332:934). Potential targets from these systems will be evaluated in clinical trials seeking to augment the benefits of antiretroviral therapy for dementia.

G. Requirements for **social support** change with the development of AIDS dementia and the consequent dependent status of the patient. Typically a caregiver must be available, and thus independent lifestyles must be altered for the safety and comfort of the patient. Financial and legal issues should be addressed as early as possible to avoid complications caused by the mental decline. Whereas institution of appropriate therapy often gives some degree of improvement, development of AIDS dementia remains an ominous sign in the course of HIV, and the outlook for prolonged independent life is guarded.

III. **Psychiatric disease** is commonly encountered in HIV and requires concurrent evaluation and therapy.

A. **Depression** is the most common and serious psychiatric problem encountered. Direct discussion of mood should be a regular part of support for the HIV patient. Changes in sleep patterns and appetite commonly accompany affective disorders. A sense of futility, hopelessness, and loss of self-worth are serious indicators of affective disorder. When such signs are seen, direct questioning about suicidal ideation or plans is indicated so that appropriate support is assured.

   1. **Therapy** should include both supportive psychotherapy and medical therapy.

      a. For **mild to moderate** depression, the selective serotonergic reuptake-inhibiting drugs appear to offer the best balance of tolerability and efficacy. **Fluoxetine**, 20 mg per day, **sertraline**, 50 to 200 mg per day, or **paroxetine**, 20 mg per day, are reasonable alternatives. Their side-effect profile typically includes nausea, nervousness, headache, insomnia, and sexual dysfunction. They are often administered early in the day because of the activating properties.

      b. **More severe** depression may respond better to tricyclic drugs with broader mechanisms (and more side effects). **Nortriptyline** (25 to 100 mg per day) and **desimpramine** (titrate to 100 to 200 mg per day) are efficacious and have slightly fewer of the typical anticholinergic, orthostatic, and sedative side effects typically associated with tricyclic antidepressants (TCAs) such as amitriptyline. When insomnia or pain are issues, the tertiary tricyclics remain the standard for therapy, including **amitriptyline** (50 to 200 mg per day) and **imipramine** (50 to 200 mg per day).

   2. **Psychiatric referral** is appropriate unless mild depression responds to first-line therapy, or in any case in which suicidal ideation is discovered.

B. **Anxiety** is an extremely common problem, particularly notable shortly after diagnosis or after progression of HIV. Although supportive care and education are essential and helpful, sometimes the symptoms of anxiety require pharmacotherapy as well. Benzodiazepines (e.g., diazepam, 2 to 5 mg t.i.d., or lorazepam, 0.5 to 2 mg t.i.d.) are helpful for short-term therapy in a crisis situation, but should be avoided for chronic therapy because tolerance and dependence develop. More prolonged and disruptive anxiety may be treated with buspirone, 5 to 10 mg t.i.d. This drug has a slow onset of action over several weeks.

C. **Psychotic** reactions are infrequent, but dramatic complications seen in HIV. They are most typically a part of the ADC when there is no antecedent history of manic or psychotic disorder. They are occasionally precipitated by changes of antiretroviral therapy. However, the approach to them should be to use continued antiretroviral therapy appropriate to AIDS dementia in conjunction with a minimum of symptomatic antipsychotic medicine. Rather low doses of **haloperidol** (2 to 5 mg per day) are often helpful, but all of the neuroleptic drugs are particularly prone to cause extrapyramidal symptoms in this setting. Consequently, low doses are advised and may require concomitant benztropine. Some success in treatment of psychotic symptoms with **valproic acid** (starting at 250 mg b.i.d. and titrating upward) or **carbamazepine** (starting at 200 mg b.i.d. and titrating) avoids the risk of extrapyramidal syndrome. A controlled environment such as a psychiatric ward may be essential to the safe care of the psychotic patient. Fortunately, these episodes tend to be limited and to respond to symptomatic care.

IV. **Myelopathy** frequently affects the spinal cord of AIDS subjects. Symptomatic myelopathy occurs in 5% to 10% of AIDS patients. Although it is commonly seen in conjunction with ADC and is generally seen with advanced immunodeficiency with the $CD4^+$ count <200 cells/mm^3, myelopathy appears to be an independent pathophysiologic entity. Some patients have only the myelopathy with no evidence of encephalopathy, and the myelopathy may progress so as to threaten gait without evidence of dementia. Pathologically, a **vacuolar myelopathy** is seen with the heavily myelinated lateral and dorsal tracts in the spinal cord, disrupted by vacuoles in the myelin sheaths of axons. Symptomatically, patients develop a spastic paraparesis, evidence of neurogenic bladder, and variable sensory loss (often in conjunction with peripheral neuropathy).

A. The **differential diagnosis** for myelopathy should include the broad spectrum of conditions resulting in spinal cord compromise.

   1. It is important that **spinal-compressive lesions** be ruled out by examination (evidence of a spinal level) and generally by MR imaging of the spine.

   2. B_{12} **deficiency** occurs more commonly in HIV than in the general population and may be a contributing factor. Serum B_{12} measurements, and if indicated, serum homocysteine and methylmalonic acid levels, will rule out this treatable cause of myelopathy.

3. Human T-cell leukemia virus type 1 (HTLV-1) is associated with a progressive myelopathy, may be contracted by the sexual route, and is occasionally a coinfection with HIV-1. Thus consideration of HTLV-1–associated myelopathy (HAM) is appropriate by testing for this virus serologically. Therapy for HAM is controversial, but consideration of corticosteroids, danazol, or interferon therapy become appropriate.

4. **Syphilis, tumors of the cord, spondylitic changes, and other concurrent viral infections (varicella zoster, JC virus, CMV)** can rarely mimic HIV-associated myelopathy when they involve the cord.

B. **Therapy** for myelopathy consists of the best antiretroviral therapy available. In some cases, quite high HIV RNA levels reflect active central viral replication, but in many cases, the pathologic studies lacks substantial evidence of replicating virus. It is thus believed that the mechanism of the neuropathology is probably indirect. If there is any chance of functional B_{12} deficiency, parenteral replacement should be instituted with 1,000 mg B_{12}. Baclofen (start 5 mg t.i.d. and titrate as needed to 40 to 80 mg per day in divided doses) or diazepam (start 2 mg b.i.d. and titrate) may reduce flexor spasms associated with spasticity and permit freer movement.

V. **Peripheral neuropathy** complicates HIV infection in 20% to 50% of cases. Several syndromes are associated with HIV infection, including a distal sensory polyneuropathy, a demyelinating motor neuropathy, and uncommon autonomic neuropathy.

A. The most common is a **distal sensory neuropathy**, which has a highly characteristic clinical appearance. Neuropathy develops in a symmetric pattern and is associated with pain or paresthesia in the feet. This pain is associated with a variable degree of boot-pattern numbness. On examination, the ankle jerks are usually decreased, and there is distal sensory loss. Weakness is absent or a minor finding. Deviation from this pattern should raise the suspicion of an alternate cause for the neuropathy.

1. The same clinical picture may develop **because of neurotoxicity of nucleoside antiretroviral therapy** including ddC, ddI, and d4T. It appears that ZDV is not toxic to the peripheral nerve, and 3TC appears relatively nontoxic. Clinical neuropathy develops earlier and to a greater degree when underlying neuropathy already exists, as in the case of alcohol abuse, diabetes, or nutritional deficiency. Typically neuropathy develops 3 to 8 months into therapy with a potentially toxic drug, but dose and neuropathic predisposition make the timing quite variable. Relief of the neuropathy by drug discontinuation is the most convincing evidence that a neuropathy is drug induced. Often neurotoxic neuropathy continues to worsen for a few weeks after drug discontinuation ("run-on"), but improvement should be under way in 4 to 8 weeks in most cases.

2. Evaluation for distal sensory neuropathy should include a careful history for toxic exposures.

a. Polypharmacy in advanced HIV sets up the potential for multiple drug-induced neuropathies.

b. Nutritional deficiency should be considered, particularly B_{12} or folate deficiency.

c. Sometimes myelopathy with sensory loss is mistaken for peripheral neuropathy. Examination will generally reveal other myelopathic signs.

d. CMV radiculomyelopathy may also be seen with distal pain, but has a more subacute course, with motor loss and sacral sensory loss not seen in the distal sensory neuropathy.

3. Diagnostic studies

a. Although **nerve-conduction studies** will help to confirm sensory neuropathy, they are generally of little help in diagnosing or monitoring the syndrome and thus should be used primarily when the picture is atypical.

   b. **Quantitative sensory evaluation** allows more precise description of the deficit, but is primarily of use in clinical research. CSF examination may be indicated in atypical pictures, but is generally unrevealing in the straightforward distal sensory neuropathy.

   c. **Nerve biopsy** reveals primary axonal loss with a variable degree of myelin loss and inflammation. Biopsy is unnecessary in most cases, but may be helpful in diagnosing alternate neuropathic processes in atypical cases.

4. **Symptomatic therapy** for distal sensory neuropathy is similar to that used for other neuropathic pain syndromes. For minor pain, patients often find they can tolerate the symptom with knowledge that it is unlikely to progress to a paralyzing or severely disabling syndrome.

   a. **Nonsteroidal antiinflammatory drugs** are occasionally of some help and should be tried for mild symptoms.

   b. **TCAs** are generally regarded as optimal symptomatic therapy.

      (1) In other pain states, the tertiary TCAs (e.g., **amitriptyline**, 25 to 100 mg per day, or **imipramine**, 25 to 100 mg per day) have generally been most effective. Because relatively low doses provide most of the efficacy for pain management, the substantial anticholinergic side effects are generally tolerable. These drugs may be given once a day at bedtime to enhance sleep and the increased appetite and the weight gain associated is often welcome in advanced HIV patients.

      (2) If the side-effect profile (dry mouth, sedation, or orthostatic blood pressure changes) is intolerable, sometimes a secondary TCA (desipramine, 25 to 100 mg per day, or nortriptyline, 10 to 75 mg per day) provides almost comparable pain relief with fewer side effects. Whereas serotonin specific reuptake inhibitor (SSRI) antidepressants are effective for mild to moderate depression with fewer side effects than TCAs, they are inferior to the older drugs in treatment of pain syndromes.

   c. Other agents including carbamazepine, phenytoin, baclofen, valproic acid, and clonazepam are sometimes helpful, but none has been carefully studied for HIV-associated neuropathic pain.

   d. Sometimes the pain of this neuropathy is severe and does not respond to alternate therapy, making long-term narcotic therapy necessary. Generally the narcotic dose can be titrated for an outpatient by using sustained-release morphine (MS Contin), transdermal fentanyl, or methadone. Because a significant number of HIV-infected subjects also have a history of drug-seeking behavior, it is helpful to have clear guidelines regarding use of narcotics and to use them in a conservative fashion. However, unnecessary suffering of patients with advanced disease should be relieved by appropriate use of narcotics when other therapies fail (see Chapter 10).

5. **Restorative therapy** is not available for neuropathic damage.

B. **Inflammatory demyelinating neuropathy** is occasionally associated with HIV infection. In contrast to the late-stage presentation of a many neurologic complications, demyelinating neuropathy may occur at seroconversion or when the CD4+ count is well preserved. The acute clinical picture is the same as the Guillain–Barré syndrome with ascending weakness or facial weakness progressing subacutely over days to a few weeks, associated with loss of reflexes and increased CSF protein. The syndrome in HIV may be associated with modest pleocytosis, contrasting with Guillain–Barré outside HIV. Therapy is unnecessary for mild cases, but plasmapheresis hastens recovery when gait is threatened. Intravenous γ-globulin is an alternative that has been effective in some cases.

C. **Mononeuropathies** also are seen during HIV infection and probably have a variety of origins.

1. Both **HIV** and **CMV** have been implicated. The diagnosis of CMV may be aided by nerve biopsy, as well as a search for other evidence of CMV by careful ocular examination and CMV buffy-coat cultures. If CMV is implicated, ganciclovir, 5 mg per kg, every 12 hours i.v., or foscarnet, 90 mg per kg, every 12 hours i.v. may be effective (see Chapter 25).
2. **Compressive neuropathies** in nerves previously damaged by HIV axonal neuropathy may cause some mononeuropathies.
3. Rarely **lymphoma** may infiltrate nerves to cause dysfunction, and Kaposi's sarcoma often locally compromises nerve function.

D. **Radiculomyelopathy** is most commonly the result of **CMV** in advanced HIV with CD4+ <100 cells/mL^3. It is important to recognize and treat this highly characteristic clinical syndrome as quickly as possible.
1. A subacute lumbosacral radiculomyelopathy develops with leg weakness, distal and sacral anesthesia, bladder and bowel dysfunction, and back and leg pain.
2. The **CSF** is characteristic, with a polymorphonuclear pleocytosis. CMV is occasionally cultured from CSF in this syndrome, whereas quantitative CMV PCR routinely reveals high titers of CMV DNA.
3. If **aggressive CMV therapy** is instituted, the syndrome may be arrested, and some degree of recovery of function may occur in the subsequent several months. Induction therapy with ganciclovir or foscarnet should be given at a minimum (see Chapter 25). Combination therapy may be indicated, particularly if the syndrome develops in a subject already receiving therapy for another CMV complication such as retinitis.

VI. **Myopathy** is seen during HIV, causing weakness, muscle pain, and increased creatine kinase levels. The major differential consideration is between a **polymyositis** developing in AIDS versus the **toxic myopathy associated with ZDV** (see Chapter 18).
A. ZDV-associated myopathy may be a mitochondrial myopathy, with morphologic changes more frequently apparent than clinical weakness from myopathy. In patients receiving ZDV with clinical weakness and myopathic pain, a ZDV drug holiday should be tried. If a clear improvement occurs in 2 to 6 weeks, ZDV should be avoided subsequently.
B. Polymyositis may occur at any stage of HIV and may lead to severe weakness. The diagnosis should be established with a muscle biopsy. If an inflammatory myopathy is demonstrated, it may be successfully treated with corticosteroid therapy. Caution must be exercised, and steroid therapy should be used only to reverse clinically significant weakness or substantial pain.

VII. **Headache and pain management** are problems regularly confronted by the physician treating HIV patients. Because of the possibility of secondary complications, which occur much more frequently in immunosuppressed patients, particular care must be exercised in treating these patients. Interpretation of pain symptoms may be complicated by a history of drug-seeking behavior or drug abuse, which may have been causative in acquiring HIV and must be considered in evaluation of the subjective complaints of pain.
A. **Tension headaches and migraines** are typical problems occurring frequently and requiring symptomatic therapy. Generally acetaminophen, aspirin, or ibuprofen is adequate for the care of intermittent tension headaches. Migraines are associated with throbbing pain, visual changes, nausea, and often a family history of "sick headaches." Although the previously described therapies also may help some migraines, symptomatic therapy with **ergots** (e.g., ergotamine, 1 mg p.o. immediately, repeated every one-half hour to a maximum of 5 mg per attack or 10 mg per week) as early in the headache as possible will provide relief. **Sumatriptan** (25 to 50 mg p.o. or 6 mg sq) is particularly effective for migraine and may even abort an established migraine. Sometimes a narcotic (morphine, 5 to 10 mg, or meperidine, 75 to 100 mg) occasionally with an antiemetic [prochlorperazine (Compazine), 10 mg p.o. or 25 mg per rectum] is required when severe pain and nausea are established. For frequent migraines, a choice of a **TCA** (amitripty-

line, 25 to 100 mg per day) or **β-blocker** (e.g., propranolol, 40 to 120 mg per day) can reduce severity and frequency of migraine. **Methysergide** (4 to 8 mg per day in divided doses, no longer than 6 months at a time) is often effective in refractory cases, but must be used with caution and for a limited duration because of retroperitoneal fibrosis associated with its chronic use.

B. Aseptic meningitis often occurs with primary HIV infection and may recur periodically during the otherwise asymptomatic period of this chronic infection. A sterile CSF is associated with lymphocytic pleocytosis, moderate protein increase, and little or no hypoglycorrhachia. Headache and stiff neck often accompany this syndrome, which is generally self-limited, requiring only symptomatic therapy. It may herald the diagnosis of HIV, requiring consideration of early or aggressive therapy.

C. Sinusitis is a common and recalcitrant problem suffered by AIDS patients, which may result in chronic headaches. Care in diagnosing it and persistence in therapy are required. Consultation with an otolaryngologist for surgical drainage may be required, if antibiotic therapy fails to improve refractory sinusitis (see Chapter 26).

D. Zidovudine has been associated with increased headache, particularly in the first few weeks of therapy. Patients that persist through this period generally find that excessive headaches are not associated with long-term use of ZDV.

E. Secondary intracranial opportunistic complications are always a serious consideration when severe, chronic, or new types of headaches are experienced by an AIDS patient. Careful neurologic examination, brain imaging with CT or MR scans, and consideration of lumbar puncture are appropriate in this context. **Cryptococcal meningitis** should particularly be considered, but other intracerebral processes must be considered and sought in the face of changing headache patterns in the immunosuppressed host.

VIII. Toxoplasma encephalitis is one of the most common neurologic complications in advanced HIV infection. Toxoplasma encephalitis has a subacute onset with clinical deterioration over days to a few weeks, associated with change in mental status, fever, headache, and a variety of focal neurologic symptoms. Movement disorders, seizures, and deteriorating gait are often seen (see Chapter 22).

IX. Cryptococcal meningitis occurs in ~10% of AIDS patients and thus is an important treatable complication (see Chapter 24).

A. Diagnosis is made quite easily when *Cryptococcus* is suspected. The **presentation** may be quite variable, but **headache, fever and malaise** are generally associated with this complication. Unlike meningitis in the immunocompetent, stiff neck is often not detected. Focal neurologic findings and seizures occur, but are uncommon. Thus when unexplained headache, nausea and vomiting, or change in mental status occurs, it is important that cryptococcal meningitis be considered. It almost uniformly occurs with CD4+ counts <200 cells/mm^3, but the counts need not be extremely low.

B. Serum cryptococcal antigen is generally detected, and when contraindication for lumbar puncture (LP) exists, or when the patient refuses LP, this test may give considerable reassurance that cryptococcal meningitis is unlikely. However, **CSF examination** is important when the diagnosis is considered, both to determine with greater certainty the presence of this disease and to provide a measure of its severity.

  1. Cryptococcal **antigen detection,** or visualization of the encapsulated yeast by using India ink or both, provide rapid documentation of cryptococcal meningitis.

  2. Other CSF values may be surprisingly normal, but proteins generally are increased, whereas glucose values are decreased. Cellular reaction may be minimal, but is also variable.

  3. An **opening CSF pressure** that is substantially increased is an important sign of severe disease and also gives prognostic information (Graybill et al. *Clin Infect Dis* 2000; 30:47).

4. **Although brain imaging** with CT or MR generally does not contribute to making the diagnosis, it is important in progressive neurologic symptoms to exclude alternate CNS processes that are also possible.

C. **Therapy** is discussed in Chapter 24.

X. **Progressive multifocal leukoencephalopathy** (PML) occurs in ~5% of AIDS patients as a result of JC virus infection in the brain. JC virus is a ubiquitous papova virus that causes disease only in immunodeficiency.

A. Presentation of PML is suggested by clear-cut focal or multifocal neurologic disease developing subacutely over a period of weeks to a few months. Typical presentations include **visual changes (hemianopsia), hemiparesis, ataxia, or cerebellar syndrome.** Headache is rare, and there is no evidence of meningismus with this encephalitis. Seizures surprisingly are seen in some cases of PML in HIV.

B. **Evaluation** should include brain imaging early in the course.

1. **Brain MR scanning** is most helpful, demonstrating definite T_2 bright white-matter lesions with minimal or no contrast enhancement. This white-matter disease also may be visualized on CT scans when advanced, but MR is more sensitive to such white-matter disease.

2. **CSF** examination shows a rather normal HIV patient's CSF (few cells, minimal protein increase, and normal glucose) and no increased intracranial pressure. If **PCR for JC virus** is available, it is helpful in suggesting the diagnosis. Recent studies (McGuire et al. *Ann Neurol* 1995; 37:395) found a sensitivity of 92% and specificity of ~92%, suggesting that PCR is a very good test for PML.

3. Definitive diagnosis still requires a **brain biopsy**; however, this is rarely needed in patients with positive CSF PCR for JC virus and a compatible MR scan.

C. **Maximal antiretroviral therapy** has proven to be the most effective treatment for this rapidly lethal disease. Mean survival without effective antiretroviral treatment is ~4 months after diagnosis, with a small fraction having much more prolonged survival. With effective treatment of HIV, survival has been prolonged to more than two years and indefinitely in some patients (Clifford et al. *Neurology* 1999;52:623).

XI. **Cytomegalovirus** (CMV) causes several important neurologic complications of HIV. The most common of these is CMV **encephalitis**. Others include **radiculomyelopathy** and **peripheral neuropathies**, which have already been described.

A. **CMV encephalitis** is seen in ~20% of AIDS autopsies, but causes a recognizable clinical syndrome in a small number of cases. Both ADC and CMV encephalitis may be seen with a similar progressive encephalopathy with diminishing cognitive and motor function, but CMV has a more aggressive course than HIV encephalitis, with death occurring in a matter of weeks. When sought, CMV disease is almost always found in other organ systems when the brain is involved. Adrenal involvement is common, leading to electrolyte disturbances (hyponatremia most commonly) and potential adrenal insufficiency. The eye is commonly involved. CMV viremia is often present, and pulmonary and GI disease caused by CMV also may be present. This encephalitis often involves the brainstem and the lower cranial nerves, causing diplopia, ataxia, facial weakness, deafness, and bulbar symptoms in a significant number of cases.

B. **Diagnosis** has been very difficult because the virus is generally not recovered from the CSF. Focal brain lesions are generally not present, so brain biopsy has rarely been undertaken to diagnose this disease.

1. It now appears that **CMV DNA** (Arribas et al. *J Infect Dis* 1995; 172:527) is always present in the CSF by **PCR** testing when CMV encephalitis occurs and is absent when the brain is not invaded. However, it may be necessary to demonstrate higher-titer CMV to suggest that a clinical encephalopathy is caused by CMV encephalitis, as minor focal CMV lesions that are clinically of less importance still are associated with CMV DNA in the CSF. Viremia alone, or CMV retinitis or both,

are not necessarily associated with a positive CSF CMV PCR. Exclusion of alternative diagnoses, a clinical picture of a progressive encephalopathy, and CMV DNA in the CSF provide a presumptive diagnosis of CMV encephalitis.

2. Brain imaging with **MR** or **CT** may reveal a periventricular encephalitis, but this is most commonly absent. Brain MR cannot be relied on to suggest this diagnosis.

C. **Therapy** with currently available drugs including **foscarnet** and **ganciclovir** is difficult. Encephalitis appears to be less responsive than the radiculomyelitis, perhaps because the blood–brain barrier remains more intact in this disease. Because encephalitis often develops in patients already receiving antiviral therapy, it is generally recommended that a new drug be introduced and or intensity of therapy be increased. Better data exist for foscarnet penetration to the CSF, so this drug may be preferred. Many experts are currently treating with a maximal combined regimen of both ganciclovir and foscarnet. Induction with ganciclovir, 5 to 7.5 mg per kg i.v., every 12 hours, and foscarnet, 90 mg per kg i.v., every 12 hours, should be introduced if tolerated. Both drugs doses must be adjusted for impaired renal function. After a clinical response is established or in ~4 weeks, maintenance therapy may be substituted with doses of ganciclovir, 6 to 10 mg per kg per day, and foscarnet, 120 mg per kg per day (see Chapter 25). Without treatment, CMV encephalitis is rapidly fatal over a period of weeks. Long-term survival with clinical improvement has been observed with early and aggressive therapy, and unproved with antiretroviral treatment.

XII. **Primary CNS lymphoma** occurs in ~5% of patients with advanced AIDS. This complication is most often confused with Toxoplasma encephalitis.

A. The **clinical presentation** of CNS lymphoma is that of a subacute progressive focal brain lesion(s). It is somewhat more likely than toxoplasmosis to be seen as a solitary lesion, but is not infrequently multicentric. Clinical signs are consistent with a mass lesion of the brain, commonly with mental-status changes. Motor signs such as hemiparesis are common, as are changes in mental status. Seizures are often encountered. Posterior fossa signs and symptoms are seen in a minority of subjects.

B. **Diagnosis** is helped by a discovery of single or multiple mass lesions on brain imaging with **CT** or **MR.** The lesions generally, but not always, enhance when contrast is administered, sometimes having ring enhancement. The lesions are radiologically indistinguishable from Toxoplasma encephalitis in some cases.

1. There is some experience with use of thallium-201 single-photon-emission CT **(SPECT)** scanning or positron-emission tomography (PET) imaging in which the tumor takes up the radioisotope and the infectious causes of the mass remain hypometabolic (Hoffman et al. *J Nucl Med* 1993;34:567).

2. **CSF** generally shows moderate protein elevation, but rarely are tumor cells detected by cytologic examination of CSF. Primary CNS lymphomas are uniformly B-cell tumors positive for Epstein–Barr virus (EBV). **CSF PCR for EBV DNA** is highly suggestive of lymphoma when an appropriate clinical lesion is present (Arribas et al. *J Clin Microbiol* 1995;33:1580). However, this test has both false positives and negatives and thus cannot be relied on for diagnosis in isolation.

3. **Brain biopsy** is often required to establish the diagnosis of CNS lymphoma. Stereotaxic guided-needle biopsy of malignant lesions has been quite successful in establishing this diagnosis with a definite, but tolerable risk of hemorrhage.

C. **Therapy** for primary CNS lymphoma is palliative at this point. Radiotherapy is recommended if other complications of HIV have not independently led to a poor performance status. Corticosteroid therapy may be useful for transient amelioration of symptoms, but should be avoided when a therapeutic trial for response to *Toxoplasma* therapy is in progress. The role of adjunctive chemotherapy is under investigation (see also Chapter 29).

14. GASTROINTESTINAL ASPECTS

Virtually all persons with human immunodeficiency virus (HIV) infection develop gastrointestinal complaints during the course of their illness. The gastrointestinal tract is vulnerable because it is directly contiguous with the outside environment, is rich in lymphoid tissue, and may harbor pathogenic organisms from prior infections. It is common for patients to have multiple coexisting infections of the digestive tract. Despite the vulnerability of the gut to HIV-associated disorders, the clinician must be cognizant that not all gastrointestinal (GI) symptoms are related to HIV.

I. Esophageal disease

   A. **Differential diagnosis.** *Candida*, cytomegalovirus (CMV), and herpes simplex infections of the esophagus are frequent in persons infected with HIV. Each may be the initial and acquired immunodeficiency syndrome (AIDS)–defining opportunistic infection. Idiopathic esophageal ulcers are also common and may be caused by HIV itself.

   B. **Clinical presentation.** Dysphagia, odynophagia, and substernal chest pain are the symptoms of esophageal disease. Dysphagia is difficulty with swallowing and is the most common symptom of candidal esophagitis. Patients complain that foods stick or drag after swallowing. Dysphagia for liquids is uncommon. Odynophagia is pain with swallowing and is a manifestation of esophageal ulceration. Candidal esophagitis and reflux esophagitis may both cause diffuse substernal pain with swallowing. Viral esophagitis, which causes discrete ulcerations, causes localized pain with swallowing. Food, water, and saliva may be painful to swallow. Viral esophagitis also causes esophagospasm with spontaneous substernal chest pain.

   C. **Empiric treatment.** Candidal esophagitis is the most common cause of infectious esophagitis in the patient with HIV infection. Because the presence or absence of thrush does not predict endoscopic findings, patients should be treated empirically for fungal infection before an expensive and invasive evaluation is undertaken. Patients with fungal esophagitis will have marked symptomatic improvement within days with an appropriate antifungal medication. A specific diagnosis should be sought when patients do not respond quickly to antifungal therapy. Acid suppression should be used in all patients with symptoms of gastroesophageal reflux. Patients taking large numbers of medications are also at risk of developing pill-induced esophagitis. Pill-induced ulcers will heal without specific treatment, but they are better prevented by instructing patients always to drink copious amounts of fluids when taking medications.

   D. **Evaluation.** Patients with esophageal symptoms who have failed to respond to empiric treatment with antifungal agents need further evaluation.

      1. **Radiographs.** Contrast-enhanced radiographs can yield a diagnosis of esophagitis and may suggest an origin, but radiographs cannot yield a definitive diagnosis.

      2. **Cytology.** A cytology brush protected by a nasogastric tube can be passed into the esophagus and mucosal brushings obtained. The tissue samples are stained and cultured for fungal and viral infections. The disadvantages of this technique are a large sampling error and missed diagnosis (*Candida* may be detected, whereas concomitant CMV infection is missed), and false negative results (idiopathic ulcers cannot be diagnosed with this method).

The author acknowledges the contribution of Mary F. Chan to the previous edition's version of this chapter.

3. **Endoscopy and biopsy.** Endoscopy with mucosal biopsy remains the gold standard for diagnosing infectious esophagitis. The highest yield is obtained when jumbo biopsy forceps are used with a therapeutic endoscope. If candidal esophagitis is found in patients for whom antifungal therapy has failed, mucosal biopsies can then be cultured and antibiotic sensitivities requested. Routine tissue stains with hematoxylin and eosin will exclude concomitant viral infections. If discrete ulcers are found, tissue culture and routine histopathologic studies will usually reveal a diagnosis. When they do not, a tentative diagnosis of idiopathic ulcers is made. Because this is a diagnosis of exclusion, most physicians will confirm the diagnosis by repeating the endoscopy to obtain more biopsies. On occasion, endoscopy will reveal a diagnosis that is unrelated to HIV infection, such as reflux esophagitis.

E. **Treatment**

1. **Antifungal medications.** Topical medications, such as clotrimazole troches and nystatin solution, are recommended for treatment of thrush. However, systemic therapy is recommended for fungal esophagitis.

2. **Acyclovir.** Herpes esophagitis can be treated with acyclovir, 200 to 800 mg p.o., 5 times a day. Secondary prophylaxis can be achieved with 400 mg p.o., b.i.d. Adverse effects include nausea, headache, and renal dysfunction.

3. **Ganciclovir.** Ganciclovir is recommended for treatment of CMV infection of the esophagus. Secondary prophylaxis may not always be necessary for GI infection (Blanshard et al. *J Infect Dis* 1995;172:622), although if the patient has any evidence of systemic infection, long-term suppressive treatment is indicated (see Chapter 25). All patients with CMV esophagitis must have ophthalmologic examinations. If CMV retinitis is found, the patient must receive maintenance therapy. The recommended dosage for active infection is 5 mg per kg body weight i.v., every 12 hours for 14 to 21 days; maintenance therapy is 5 mg per kg per day i.v., or 6 mg per kg i.v,. 5 times a week, or 1 g p.o., t.i.d.

4. **Foscarnet.** Foscarnet is available as an alternative treatment for CMV esophagitis for patients who do not tolerate ganciclovir and for patients infected with ganciclovir-resistant strains. Foscarnet, 60 mg per kg body weight i.v., every 8 hours or 90 mg per kg body weight i.v., every 12 hours for 14 to 21 days is recommended for treatment of esophagitis.

5. **Corticosteroids.** Idiopathic esophageal ulcers have successfully been treated with oral, intravenous, and intralesional corticosteroids. A 4-week taper of prednisone is recommended beginning with 40 mg per day p.o. and tapering by 10 mg each week (Wilcox et al. *Am J Med* 1992;93:131).

6. **Thalidomide** has been demonstrated to have considerable activity in patients with idiopathic oral or esophageal ulcerations. Because of its profound teratogenicity, thalidomide should be used carefully in this circumstance (see chapter 20).

7. **Nonspecific treatment**

   a. **Acid suppression.** Histamine-2 receptor (H_2R) antagonists and proton-pump inhibitors may provide symptomatic relief in patients with esophageal ulcers of any origin. H_2R antagonists should be given in divided doses twice a day to achieve 24-hour acid suppression. Proton-pump inhibitors can be given once a day. Acid suppression will decrease the bioavailability of ketoconazole and is not recommended when this drug is used.

   b. **Cytoprotection.** Sucralfate, 1 g p.o., q.i.d., or 2 g p.o., b.i.d., may provide cytoprotection in ulcerative esophagitis. A slurry preparation is preferred. Sucralfate may interfere with the absorption of many other medications, thus limiting its use in HIV infection.

   c. **Analgesia.** Esophageal ulcers may cause such severe odynophagia that patients refuse to eat. Analgesia with opiates may be required to maintain nutritional status in the more severe cases.

   d. Nutrition support. Patients who do not maintain adequate oral intake because of severe esophageal pain can be supported with nasogastric or nasointestinal tube feedings until a clinical response to specific therapy has been achieved.

II. Diarrhea. Diarrhea is the most common GI complaint of people infected with HIV. Drug-associated diarrhea, especially with the use of the protease inhibitors, is common. Secondary infections account for additional cases. As many as 20% of cases are idiopathic and may represent unrecognized opportunistic infections or HIV-associated enteropathy. Diarrhea results from either small intestinal or colonic pathologic conditions. A careful history and physical examination will direct the evaluation and treatment strategy of AIDS-associated diarrhea. Small-intestinal disease produces a large-volume diarrhea that is frequently associated with dehydration and serum electrolyte abnormalities. Abdominal pain, gaseous distention, nausea, and vomiting also may be present. Tenesmus and fecal leukocytes are absent. Colonic diarrhea is less voluminous, and dehydration is uncommon. Tenesmus and left lower quadrant pain are common. When the colonic mucosa is disrupted, fecal leukocytes and hematochezia are frequently present; however, the absence of leukocytes and red blood cells does not exclude colonic disease. The medical history must elicit the frequency, volume, color, and consistency of bowel movements. Nocturnal bowel movements and fecal incontinence indicate more significant diarrhea. Fever, fecal leukocytes, and hematochezia are caused by invasive organisms, and if present, should prompt the physician to pursue further diagnostic testing when stool studies are unrevealing.

   A. Differential diagnosis
      1. Bacterial infections. Although not specifically associated with HIV infection, *Salmonella, Shigella,* and *Campylobacter* cause more severe diarrhea with longer durations of illness in the immunocompromised host. These infections are also more likely to cause bacteremia or septicemia. *Clostridium difficile* is not specifically associated with HIV infection and is surprisingly uncommon, given the number of hospitalizations and antibiotic courses required by patients with AIDS. However, it is a treatable cause of diarrhea and must always be considered in the differential diagnosis of AIDS-associated diarrhea.
      2. Parasitic infections. Cryptosporidium, Isospora, Giardia, and microsporidia all infect the small intestine. *Entamoeba histolytica* is uncommon but when present involves the cecum, ascending colon, and terminal ileum. *Entamoeba dispar* is commonly found on ova and parasite examinations in patients with HIV infection, but it is not pathogenic.
      3. Mycobacterial infections. *Mycobacterium avium* complex (MAC) is found in macrophages in the lamina propria of the small intestine or colon. *Mycobacterium tuberculosis* may cause granulomas and ulcerations throughout the GI tract, but is most commonly found in the cecum and terminal ileum, where there is an abundance of lymphoid tissue.
      4. Viral infections. Cytomegalovirus is the most important viral cause of AIDS-associated diarrhea. CMV may affect any part of the GI tract; colitis and esophagitis are quite common. Herpes simplex may cause proctitis. Adenovirus infects small-intestinal mucosa. HIV has been cultured from intestinal mucosa when no other cause of diarrhea is found, but a causative role in diarrhea has not been documented.
      5. Drug-associated diarrhea. Diarrhea, with or without abdominal cramping, bloating or flatulence, is a common complaint among patients receiving protease inhibitors. This is especially true with use of nelfinavir, where diarrhea occurs in up to 20% of patients and may be severe enough to require drug discontinuation in 4% to 5% of patients.
      6. Idiopathic diarrhea. No etiology is found in 20% of patients with AIDS-associated diarrhea. Some of these patients may have unrecognized opportunistic infections. Idiopathic diarrhea is often labeled HIV enteropathy, but the pathogenic role of HIV infection in diarrhea has not been elucidated.

B. Evaluation

1. Noninvasive evaluation. The initial evaluation of AIDS-associated diarrhea is stool analysis, including culture for enteric pathogens, examination for ova and parasites, assay for *C. difficile* toxin, and Gram stain for fecal leukocytes. Because routine ova and parasite examinations do not look for Cryptosporidium, microsporidia, and Isospora, their identification must be specifically requested. Blood cultures are helpful when fever is present to exclude bacteremia with enteric pathogens and to exclude disseminated MAC. If disseminated MAC is diagnosed and treated, but diarrhea persists, then other causes of diarrhea should be excluded.

2. **Sigmoidoscopy.** When colonic diarrhea is suspected and when stool analysis is nondiagnostic, sigmoidoscopy is recommended. Sigmoidoscopy is a safe office procedure that does not require intravenous sedation. If performed on an unprepped patient, stool aspirate can be sent to the laboratory for evaluation and culture. Caution must be taken when a patient with significant diarrhea is given a cathartic preparation for the examination. Dehydration, orthostasis, and near syncope can be precipitated. A biopsy should be performed on abnormal-appearing mucosa for histopathologic study and, if indicated, for culture. If the colonic mucosa to 60 cm from the anal verge is normal, then random biopsies of the rectum are recommended. Rectal tissue may reveal MAC, viral inclusions, parasites, or a nonspecific microscopic colitis.

3. **Upper GI endoscopy.** Esophagogastroduodenoscopy (EGD) is indicated to evaluate diarrhea when small-intestinal diarrhea is suspected, malnutrition is present with diarrhea, or sigmoidoscopy is negative and diarrhea persists. EGD is invasive and expensive and should be performed only if stool studies are negative. Complications of endoscopy include cardiopulmonary reactions to sedative medications, bowel perforation, and bleeding. As with sigmoidoscopy, a biopsy should be performed on any abnormal-appearing mucosa, and random small-bowel biopsies should be obtained if the intestine appears normal. This is very important, as cryptosporidiosis, microsporidiosis, giardiasis, and MAC do not cause mucosal disruption.

4. **Colonoscopy.** Colonoscopy is rarely indicated in the evaluation of AIDS-associated diarrhea. When colonoscopy is performed, the endoscopist should intubate and perform biopsies of the ileum, unless gross pathologic conditions are found in the colon.

C. Treatment

1. **Nonspecific management**. Regardless of the origin of AIDS-associated diarrhea, many nonspecific measures are effective in managing symptoms and improving quality of life. Antidiarrheal agents can be safely administered to the stable patient before a specific diagnosis is made. When the patient has fever, severe abdominal pain, peritonitis, hematochezia, or emesis, an evaluation should precede administration of antimotility drugs so as not to precipitate toxic megacolon and perforation.

   a. **Luminal agents.** Dietary fiber and fiber supplements improve the consistency of watery diarrhea. Bacterial fermentation of fiber also provides short-chain fatty acids as energy substrate for colonocytes. Short-chain fatty acids are essential for reparative processes in the colon. The so-called BRAT diet, Bananas, white Rice, Apples, and white Toast, provides soluble fiber and is good for short-term control of diarrhea. However, the BRAT diet is an incomplete diet and should not be consumed as sole-source nutrition for extended periods. Psyllium and methylcellulose are commercially available forms of soluble fiber and are marketed under many brand names as laxatives. Patients should be reassured that these products can be very effective in managing diarrhea. The dose should be titrated to effect. Cholestyramine is a resin binder that is also effective as an intraluminal antidiarrheal agent. The disadvantage of cholestyramine is that it also binds many medications; therefore it should never be taken concomitant with other drugs. The complexity of the medication schedule of the typical person with HIV infection limits the practicality of cholestyramine for this population.

b. **Antimotility agents.** Opioids and anticholinergic medications decrease bowel motility and are very effective antidiarrheal agents. Their use is limited by side effects such as nausea, vomiting, drowsiness, dry mouth, and difficulty voiding. Fear of addiction should not be a reason to avoid opioids. Loperamide is a synthetic opioid with few central nervous system side effects, making it the drug of choice for the initial treatment of diarrhea. Tolerance to the antidiarrheal effect has not been reported. The recommended dose is 4 mg (two capsules) followed by 2 mg after each unformed stool. Daily dosage should not exceed 16 mg (eight capsules). Diphenoxylate with atropine is recommended for patients for whom loperamide fails. Diphenoxylate is chemically related to meperidine and is classified as a Schedule V controlled substance. Atropine is an anticholinergic drug. Each tablet and 5 mL of liquid contain 2.5 mg of diphenoxylate hydrochloride and 0.025 mg of atropine sulfate. The recommended dosage is two tablets p.o., q.i.d., or 2 teaspoons (10 mL) p.o., q.i.d. Tincture of opium also is effective for people who do not tolerate the anticholinergic side effects of atropine. Most patients will require 0.6 mL p.o. or s.l., q.i.d. The maximum dose should not exceed 1 mL p.o., q.i.d. All other narcotic analgesics are also effective antidiarrheal agents and can be efficiently used to treat diarrhea and pain (i.e., HIV neuropathy).

c. **Hormonal therapy.** Octreotide is a long-acting, synthetic analog of somatostatin. Octreotide has many GI effects. It inhibits the release of vasoactive intestinal peptide and several other gut hormones. It enhances net water and electrolyte absorption, and it slows GI transit. Octreotide has been shown to be effective for some patients with AIDS-associated secretory diarrhea. It decreases stool volume and improves stool consistency. There are several major drawbacks to its use. It is a parenteral medication that must be injected s.q. every 8 to 12 hours, and the injections can be painful. It is expensive and does not have a Food and Drug Administration (FDA)-approved indication for AIDS-associated diarrhea; therefore many insurance companies will not pay for it. It causes steatorrhea by significantly decreasing pancreatic exocrine function. The steatorrhea may result in worsening malnutrition. Exogenous pancreatic enzyme replacement may ameliorate this effect. Long-term use can lead to gallstone formation, organomegaly, and carpal tunnel syndrome. When diarrhea is a debilitating symptom that has not responded to other treatment modalities, octreotide should be tried. Recommended starting dosage is 100 mg s.q. every 8 hours. The dose can be titrated as needed every 3 days to a maximal dose of 500 mg s.q. every 8 hours. If no response is seen within 2 weeks, the medication should be discontinued (Cello JP et al. *Ann Intern Med* 1991;115:705).

d. **Oral-rehydration formula.** The World Health Organization (WHO) recommends oral rehydration formula for children with diarrhea to replete lost fluid and electrolytes. The WHO formulation has been studied and used extensively in children. Studies of its use in adults with AIDS-associated diarrhea are not available. Oral rehydration therapy takes advantage of the sodium–glucose cotransporter present in the brush border of intestinal epithelium. Thus sodium is actively transported across the intestine, whereas water follows passively by solvent drag. Several oral-rehydration formulas are available in the United States. Each formula is an isotonic glucose or starch-based electrolyte solution. The concentration of sodium is the most important factor. The WHO formula has a sodium concentration of 90 mM based on balance studies in patients with cholera. The WHO solution is made by mixing 3.5 g of sodium chloride, 2.9 g of sodium bicarbonate, 1.5 g of potassium chloride, and 20 g of glucose (40 g sucrose can be substituted) in 1 L water. This roughly translates to 1 tsp table salt, ¼ tsp baking soda, ⅛ tsp salt substitute, and 8 tsp sugar in 1 L water. Sports drinks have limited sodium concentrations and are inappropriate for electrolyte replacement. Most oral-rehydration solutions are isoosmolar. Replacement of glucose with polymeric forms of carbohydrate, such as rice-syrup solids, provides a hypotonic solution that may be more effective than glucose-based solutions in decreasing stool volume.

  e. Total parenteral nutrition (TPN). Bowel rest and parenteral nutrition are not indicated in the treatment of AIDS-associated diarrhea. However, parenteral nutrition may provide adjunctive therapy for the malnutrition that so commonly accompanies severe diarrhea. Fluid and electrolyte balance can be achieved with TPN.

2. Specific antimicrobial therapy

  a. Cryptosporidiosis. No available antibiotic has been shown to be effective against Cryptosporidium. Paromomycin, 500 to 750 mg p.o., q.i.d., has been tried with some success.

  b. Microsporidia. Albendazole, 400 mg p.o., b.i.d., may be effective against Septata intestinalis and Enterocytozoon bieneusi.

  c. Isopora. Trimethoprim (TMP)–sulfamethoxazole (SMX) is effective against Isopora belli. Recommended dosage is 160 mg TMP and 800 mg SMX, p.o., q.i.d. for 10 days and then b.i.d. for 3 weeks.

  d. Giardiasis. Giardia is treated with metronidazole, 250 mg p.o., t.i.d. for 5 days, or paromomycin, 25 to 35 mg per kg per day in three doses for 7 days.

  e. *Entamoeba histolytica.* The drug of choice for severe intestinal disease or hepatic abscess is metronidazole, 750 mg p.o., t.i.d. for 10 days.

  f. *Mycobacterium avium* complex. Disseminated MAC is treated with clarithromycin, 500 mg p.o., b.i.d., or azithromycin, 500 mg p.o., daily, and one or more of the following: ethambutal, 15 to 25 mg per kg p.o. daily; clofazimine, 100 to 200 mg p.o. daily; ciprofloxacin, 750 mg p.o., b.i.d.; or rifabutin, 300 to 450 mg p.o. daily.

  g. *Mycobacterium tuberculosis.* Treatment of GI tuberculosis is the same as that for pulmonary disease. A four-drug regimen is recommended for initial treatment until antibiotic sensitivities are available. Medications and dosages recommended are isoniazid, 300 mg p.o. daily, plus rifampin, 600 mg p.o. daily, plus pyrazinamide, 15 to 25 mg per kg p.o. daily, and ethambutol, 15 to 25 mg per kg per day p.o., or streptomycin, 15 mg per kg per day.

  h. Cytomegalovirus. Ganciclovir or foscarnet is recommended in the same dosages as those for esophageal disease (see Sections I.E.3. and I.E.4).

III. Gastric disease. The stomach is variably involved in persons infected with HIV. Gastric lymphoma is one of the more common and serious conditions. The diagnosis can be made with upper endoscopy and biopsy. Treatment is chemotherapy or surgery. Peptic ulcers are no more common in people with AIDS than in the general population, and they respond to acid suppression and *Helicobacter pylori* eradication. Atypical presentations of secondary infections include luetic gastritis and gastric tuberculosis and are treated with appropriate antibiotics for syphilis and disseminated tuberculosis.

IV. Hepatobiliary diseases. Abnormal liver tests are common in HIV infection. The differential diagnosis is extensive and includes chronic viral hepatitis, adverse drug reactions, sclerosing cholangitis, infiltrative liver disease (i.e., tuberculosis or Kaposi's sarcoma), bacillary angiomatosis, and steatohepatitis. Transaminase and bilirubin elevations indicate hepatocellular injury. Elevated alkaline phosphatase with or without bilirubin elevation indicates cholestasis or infiltrative disease. Many medications used in HIV infection cause abnormal liver tests, including TMP-SMX, pentamidine, isoniazid, rifampin, pyrazinamide, paraaminosalicylic acid, and ketoconazole. All potential hepatotoxic drugs should be withdrawn, if possible, when abnormal liver tests are found in the asymptomatic patient and must be stopped in all symptomatic patients. If the liver tests remain abnormal after hepatotoxic drugs are discontinued, an evaluation should be performed. A pattern of hepatocellular injury warrants an evaluation for the viral hepatitides including A, B, C, and D, CMV, Epstein–Barr virus, and herpes simplex virus. Cholestatic liver disease should initially be evaluated with ultrasound to exclude bile-duct obstruction, gallstones, focal mass lesions, and fatty liver. AIDS cholangiopathy can be diagnosed with endoscopic retrograde cholangiography. The papillary-stenosis variant can be treated with endoscopic sphincterotomy. Biopsy of focal mass lesions can be performed with radiologic guidance. If serologic and radiologic examinations are unrevealing, a percutaneous liver biopsy can be performed. Treatment strategies will be guided by the pathology.

V. **Hepatitis virus infection.** All HIV patients should be tested for hepatitis A, B, and C, and non-immune patients should be vaccinated against hepatitis A and B. **Co-infection with hepatitis C virus (HCV) and HIV** is relatively common, especially in hemophiliacs and intravenous drug users. HIV infection appears to accelerate the natural course of HCV infection, although HCV infection does not appear to affect HIV course. Co-infection with hepatitis C may increase the risk of hepatotoxicity from potent antiretroviral therapy, especially ritonavir (Sulkowski et al. *JAMA* 2000; 283:74). Progressive liver disease from hepatitis C has emerged as an important cause of morbidity and death in patients with HIV infection. Patients with persistent transaminase elevation and evidence of inflammation and fibrosis on biopsy (but without cirrhosis) are candidates for treatment of their HCV infection. Treatment with the combination of interferon (3 million units sc three times weekly) and ribavirin 800-100 mg PO daily is safe and effective in HIV-negative patients, and response rates among co-infected patients appear similar. Patients with higher CD4+ cell count appear to respond better.

VI. **Pancreatic disease.** Pancreatitis may be caused by medications used to treat AIDS and related illnesses. Pentamidine, dideoxyinosine, dideoxycytidine, and TMP-SMX are the drugs that commonly cause pancreatitis. Treatment is discontinuation of the medication and supportive therapy. Acute pancreatitis also has been caused by CMV, Cryptosporidium, and *Cryptococcus*. CMV infection of the pancreas is a difficult diagnosis to make antemortem. Asymptomatic hyperamylasemia is common and does not require specific therapy. Kaposi's sarcoma and lymphoma have both been reported to involve the pancreas and are treated with chemotherapeutic agents (see also Chapter 19).

15. THE KIDNEY IN HIV DISEASE

Renal disorders are common in patients infected with human immunodeficiency virus (HIV), and they significantly contribute to both morbidity and mortality. Diseases range from common presentations such as fluid and electrolyte disorders and acute tubular necrosis (ATN) to the rare occurrences of crystalline nephropathies and the microangiopathies: hemolytic uremic syndrome/thrombotic thrombocytopenic purpura (HUS/TTP). HIV also is associated with a specific, aggressive glomerulonephropathy [the HIV-associated nephropathy (HIVAN)] heralded by proteinuria, the nephrotic syndrome, and progression to end-stage renal disease (ESRD). Primary renal diseases seen in the general population also may afflict HIV-infected patients, and many of the drugs used to treat a variety of infectious complications are nephrotoxic.

I. Renal diseases coincidental with HIV infection

A. Acute renal failure may occur in critically ill patients with disseminated infection or malignancy. It does not usually occur in patients with asymptomatic HIV infection. The clinical course is often similar to that in those without HIV, with patient survival and recovery of renal function depending on the underlying cause. Patients may have oliguria (urine output <500 mL per 24 hours) or may be nonoliguric. Therapy is often supportive with appropriate attention to volume status, electrolytes including calcium and phosphorus, blood pressure, acid–base status, and adjustment of drugs with significant renal metabolism and clearance. Prognosis with conservative or dialytic therapy is poor. Indications for dialysis are similar to those of acute renal failure in patients without HIV infection, and initiation should be considered for uremia, extreme volume overload not responding to diuretic therapy, profound acidosis, and life-threatening hyperkalemia. Table 1 lists common causes of acute renal failure in HIV-infected patients; specific disorders are discussed subsequently. With growing numbers of HIV-infected patients in the United States surviving into middle age because of effective antiretroviral therapy, systemic disorders that affect the kidney may come to clinical attention, including diabetes mellitus, polycystic kidney disease, obstructive uropathy, and primary and secondary forms of glomerulonephritis (GN). Patients with these diseases may develop acute renal failure but more commonly progress to ESRD over a long period.

1. **ATN** may occur from a variety of insults, but common causes include ATN resulting from nephrotoxic drugs, hypovolemia, shock, and sepsis. Hypovolemia results from the nausea, vomiting, diarrhea, and poor oral intake of fluids seen commonly in symptomatic HIV-infected patients. Sepsis, with or without shock, may produce renal dysfunction, which can progress to renal failure. Table 2 lists drugs commonly used in HIV-infected individuals that may produce ATN and acute renal failure. Cidofovir (see Chapter 25) should be specifically noted because of its propensity to cause renal failure if not used cautiously. It should be avoided in patients with ≥ 2 proteinuria or with serum creatinine ≥ 1.5 mg per dl. The diagnosis of ATN is made by careful assessment of volume status, urine and serum measurement of electrolytes, blood urea nitrogen (BUN), creatinine, and examination of the urine sediment. Occasionally hemodynamic monitoring is necessary.

2. **Interstitial nephritis** usually results from an idiosyncratic drug reaction and may produce renal dysfunction or acute renal failure. Typical findings include fever, rash, peripheral eosinophilia, as well as the presence of urine eosinophils documented on urine stained with Hansel's stain. These findings may be absent, and a high index of suspicion is

Table 1. Acute renal failure

PRERENAL LESIONS
  Volume depletion (hemorrhage, vomiting, diarrhea, third-space fluid)
  Severe liver dysfunction
  Cardiac failure

RENAL PARENCHYMAL DISORDERS
  Acute tubular necrosis (drugs, sepsis, shock, rhabdomyolysis)
  Interstitial nephritis (drugs, infectious, infiltrative)
  Glomerulonephritis
  Systemic disorders affecting the kidney (diabetes, polycystic kidney disease)

POSTRENAL OBSTRUCTION
  Tumors
  Nephrolithiasis
  Intratubular precipitation
  Hemorrhage/clots
  Retroperitoneal fibrosis

---

often required for diagnosis in patients taking drugs such as sulfon-amides (trimethoprim–sulfamethoxazole), penicillins, or nonsteroidal antiinflammatory drugs (NSAIDs). Therapy consists of removal of the offending agent and possibly a short course of prednisone, but the use of immune-suppressing medications remains controversial. A presentation similar to that of drug-induced interstitial nephritis may occur with cytomegalovirus (CMV) infection. This may be distinguished by the presence of nephrocalcinosis (Seney et al. *Am J Kidney Dis* 1990;16:1; *Kidney Int Suppl* 1995;35:S13). A plasmacytic interstitial nephritis with nonnephrotic-range proteinuria, azotemia, and generalized lymphade-nopathy responsive to steroids has been described in HIV-infected patients.

3. **Postinfectious GN** may be seen with the indolent occurrence of renal dysfunction or a more aggressive course with acute renal failure, often associated with crescent formation in the glomeruli on renal biopsy. Renal disease may result from a number of infections including endocarditis, infected indwelling intravascular catheters, and visceral abscesses

Table 2. Nephrotoxic drugs

Amphotericin B
Acyclovir
Aminoglycosides
Cephalosporins
Cidofovir
Cyclosporin A
Dapsone
Foscarnet
Indinavir
Nonsteroidal antiinflammatory drugs (NSAIDs)
Penicillins
Pentamidine
Radiocontrast agents
Rifampin
Sulfadiazine
Trimethoprim/sulfamethoxazole

(pulmonary and abdominal). Disease is mediated by glomerular injury from immune complex deposition, and therapy centers on treatment of the underlying infection. Poststreptococcal disease may be seen in normal hosts as well as in those infected with HIV. Renal dysfunction and rarely renal failure occur 2 to 6 weeks after a pharyngeal or cutaneous group A streptococcal infection. Therapy is supportive; rarely is dialysis required.

4. **Crystal-induced renal failure** may result from intratubular precipitation of sulfadiazine or indinavir, but is rare. Therapy is preventive by ensuring adequate volume expansion before administration. Acute urate nephropathy may occur with hyperuricemia after chemotherapy for lymphoproliferative disorders as part of the tumor-lysis syndrome. This may be prevented with the use of allopurinol, 600 mg initially, followed by 100 to 300 mg per day p.o. before the administration of chemotherapy. Urine alkalinization to a pH of 6.5 to 7.0 also may be beneficial.

5. **Hemolytic uremic syndrome/thrombotic thrombocytopenia purpura** consists of microangiopathic hemolytic anemic, thrombocytopenia, fever, mental-status changes, and renal dysfunction. Renal failure results from hemoglobinuria and glomerular thrombosis. HUS/TTP is often preceded by a viral syndrome (including primary HIV infection), frequently involving the gastrointestinal tract, but can occur with vasculitidies, malignant hypertension, disseminated malignancies, and in association with certain drugs (mitomycin, cyclosporin A; valaciclovir). Certain strains of enterohemorrhagic *Escherichia coli* have been associated with HUS. Treatment consists of plasmapheresis and dialytic therapy if necessary. If HUS/TTP occurs in association with HIV infection, some reports have noted improvement of hematologic parameters with antiretroviral therapy (Pottage et al. *JAMA* 1988;260:3045; Salem et al. *South Med J* 1991;84:493). When HUS/TTP occurs with AIDS, the prognosis is poor.

6. **Glomerulonephritis.** Primary GN, such as membranous or proliferative lesions seen in the general population, may occur in patients infected with HIV. Secondary forms of GN may occur in patients exposed to parenterally transmitted infections. Membranous GN may result from immune-complex injury induced by hepatitis B or *Treponema pallidum*. Appropriate serologic tests and a screening VDRL may suggest such a cause. The syndrome of cryoglobulinemia and membranoproliferative GN has been described in association with hepatitis C infection (Johnson et al. *N Engl J Med* 1993;328:465). Intravenous-heroin users may develop a focal sclerosis lesion similar in many respects to HIVAN, thought to be the result of impure admixtures of these preparations (Friedman et al. *Am J Kidney Dis* 1995;25:689).

B. **Infections of the kidney.** Many agents may produce direct parenchymal infection of the kidney, including CMV, *Cryptococcus, Histoplasma, Candida* sp., *Mycobacterium tuberculosis, Aspergillus* sp., as well as more common disseminated bacterial infections. Symptoms are often predominated by the systemic nature of these illnesses, and renal dysfunction is usually mild and often overlooked. Rarely significant azotemia may occur from an exuberant tubulointerstitial disease with acute renal failure. Diagnosis relies on a high index of suspicion with careful attention to examination of the urinary sediment and specific cultures. Therapy is supportive and aimed at the underlying infection.

C. **Infiltrative diseases.** Infiltration of the kidney by disseminated malignancy has been reported with lymphoproliferative diseases and Kaposi's sarcoma. When this occurs, renal function is rarely impeded. Massive infiltration rarely results in renal failure, usually in association with nephromegaly. Diagnosis relies on a high index of suspicion with careful attention to examination of the urinary sediment and possibly renal biopsy. Therapy is supportive and aimed at the underlying malignancy.

Minimal-change glomerulonephropathy has been described in an association with lymphoma. Clinical manifestations of the nephrotic syndrome may be present, including significant proteinuria (>3.5 g per 24 hours), hypoalbuminemia, hypercholesterolemia, and edema, and often regress with successful therapy for the malignancy. Systemic amyloidosis with renal involvement can be seen in association with lymphoproliferative processes and in chronic inflammatory conditions. Nephromegaly and the nephrotic syndrome are usually present. Treatment is usually supportive and aimed at treatment of the underlying conditions.

   D. **Fluid, electrolyte, and acid–base disorders.** Disorders of fluid and electrolytes, including hyponatremia, hyperkalemia, and acidemia, are extremely common in patients infected with HIV.

      1. **Hyponatremia** occurs frequently in hospitalized patients. Extrarenal losses (vomiting and diarrhea) are common, resulting in hypovolemic hyponatremia. Treatment consists of intravascular replacement of sodium and water with isotonic (0.9% saline) solutions. The syndrome of inappropriate antidiuretic hormone secretion (SIADH) may occur in association with central nervous system (CNS) or pulmonary infections [e.g., tuberculosis (TB)], or caused by drugs. Treatment of chronic SIADH consists of fluid restriction and oral demeclocycline, 300 to 600 mg per day. If hyponatremia is acute or patients are symptomatic, fluid restriction, in combination with more aggressive measures to increase serum sodium levels, should be undertaken. Abnormalities in adrenal glucocorticoid and aldosterone biosynthesis have been described and may contribute to the hyponatremia seen in HIV-infected patients.

      2. **Hyperkalemia** most commonly occurs with acute or chronic renal insufficiency. Drug-induced hyperkalemia may result from trimethoprim, angiotensin-converting enzyme inhibitors, pentamidine, and NSAIDs. Disseminated infection involving the adrenal glands (TB, histoplasmosis, or CMV) may occasionally result in adrenal crisis with hyperkalemia and hypotension. Therapy consists of potassium restriction, liberalized sodium and alkali intake, and loop-acting diuretics (e.g., furosemide). If hyperkalemia is acute or severe and cardiac toxicity is present, intravenous calcium chloride (10 mL of a 10% solution or 1 g) and dialytic therapy may be necessary.

      3. **Hypocalcemia and hyperphosphatemia** commonly accompany acute and chronic renal insufficiency. Calcium carbonate as a phosphate binder (500 to 1,000 mg, p.o.) with meals is the initial therapy. Aluminum hydroxide, 15 to 30 cc p.o. every 4 to 6 hours, also is effective as a phosphorus binder but is not recommended for long-term use or in those patients receiving dialysis.

      4. **A Fanconi-like syndrome** with proximal tubular damage is a frequent side-effect of adefovir, the nucleotide reverse transcriptase inhibitor, which was investigated in patients as an antiretroviral agent. It produced hypophosphatemia, glycosuria, proteinuria and ultimately elevated serum creatinines. It usually reversed on cessation of therapy.

II. **Renal diseases causally related to HIV infection**
   A. **HIV-associated nephropathy** (HIVAN) is a pathologically unique glomerulonephropathy associated with HIV infection occurring in 2% to 10% of HIV-infected individuals (Rao et al. *N Engl J Med* 1984;310:669). Genetic factors appear to play a role, with clinical nephropathy occurring with much greater frequency in black men.

      1. The clinical presentation of HIVAN consists of (a) heavy proteinuria (90% have nephrotic range), usually with a benign urinary sediment; (b) rapid deterioration in renal function with progression to ESRD commonly occurring in 6 to 12 months; (c) minimal to no increase in systemic blood pressure; and (d) normal to increased kidney size. On biopsy, the histology is similar to that of idiopathic focal segmental glomerulosclerosis (FSGS). However, in distinction, HIVAN exhibits sclerosis of the whole

glomerular tuft with what has been described as a collapsed glomerulus. This is associated with severe tubular injury with microcyst formation and tubular degeneration (Bourgoignie et al. *Kidney Int Supple* 1991;35:S19). Numerous tubuloreticular structures also are present in the endothelial cells of the glomerulus, demonstrated by electron microscopy.

2. Diagnosis is established on renal biopsy. Therapy has been largely empiric. Antiretroviral therapy may retard progression of disease if started early in those with minimal renal dysfunction and mild proteinuria. Case reports have documented improvement in renal insufficiency with prednisone, 60 mg per day for 2 to 6 weeks followed by a taper, but at the expense of increased infectious complications (Smith et al. *Am J Med* 1994;97:145). Prognosis is generally related to the stage of HIV disease rather than to the degree of renal dysfunction. Patients with asymptomatic HIV infection had a >2-year survival with dialysis in one study (Ortiz et al. *Kidney Int* 1988;34:248). Patients with advanced HIV disease generally do very poorly with renal-replacement therapy, with survival rates usually measured in months.

B. **Immunoglobulin A (IgA) nephropathy**. An association of IgA nephropathy has been noted in patients infected with HIV (Kimmel et al. *Kidney Int* 1993;44:1327). In contrast to HIVAN, IgA nephropathy more commonly afflicts white and Hispanic patients. The clinical presentation is less aggressive than HIVAN, with mild azotemia, proteinuria, and hematuria. Disease progression is variable, with some individuals having spontaneous remissions and others progressing to ESRD. Diagnosis is established by renal biopsy with the demonstration of mesangial deposits of IgA. Epithelial crescents may be present, as well as tubuloreticular structures similar to those seen in HIVAN. Treatment is largely supportive, with dialysis reserved for those with advanced renal insufficiency. Proliferative GN, idiopathic minimal-change disease, and mesangioproliferative GN are uncommon.

III. **HIV infection during renal-replacement therapy**. In addition to transmission of HIV from unprotected sexual practices and i.v. drug use, patients receiving dialysis may acquire HIV infection through exposure to blood products used for treatment of chronic anemia or transplanted allografts. Healthcare providers working in a hemodialysis setting should adhere to strict universal precautions to avoid the danger of possible transmission (Velandia et al. *Lancet* 1995;345:1417). There are no recommendations for routine testing of dialysis populations for HIV.

IV. **Renal-replacement therapy in HIV-infected patients**. HIV-positive patients in whom ESRD develops have been successfully treated with both peritoneal dialysis (PD) and hemodialysis (HD), and HIV positivity is not a contraindication to dialysis. Given the limited resources of renal allografts, the life expectancy of HIV patients, and the dangers of immunosuppression, renal transplantation is not generally undertaken. PD has several potential advantages, including less risk of endovascular infection, less risk to a population of patients with a higher incidence of communicable diseases (e.g., TB), and benefits to health-care workers who are less commonly exposed to body fluids of HIV-infected patients. PD may be complicated by increased dietary protein requirements that HIV-positive patients often cannot meet because of poor oral intake, with an associated wasting syndrome. Bacterial and fungal peritonitis may occur in patients receiving PD. Patients that develop dementia or are physically unable to do PD exchanges are not candidates for PD; for these patients, HD is the only option.

16. OPHTHALMOLOGIC ASPECTS

Ocular involvement occurs in many patients with acquired immunodeficiency syndrome (AIDS) and can be a significant source of morbidity. Opportunistic intraocular infections can develop in patients with AIDS along with severe or atypical manifestations of common ocular conditions because of their immunocompromised status. Ocular manifestations can be classified by whether the anterior segment (lids, lashes, periocular skin, cornea, anterior chamber, iris, or lens), posterior segment (vitreous, retina, or choroid), or orbit are involved. Neuro-ophthalmologic aspects of AIDS are covered in the neurologic chapter.

I. Anterior segment
A. Infections
1. **Herpes simplex keratitis** has a prolonged course, with frequent recurrences and increased risk of secondary bacterial infection in patients with AIDS.
   a. **Diagnosis.** Symptoms include pain, redness, decreased vision, and photophobia. Slit-lamp examination demonstrates either a dendritic epithelial defect that stains with fluorescein or a disciform area of stromal and endothelial edema. Corneal anesthesia is frequently present.
   b. **Treatment** involves topical antivirals such as 1% trifluorothymidine drops every 2 hours while awake, or 3% vidarabine ointment 5 times per day. Topical steroids (Section I.E) should be used if there is severe, concomitant anterior chamber inflammation but should be given no more frequently than topical antivirals to avoid exacerbating the viral infection. Cycloplegics (Section I.E) can be given for photophobia. Sequelae include posterior synechiae, glaucoma, severe uveitis, and corneal scarring.
2. **Varicella-zoster** can cause blepharitis, conjunctivitis, keratitis, and uveitis that may appear similar to herpes simplex on slit-lamp examination, with minor differences in the appearance of the dendrites.
   a. **Symptoms** usually include an antecedent or concurrent rash with herpetic vesicles on the skin in the distribution of the ophthalmic division of the trigeminal nerve or its branches (frontal, nasociliary, or lacrimal); occasionally there is extensive multidermatomal involvement. Vesicles on the tip of the nose indicate involvement of the nasociliary nerve, with a high probability of ocular involvement. Ocular varicella-zoster is both more common and more severe in patients with AIDS than in immunocompetent individuals with a higher incidence of corneal involvement and uveitis.
   b. **Treatment** of the ocular disease is similar to that for herpes simplex keratitis but also includes systemic treatment with acyclovir, 800 mg p.o. 5 times per day, famciclovir, 500 mg p.o. t.i.d., or valaciclovir, 400 mg p.o. t.i.d. Acyclovir, 10 mg per kg i.v. every 8 hours, may be needed for more severe cases. Sequelae are similar to those of herpes simplex keratitis but also include postherpetic neuralgia in ~40% of eyes, iris atrophy, and facial scarring. The occurrence of zoster ophthalmicus in an otherwise apparently healthy young patient should raise the suspicion of human immunodeficiency virus (HIV).
3. **Corneal ulcers** may be bacterial or fungal and are often bilateral, recurrent, and polymicrobial. Contributing factors include dry eyes, poor lid hygiene, immunocompromised status, i.v. drug use, and exposure keratopathy.

      a. Symptoms include pain, decreased vision, foreign-body sensation, and redness. Findings include a corneal intrastromal cellular infiltrate with an overlying epithelial defect that stains with fluorescein and anterior chamber cell and flare with a hypopyon (inferior layering of inflammatory cells). Corneal scraping is performed to obtain material for cultures and stains.

      b. Treatment often requires hospital admission for frequent topical antibiotics or antifungals or both. Broad-spectrum topical combination therapy is used until culture and Gram-stain results are available. Frequently used regimens include fortified aminoglycosides (gentamicin; tobramycin or amikacin) every 1 hour, combined with fortified cephalosporins or vancomycin (cefazolin, ceftazidime, or vancomycin, 50 mg per mL) every 1 hour. Occasionally, commercially available preparations of fluoroquinolones (ciprofloxacin 0.3% or ofloxacin 0.3%) may be used on an outpatient basis for small, noncentral ulcers in compliant patients. Topical cycloplegia is used for comfort and to prevent the formation of posterior synechiae (Section I.D). Fortified antibiotic drops are administered at least hourly for the first 48 hours and are tapered based on the clinical response. Patients suspected of having a fungal keratitis are treated in a similar fashion with 5% natamycin (best for superficial infections), 0.15% amphotericin B, or 1% miconazole or clotrimazole. Fluconazole, 200 mg per day p.o., may be used in addition to topical therapy in severe cases.

    4. Microsporidiosis is caused by a protozoan (Encephalitozoon hellem or cuniculi) that can affect multiple organ systems, including the cornea.

      a. Ocular symptoms include severe foreign-body sensation, blurred vision, and photophobia. Findings are minimal conjunctival or intraocular inflammation, with extensive coarse punctate keratitis. Conjunctival scrapings or a tissue biopsy may be required for diagnosis.

      b. Treatment options are topical fumagillin, 3 to 10 mg per mL every hour, tapering to every 4 hours, or 0.1% propamidine isethionate 6 times per day.

    5. Molluscum contagiosum is caused by a pox virus and is seen as umbilicated papules on the skin, lids, lid margins, and rarely on the conjunctiva or limbus. Patients may be asymptomatic or may complain of redness, tearing, or foreign-body sensation. Slit-lamp examination may show follicular conjunctivitis, punctate keratopathy, filamentary keratitis, punctal scarring, or superficial vascular pannus. Initial treatment consists of lubrication with artificial tears every 1 to 6 hours. Recalcitrant cases can be treated with excision, curettage, or cryotherapy, but there is a high recurrence rate.

B. Surface disease

    1. Seborrhea and blepharitis are common inflammatory conditions of the lid and lid margins that are more frequent and more severe in patients with AIDS. Symptoms include morning crusting and visual blurring, redness, and foreign-body sensation. Slit-lamp examination will show thickened, irregular, or erythematous lid margins with plugged meibomian glands, telangiectasias, and scruff or collarettes on the lashes. Treatment involves lid hygiene with warm compresses and lid scrubs with warm water and baby shampoo twice daily. Topical antibiotics such as erythromycin or combination (Polysporin) ophthalmic ointment can be used at bedtime. Artificial tears can be used for comfort. Rarely systemic antibiotics (e.g., doxycycline, 100 to 200 mg per day p.o.) can be used for 3 to 6 months for recalcitrant cases with severe meibomitis.

    2. Dry-eye syndrome is more common in patients with AIDS and symptoms include redness, tearing, burning, foreign-body sensation, and transient visual blur. Findings include a decreased tear lake, rapid tear break-up, decreased tear production on Schirmer's testing, and fluorescein and/or rose bengal staining of the interpalpebral cornea and conjunctiva. Dry eyes can predispose patients to corneal ulceration. Treatment involves lubrication with artificial tears every 1 to 6 hours as needed. Punctal occlusion with silicone plugs or by cautery can be used to decrease tear outflow. Coexisting seborrhea and blepharitis must be treated.

C. Malignancies

1. **Kaposi's sarcoma** is a common ocular finding that is present in up to one quarter of all patients with Kaposi's. Ocular Kaposi's is most commonly found on the lids but also can be seen on the periocular skin, conjunctiva, and rarely in the orbit. The characteristic lesions can appear as reddish or purplish plaques or papules that can mimic subconjunctival hemorrhages. Usually no specific treatment is required for ocular Kaposi's, although low-dose x-ray radiotherapy (800 to 1200 cGy in fractions) will cause regression in ~85% of cases. In addition, local excision combined with extensive cautery, intralesional interferon chemotherapy, or cryotherapy can be used for isolated lesions causing ocular problems, such as exposure keratopathy. Systemic treatment for visceral Kaposi's (see Chapter 28) with various chemotherapy regimens or interferon often reduces the ocular disease.

2. **Non-Hodgkin's lymphoma** can occasionally be seen with unilaterally or bilaterally swollen eyelids (see Section III.A.1 on the orbit).

D. HIV-induced microangiopathy can be observed in conjunctival blood vessels. Comma-shaped capillaries and segmentation of capillary blood flow are visible manifestations of the erythrocyte sludging that can occur with HIV. The observation of conjunctival microangiopathy in an otherwise healthy individual should raise the suspicion for HIV.

E. Anterior uveitis (iritis, iridocyclitis) is inflammation involving the anterior structures of the eye. Patients may have photophobia, redness, tearing, pain, floaters, and blurred vision. Slit-lamp examination may reveal ciliary flush, keratic precipitates (clumps of leukocytes on the posterior surface of the cornea), anterior-chamber cell and flare, iris nodules, and posterior synechiae. Symptomatic inflammation is less common than would be expected, probably because of defects in T cell–mediated immunity. **Treatment of uveitis** involves therapy for the underlying cause, along with topical cycloplegia to relax the ciliary muscle (homatropine 5% t.i.d., scopolamine 0.25% b.i.d, or atropine sulfate 1.0% b.i.d) and topical steroids such as prednisolone acetate 1.0% every 1 to 6 hours for inflammation.

1. **Infections** may cause intraocular inflammation both in association with active intraocular infection and as an immune reaction against infection elsewhere in the body (e.g., mycobacteria or syphilis). Herpes simplex and herpes zoster can cause an iritis without the characteristic corneal dendritic lesions. Identification of the infectious agent is often possible through characteristic clinical appearance, but occasionally laboratory evaluation or diagnostic procedures [e.g., aqueous tap for culture and polymerase chain reaction (PCR)] may be required. Treatment is directed at the underlying systemic condition, with topical cycloplegia and steroids as needed to control the intraocular inflammation.

2. **Drug-induced uveitis** has been observed with **rifabutin**, used for the prophylaxis and treatment of *Mycobacterium avium* complex (MAC), and **cidofovir**, an anticytomegalovirus (CMV) drug. Rifabutin has been associated with a hypopyon uveitis when administered at high doses or in combination with clarithromycin or both. Treatment involves discontinuation of the drug and administration of topical steroids and cycloplegics. Cidofovir can cause a transient, self-limited iritis, or severe hypotony.

3. **Reiter's syndrome** appears to be more common among patients with AIDS and includes conjunctivitis and occasionally iritis, arthritis, and urethritis. The uveitis is treated with topical steroids and cycloplegics.

   4. Spillover from posterior-segment infections (e.g., toxoplasmosis, CMV) can cause anterior-segment inflammation. The diagnosis can be made on the basis of concomitant vitreous inflammation and characteristic retinal findings (see Posterior Segment, Section II.A.1–8).

II. Posterior segment
A. Opportunistic diseases

   1. CMV retinitis is by far the most common posterior-segment infection in AIDS, developing in 20% (range, 15% to 40%) of patients with AIDS. It is a significant cause of morbidity in AIDS. The disease is rarely seen with CD4+ T-cell counts >50 cells/mm^3. Because CMV retinitis develops late in the course of AIDS, only 2% to 5% of patients will have CMV retinitis as the presenting sign of AIDS.

   a. Diagnosis. Symptoms include peripheral visual-field loss, floaters, and decreased vision, although occasional patients are asymptomatic. Slit-lamp examination usually reveals minimal anterior or vitreous inflammation. Stellate keratic precipitates may be quite characteristic. Fundus findings include multiple irregular, granular, white–yellow intraretinal lesions with hemorrhages. Currently fundus findings are classified into three types based on appearance and disease course: (a) classic CMV, with dense retinal whitening in a perivascular pattern, vascular sheathing, and marked hemorrhage ("pizza-pie" fundus); (b) indolent or granular CMV, with subtle retinal opacification and granularity, and minimal hemorrhage, or (c) frosted-branch angiitis, with marked vascular sheathing, which may be a variant of the classic form.

   b. The location of CMV lesions within the fundus is important in determining the visual prognosis and the urgency of treatment. The most visually important area of the retina is zone 1, an area within two disc diameters (3,000 microns) from the center of the fovea and one disc diameter from nasal edge of the optic nerve (Fig. 1). This region can be seen with the direct ophthalmoscope. Zone 2 is the

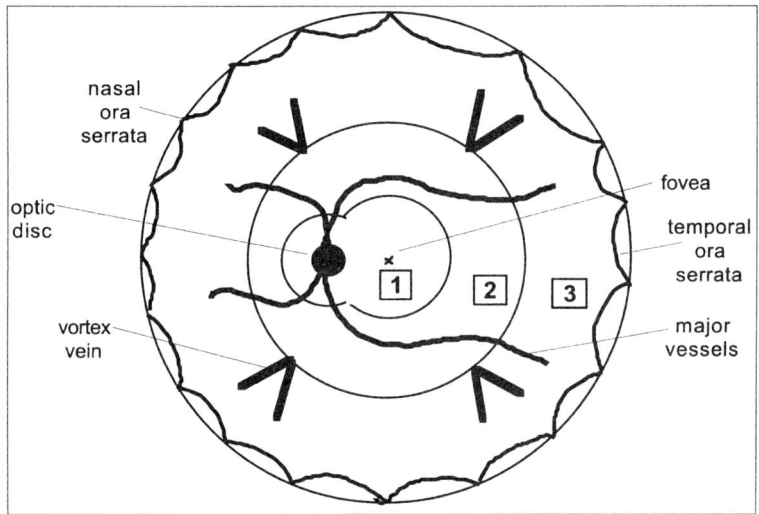

FIG. 1. Retinal zones for the CMV retinitis. Zone 1: area within 3,000 mm from the fovea and 1,500 mm from the optic disc. Zone 2: anterior border of zone 1 to the ampullae of the vortex veins. Zone 3: anterior border of zone 2 to the ora serrata.

region between zone 1 and the ampullae of the vortex veins at the equator of the globe, and zone 3 is the residual retina anterior to zone 2 (Fig. 1). Lesions in zone 1 are the most visually significant because of possible damage to the macula or contiguous spread to the optic nerve. Peripapillary CMV retinitis must be treated aggressively because involvement of the optic nerve can result in a sudden and precipitous loss of vision. Lesions in zone 2 can cause peripheral field loss. Zone 3 lesions are often asymptomatic but are significant because of the risk of posterior spread. Retinal detachment can develop from full-thickness retinal necrosis in any zone.

    c. **The differential diagnosis of CMV retinitis** is broad and includes acute retinal necrosis (ARN), progressive outer retinal necrosis (PORN), toxoplasmosis, syphilis, intraocular lymphoma, and fungal endophthalmitis (see the following). The diagnosis usually can be made based on the fundus appearance. However, if the diagnosis is in doubt, PCR analysis of aqueous or vitreous specimens may be performed for cases with an atypical appearance or a limited response to therapy. Alternatively, patients can be treated empirically with intravenous ganciclovir or foscarnet, because chorioretinal scarring should develop at the site of previously active CMV retinitis within 2 to 4 weeks after initiating this therapy.

    d. **Treatment** includes parenteral ganciclovir, foscarnet or cidofovir, or the insertion of a ganciclovir intraocular implant with concomitant oral ganciclovir. (See Chapter 25 for a complete discussion.)

    e. **Complications.** Retinal detachment will eventually occur in ~20% of patients with progressive CMV and is one of the major causes of visual loss from CMV, along with macular or optic nerve involvement. Retinal detachment is generally a late complication resulting from the development of full-thickness retinal breaks from the necrotizing retinitis. Risk factors for retinal detachment include duration of disease, activity of disease, and the extent of disease. If the detachment is localized and extramacular, consideration can be given to laser photocoagulation to "wall off" the detached area; however, most detachments will progress through the laser scars over the course of months. Definitive treatment involves pars plana vitrectomy with silicone oil and endolaser photocoagulation and occasionally a scleral buckle. Anatomic success is achieved in 80% to 90% of eyes, often with the restoration of ambulatory vision if there has not been destruction of the macula or optic nerve by CMV. A contact lens is required for full visual rehabilitation postoperatively because of the refractive change induced by the high index of refraction of the silicone oil.

2. **Varicella-zoster retinitis** can be seen in several ways, possibly related to the degree of immunosuppression.

    a. **ARN** is classically a disease of immunocompetent patients but has been seen in patients with AIDS as well. It is usually due to varicella-zoster virus (VZV), but rare cases caused by herpes simplex virus type 1 (HSV-1), HSV-2, CMV, and Epstein–Barr virus (EBV) have been reported in immunocompetent patients. ARN has been reported to occur simultaneously with or shortly after chickenpox, cutaneous zoster, and herpes encephalitis. The disease is often unilateral, but the second eye can become involved in up to two–thirds of untreated patients within several months.

        (1) **Diagnosis.** Patients have decreased vision, ocular or orbital pain, injection, visual field loss and photophobia. There is usually conjunctival injection, a significant anterior-chamber reaction, and marked vitritis. Fundus examination shows multifocal peripheral areas of white–yellow retinitis with sharply defined edges, occlusive vasculitis, and occasional optic neuritis.

Multiple holes can develop at the junction of necrotic, involved retina, and uninvolved retina, leading to retinal detachment in 70% of eyes.

   (2) **The differential diagnosis** of ARN includes toxoplasmosis, syphilitic retinitis, CMV retinitis, PORN (see the following), intraocular lymphoma, sarcoidosis, and Behçet's disease. The diagnosis of ARN is usually clearly based on the presence of the classic triad of vitritis, retinitis, and vasculitis. However, PCR analysis of aqueous or vitreous fluid or both can be performed if there is doubt about the diagnosis.

   (3) **Treatment** includes i.v. acyclovir (10 mg per kg every 8 hours for 14 days), followed by p.o. acyclovir (800 mg p.o. 5 times per day) for many months, along with topical cycloplegics and steroids (see Section I.E). Maintenance therapy with oral acyclovir appears significantly to reduce the risk of disease in the contralateral eye. High-dose systemic steroids (methylprednisolone, 250 mg i.v. every 6 hours for 3 days) started 24 to 48 hours after initiating acyclovir, followed by p.o. steroids (prednisone 1 to 1.5 mg per kg per day) are commonly used in immunocompetent patients but should be used with caution in patients with AIDS. Aspirin (325 to 650 mg per day) may theoretically decrease the occlusive vasculitis and optic neuritis in ARN, although there is no proof of its efficacy. Prophylactic retinal laser photocoagulation can create chorioretinal adhesions around retinal holes if there is sufficient resolution of the vitritis to allow a clear view. If retinal detachment develops, treatment involves pars plana vitrectomy, endolaser photocoagulation, silicone oil injection, and possibly a scleral buckle. Optic nerve sheath fenestration has been attempted in some cases of acute optic neuropathy resulting from ARN, although the efficacy of this therapy remains to be determined.

  b. **PORN** is a recently recognized disease that is probably caused by VZV. It is associated with cutaneous zoster in about two-thirds of patients.

   (1) **Clinical findings** include minimal vitreous and anterior-chamber reaction (unlike ARN), with bilateral, multifocal deep yellow–white opaque intraretinal lesions with a predilection for the posterior pole. Lesions coalesce rapidly as the disease progresses, and retinal necrosis develops within days or weeks. Retinal vasculitis occurs rarely. There can be early clearing of retinal edema around vessels, giving the appearance of perivascular sparing. Sequelae include optic atrophy, attenuation of retinal vessels, dense white chorioretinal scars, and retinal detachment (70%). No-light-perception vision develops in 67% of eyes within 1 to 6 months.

   (2) **All therapies** have had universally poor results. Antiviral therapy directed against VZV is given but there is little evidence of benefit.

3. **Bacterial endophthalmitis** can be endogenous (intravascular spread from another body site) or exogenous (i.e., caused by a perforated corneal ulcer). Treatment is the same as that in nonimmunosuppressed patients and involves par plana vitrectomy or a diagnostic vitreous tap with the injection of broad-spectrum intravitreal antibiotics or both. Intravitreal antibiotic options include vancomycin, 1.0 mg in 0.1 mL, combined with ceftazidime, 2.25 mg, or amikacin, 100 to 200 mg in 0.1 mL, along with broad-spectrum systemic antibiotics directed toward the suspected organism or source of infection for endogenous endophthalmitis. Vancomycin, 1 g i.v. every 12 hours, and ceftazidime, 1 g i.v. every 12 hours, have been shown to have good ocular penetration.

4. *Pneumocystis carinii* **choroiditis** is an intraocular infection found exclusively in patients with AIDS. The disease is often an incidental finding, because patients may have good vision even with foveal lesions. There is minimal or no anterior-chamber or vitreous reaction. Multifocal, discrete, round lesions or multilobular, yellow–white subretinal plaques are present posterior to the equator in one or both eyes, with occasional overlying serous retinal detachment or retinal pigment epithelium (RPE) mottling. The disease may be related to the use of inhaled pentamidine for prophylaxis of *Pneumocystis carinii* pneumonia (PCP), since extrapulmonary infection is not treated with inhalation therapy. Systemic treatment is administered because intraocular Pneumocystis may be an early sign of systemic pneumocystosis. The preferred therapy is trimethoprim/sulfamethoxazole (two double-strength tablets p.o. q.i.d for 21 days; see Chapter 22).

5. **Toxoplasmosis** is a relatively uncommon eye infection (<5 %) despite being the most common nonviral central nervous system (CNS) infection in AIDS. Toxoplasmosis in immunocompetent patients causes a severe vitritis with a discrete focus of intense retinitis adjacent to a pre-existing chorioretinal scar. In patients with AIDS, single or multiple lesions unassociated with previous chorioretinal scars can be seen in one or both eyes. There is usually full-thickness retinal involvement, but lesions can be restricted to only the inner or outer retina. There is more vitreous and anterior-segment inflammation than CMV retinitis but less inflammation than would be expected in immunocompetent patients. Up to half of patients with AIDS with ocular toxoplasmosis will have CNS disease, and occasionally the ocular disease may be the first indication of disseminated toxoplasmosis. Therapy involves treating the systemic infection (see Chapter 22). Topical cycloplegics and steroids (see Section I.E) can be used for anterior-segment inflammation. Prednisone (1 to 1.5 mg per kg per day) can be added with caution for patients with severe vitritis.

6. **Syphilis** has more severe ocular manifestations in patients with AIDS. Progression from primary syphilis to neurosyphilis can occur rapidly, despite treatment with doses of antibiotics that would cure immunocompetent patients.
   a. **Diagnosis.** Ocular manifestations are protean, ranging from a mild isolated iritis to a fulminant chorioretinitis mimicking ARN and include granulomatous uveitis, perivasculitis, panuveitis, papillitis, optic neuritis, and intraretinal hemorrhage. Deep yellowish plaques at the level of the RPE are characteristic of ocular syphilis in patients with AIDS.
   b. **Treatment.** Ocular syphilis is a form of neurosyphilis and must be treated aggressively with penicillin G, 12 to 24 million units i.v. for 10 to 21 days (see Chapter 28). In addition to systemic antibiotics, topical steroids and cycloplegics (Section I.E) may be indicated for ocular inflammation.

7. **Fungal infections**
   a. *Cryptococcus neoformans* is the most common fungal cause of visual loss in patients with AIDS, resulting from optic nerve or visual cortex involvement from meningitis or both; however, intraocular infection is relatively rare. Cryptococcus has been found in retinal and choroidal vessels at autopsy without associated microscopic inflammation or visible macroscopic lesions.
      (1) **Diagnosis.** Cryptococcal choroiditis or chorioretinitis appears as multifocal yellow–white lesions of the choroid or retina or both in the absence of anterior-chamber or vitreous inflammation. Vision is usually preserved unless there is direct macular or optic nerve involvement. The diagnosis is presumptive and is based on simultaneous cryptococcal infection elsewhere and improvement of the chorioretinal lesions with antifungal therapy.

        (2) **Treatment** is as for cryptococcal meningitis (see Chapter 24).

        (3) Visual loss has been associated with **increases in opening pressure** in the cerebrospinal fluid. Surgical decompression may be needed.

    b. Candida is a rare cause of intraocular infection in patients with AIDS, despite the high incidence of mucocutaneous candidiasis. Risk factors for Candida endophthalmitis are the same as those for immunocompetent patients: intravenous drug abuse, indwelling catheters, and the administration of broad-spectrum antibiotics. Fundus findings include fluffy white chorioretinal infiltrates that may extend into the vitreous with an associated vitritis. Treatment is amphotericin B, 0.4 to 0.6 mg per kg per day i.v. for a total dose of 0.5 to 1.0 g. In addition, vitrectomy and injection of intravitreal amphotericin B (5 mg in 0.1 mL) can be performed for sight-threatening infections if the patient's systemic condition is stable enough to allow surgery; otherwise, intravitreal injections of amphotericin alone can be performed at the bedside.

    c. Histoplasmosis rarely infects the eye in AIDS. There are case reports of posterior-segment involvement with creamy white intraretinal and subretinal lesions in patients with known disseminated histoplasmosis. Treatment is with amphotericin B or itraconazole (see Chapter 24).

  8. Mycobacterial choroiditis is rare despite the high incidence of systemic *Mycobacterium avium* complex (MAC) and tuberculosis (TB) infection. Multiple yellow–white choroidal nodules are seen, with little to no retinitis or vitritis. The diagnosis may be presumptive, because the appearance may be similar to that of Pneumocystis or Cryptococcus. Treatment is directed toward the systemic disease.

B. Intraocular lymphoma can present as a vitritis, which can be difficult to diagnose. There may be an initial improvement with systemic steroids; diagnosis is often made on the basis of a vitreous biopsy (see orbit, Section III.A.1.).

C. Other

  1. HIV retinopathy is the most common manifestation of systemic HIV in the eye but is usually asymptomatic. Fundus examination will reveal cotton-wool spots, which represent microinfarctions of the retinal nerve fiber layer. These are often whiter and more posterior than those seen in other conditions and must be differentiated from early CMV retinitis. Occasional microaneurysms and hemorrhages can be seen. HIV must be considered in the differential diagnosis for patients who are noted to have cotton-wool spots on fundus examination without underlying conditions such as hypertension, diabetes, or collagen vascular diseases. Occasionally scattered dot and blot hemorrhages also are seen and may be the result of HIV-induced microangiopathy, associated anemia, or thrombocytopenia. No specific therapy is indicated.

  2. Vascular occlusions (central or branch retinal vein occlusions, central or branch retinal artery occlusions) have been reported in patients with AIDS and are thought to be caused by rheologic alterations from the HIV virus. Histopathologic examination does not reveal any evidence of infectious agents in autopsy studies.

  3. Drug-induced retinal or choroidal degenerations have been reported with systemic clofazimine, didanosine, and intravitreal fomiversin. Clofazimine has been associated with a bull's-eye maculopathy with retinal degeneration, and didanosine has been associated with RPE alterations in children. Intravitreal fomiversin has been associated with visual field loss, and RPE mottling occurs at doses higher than are currently being used. An excessively high dose of intravitreal ganciclovir (40 mg) can cause retinal necrosis and blindness. Most posterior-pole changes are reversible with discontinuation of the drug.

III. Orbital. Orbital involvement from mass lesions caused by infectious or neoplastic processes can cause proptosis, motility disturbances, diplopia, periocular or lid swelling, erythema, ptosis, conjunctival injection or chemosis, decreased visual acuity, contrast sensitivity or color vision, or a Marcus–Gunn pupil. Workup includes an orbital computed tomography (CT) scan with i.v. contrast and axial and coronal cuts, or magnetic resonance imaging (MRI) with gadolinium and fat suppression. The radiologic appearance may be diagnostic, but occasionally orbital biopsies are required to establish the diagnosis.

A. Neoplastic

1. **Non-Hodgkin's lymphoma, usually large-cell,** but occasionally small-cell, is relatively common in patients with AIDS and may be the first manifestation of CNS or systemic involvement. Symptoms usually have a gradual onset, although rare cases have a fulminant course suggestive of an infectious process. Treatment is with orbital radiation to 4,000 cGy in fractionated doses, possibly with systemic steroids (e.g., prednisone, 1 to 1.5 mg per kg day) for severe inflammation and optic nerve compromise. CNS disease requires whole-brain radiation therapy, and systemic disease requires systemic chemotherapy (see Chapter 29).

2. **Kaposi's sarcoma** of the orbit is extremely rare. It can be treated with orbital radiation or systemic chemotherapy.

B. Infectious

1. Bacterial orbital cellulitis is a surgical emergency, requiring drainage of the infection and treatment with broad-spectrum i.v. antibiotics.

2. **Fungal cellulitis or sinusitis** or both can be seen with case reports of contiguous spread of **mucormycosis** and **aspergillosis** from the sinuses. Treatment usually involves surgical debridement from both an ear, nose, and throat (ENT) and ophthalmologic approach and prolonged systemic therapy with i.v. amphotericin B.

17. CARDIOVASCULAR ASPECTS

Cardiac abnormalities associated with the acquired immunodeficiency syndrome (AIDS) have been reported since the mid-1980s. It is unclear which of these abnormalities observed are primary complications of the human immunodeficiency virus (HIV) or potential complications of treatment. It is uncertain whether HIV itself poses a risk for myocardial diseases or whether patients with HIV-related cardiac disease have pre-existent cardiac disease or risk factors (e.g., hypertension, coronary artery disease, diabetes, hyperlipidemia, or tobacco or alcohol use). In addition, the cardiac disease may be the result of opportunistic infections, HIV-associated malignancies, or drug toxicities—either recreational or therapeutic. Multiple prospective studies have detailed echocardiographic evidence of asymptomatic heart disease, and it has been postulated that there would be a significant potential for AIDS patients to develop cardiovascular disease if survival improved. However, the incidence of HIV cardiac disease as documented cause of death is essentially unchanged despite survival improvement over the past 10-year period.

I. **Epidemiology.** Reports of HIV-associated cardiac disease range from 5% to 50%.
   A. Symptomatic heart disease occurs in between 5% and 7%. Echocardiographic evidence of heart disease ranges in advanced HIV disease from 35% to 54%, with pericardial effusion, decreased left ventricular (LV) function, and dilated cardiomyopathy (DCOM) the most common findings and endocarditis or malignancy the least common.
   B. Right ventricular hypertrophy is most associated with recurrent respiratory infections, especially *Pneumocystis carinii* pneumonia (PCP) and the use of ventilatory support. Nevertheless, there is increasing evidence to suggest that pulmonary hypertension occurs more frequently in the HIV population regardless of stage, CD4$^+$ count, or risk factors for HIV.
   C. Postmortem studies reveal that ~50% of AIDS patients have histopathologic evidence of heart disease, the clinical significance of which is unknown.
II. **Cardiac abnormalities**
   A. **Pericarditis**
      1. **Prevalence.** AIDS is now a common cause of pericarditis. It is estimated that between 20% and 40% of all AIDS patients have pericarditis at some time. Prospective echocardiographic studies document effusions in 13% to 32% of patients with AIDS. Most often an origin for the effusion cannot be identified. Given the increased incidence of "idiopathic" effusions present in AIDS, it is postulated that HIV itself may play a role. Approximately 25% of these "idiopathic" effusions spontaneously resolve. Approximately one third may be attributed to opportunistic infections. Other causes include inflammatory, neoplastic, metabolic, drug-induced, or connective tissue diseases. Less commonly seen causes include myocardial infarction, cardiac rupture, or amyloidosis.
      2. **Clinical features.** Patients typically have chest pain of variable intensity, usually pleuritic, that improves with sitting up. The majority have a low-grade fever. Clinical signs of tamponade may include tachycardia, tachypnea, pulsus paradoxus, and increased jugular venous pressures. A pericardial friction rub is pathognomonic. Patients with AIDS may have low-pressure tamponade and have no clinical manifestations at all. Low-pressure tamponade is seen most frequently with infiltrative heart disease such as tuberculosis or malignancy and severe volume depletion. Most often the effusions found in patients with HIV have little clinical significance, if any.

3. Diagnosis

a. The **electrocardiogram** (ECG) in pericarditis reveals diffuse ST-segment elevation, except in leads aVR and V_1, in which ST depression may be seen. A highly specific finding on ECG in pericarditis is depression of the PR. In chronic pericarditis, T-wave inversion may persist. The voltage may be reduced, depending on the size of the effusion. Electrical alternans may be seen in tamponade but will be absent in the presence of low-pressure tamponade.

b. **Echocardiogram** (ECHO) remains the gold standard for detecting effusions. Pericardiocentesis or pericardiotomy may be necessary for diagnosis or if an effusion persists despite therapy or presence of tamponade.

4. Therapy.
An aggressive approach for diagnosis of opportunistic infections or malignancy is recommended for patients with AIDS. After treatable causes have been excluded, most patients will respond to nonsteroidal antiinflammatory drugs or aspirin. If symptoms persist, then a 1- to 2-month course of prednisone may be indicated. Anecdotal reports suggest that patients with AIDS may be at increased risk for persistent or recurrent pericarditis.

B. Myocarditis

1. Prevalence. Nonspecific inflammatory myocarditis without necrosis is the most common lesion seen pathologically in HIV patients, the clinical significance of which is unknown. Autopsy studies suggest that the prevalence of focal myocarditis ranges from 11% to 50%. Clinically significant myocarditis is much less common. There is no evidence that myocarditis plays a role in the pathogenesis of dilated cardiomyopathy.

2. Clinical features. The majority of patients with HIV-associated myocarditis are asymptomatic or have subclinical disease such as sinus tachycardia. Patients have chest pain, fatigue, palpitations, dyspnea on exertion, or a combination of these mimicking an acute myocardial infarction. Rarely patients have congestive heart failure or sudden death resulting from arrhythmias.

3. Diagnosis. ECG usually reveals sinus tachycardia with nonspecific ST changes and occasional conduction defects. The chest radiograph is almost always normal. Definitive diagnosis is made by myocardial biopsy but is not warranted in most cases. A subgroup of patients may have a positive gallium scan revealing diffuse uptake.

4. Therapy. Treatment of the underlying illness and supportive cardiac care is recommended. Distinction must be made between HIV-associated myocarditis and myocarditis caused by opportunistic infections. Steroids should be used with caution.

C. Endocarditis

1. Prevalence

a. There appears to be an increased incidence of nonbacterial thrombotic endocarditis (NBTE) in AIDS. Necropsy studies reveal an incidence of 1% to 3% of NBTE in AIDS patients with abnormal cardiac findings. However, death resulting from central nervous system embolization is reported infrequently.

b. There does not appear to be an increased risk of infective endocarditis (IE) in AIDS independent of the association with intravenous drug use. Use of intravenous cocaine appears to be the highest risk factor for developing IE. Staphylococcus aureus remains the most common cause of IE. Acute right-sided endocarditis is more common than left-sided endocarditis. The tricuspid valve is affected in >50% of the cases.

2. Clinical features. Patients typically have high fevers and appear ill. Two-thirds of the patients have no clinical evidence of heart disease. Approximately one-third have respiratory symptoms such as cough and pleuritic pain. The majority of the symptomatic patients have an abnormal chest radiograph suggestive of septic pulmonary emboli. Approximately 35% will have clinical evidence of tricuspid insufficiency, characterized by presence of a gallop, a systolic regurgitant murmur with inspiration, and large V waves. Patients with IE attributable to *S. aureus* frequently have peripheral embolic stigmata. Patients with left-sided endocarditis may have rapid valvular dysfunction, resulting in congestive heart failure or arrhythmias or both. Mitral and aortic valve endocarditis are more associated with cerebral infarcts. Two-thirds of all patients with endocarditis have extravalvular sites of infection. Patients with NBTE may have embolic phenomena, but given that NBTE does not cause an inflammatory reaction, most patients are asymptomatic, and NBTE is discovered on postmortem examination.

3. **Diagnosis.** Pulmonary involvement associated with IE must be distinguished from pulmonary complications of opportunistic infections. Blood cultures are almost always positive. An ECHO may be used for supportive evidence but can never be used to exclude the diagnosis of endocarditis.

4. **Therapy.** Pathogen-directed antimicrobial therapy should be used for 4 to 6 weeks. Vancomycin plus an aminoglycoside should be started empirically in all cases of suspected IE in patients with history of intravenous drug use, given the increased incidence of methicillin-resistant *S. aureus* isolated in this patient population.

D. **Dilated Cardiomyopathy (DCOM)**

1. **Prevalence.** The incidence of echocardiographic evidence of DCOM in patients with AIDS is 25% to 40%; however, the actual incidence of symptomatic heart disease in these patients is only 3% to 6%. The incidence of DCOM by histopathology at autopsy is 1.7% to 3.7%. The presence of DCOM in patients with AIDS is a poor prognostic indicator, with a mortality rate of 50% within 6 months of diagnosis of DCOM. These deaths are not usually attributed to heart disease; therefore, no causal relation can be implied. In children, nucleoside reverse transcriptase inhibitors have been associated with the development of cardiomyopathy.

2. **Pathogenesis.** The pathogenesis of cardiomyopathy in AIDS is not well understood. Myocardial risk factors are common, especially given the higher prevalence of hypertension and diabetes in blacks and Hispanics, which may in turn contribute to the pathogenesis of DCOM independent of or in conjunction with HIV infection.

3. **Features.** The majority of patients are asymptomatic. Symptomatic patients have dyspnea on exertion and complain of decreased endurance and easy fatigability resulting from diminished cardiac output. In the advanced stage, patients have signs and symptoms of congestive heart failure.

4. **Diagnosis.** It is imperative to exclude other causes of DCOM, such as ischemic cardiomyopathy caused by coronary artery disease or hypertension, alcohol-induced cardiomyopathy, drug-induced cardiomyopathy, or rheumatic heart disease before attributing it to HIV infection. Diagnosis may be made in most patients by clinical history, physical examination, and noninvasive studies. The chest radiograph reveals cardiomegaly with pulmonary venous congestion. The ECG may show sinus tachycardia or other arrhythmias, ventricular and atrial enlargement, low voltage, various heart blocks, or only nonspecific ST changes. The echocardiogram reveals dilated cavities, normal wall thickness, decreased fractional shortening, reduced ejection fraction, and possible mitral or tricuspid regurgitation or both. The ECHO is useful in monitoring chamber size and overall ventricular function.

5. **Therapy.** Therapy should be directed at treatment of the underlying disease if possible. The mainstay of therapy is supportive cardiac care, including restricting level of activity to moderation, angiotensin-converting enzyme inhibitors, digoxin, and diuretics. Dopamine and dobutamine may

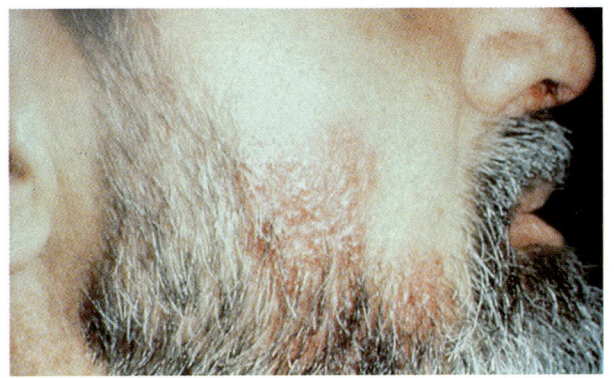

COLORPLATE 1. Seborrheic dermatitis.

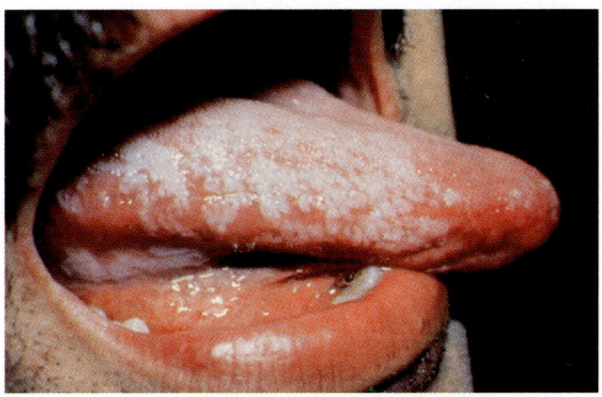

COLORPLATE 2. Oral hairy leukoplakia.

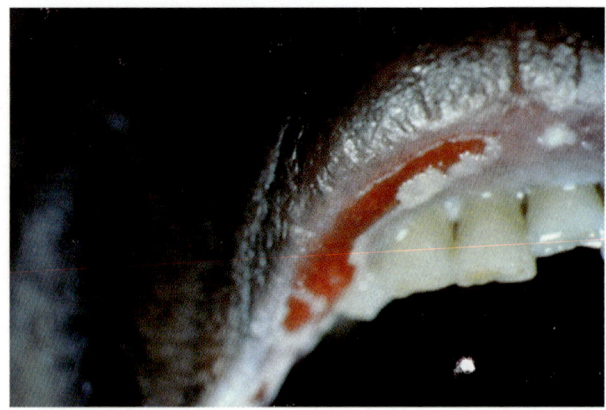

COLORPLATE 3. Erosive candidiasis of gums.

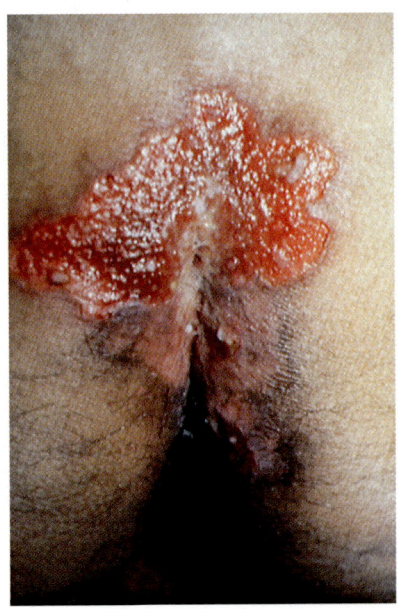

COLORPLATE 4. Perianal herpes simplex.

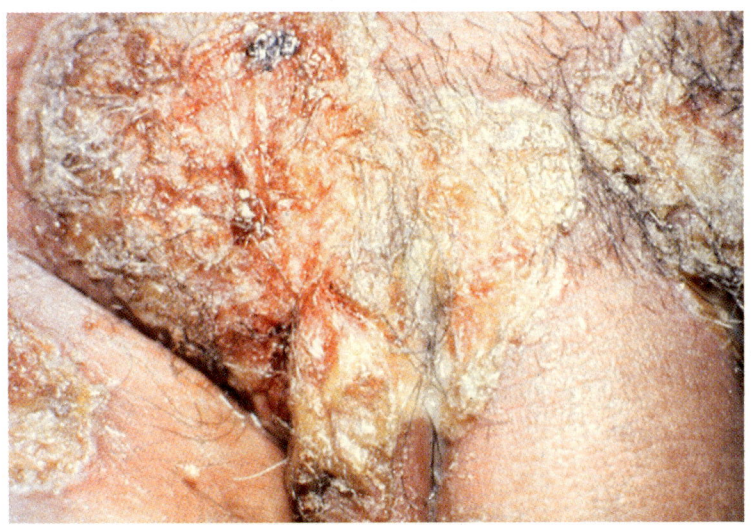

COLORPLATE 5. Extensive chronic acyclovir resistant herpes simplex infection.

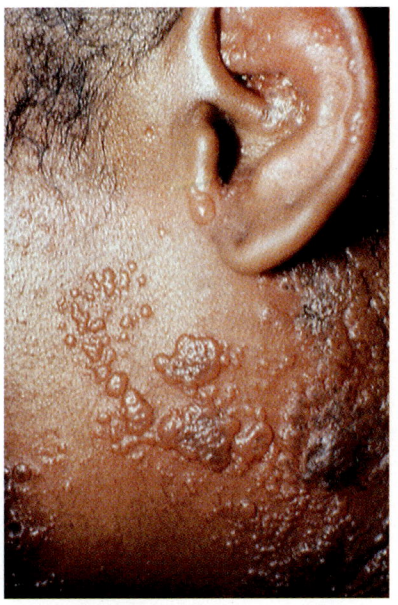

COLORPLATE 6. Herpes zoster.

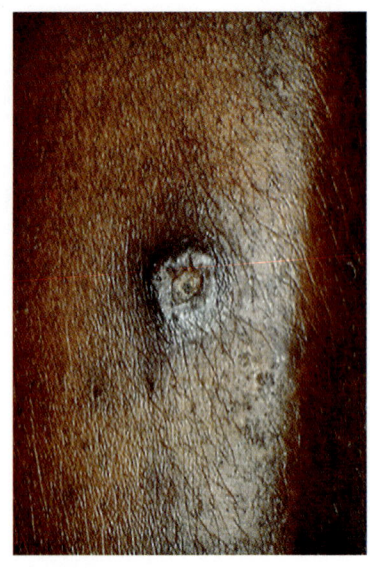

COLORPLATE 7. Acyclovir-resistant herpes zoster.

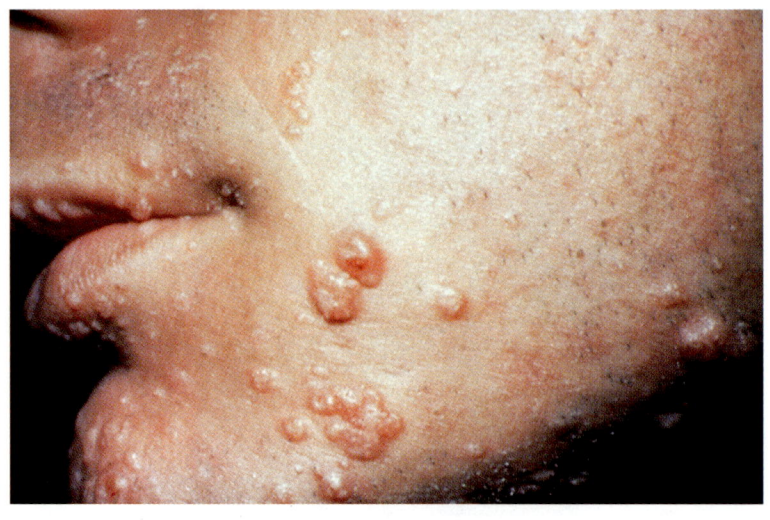

COLORPLATE 8. Molluscum contagiosum.

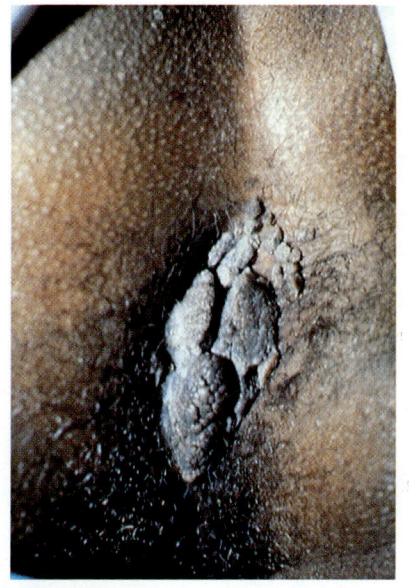

COLORPLATE 9. Perianal condylomata.

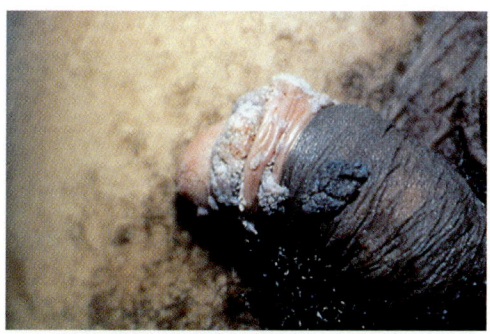

COLORPLATE 10. Penile condyloma.

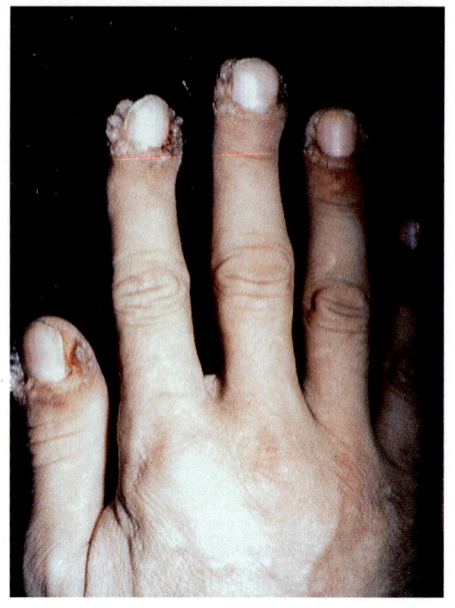

COLORPLATE 11. Human papillomavirus infection of finger.

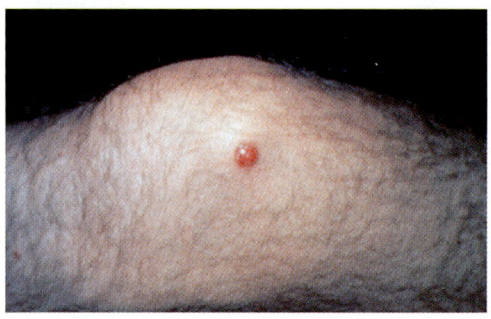

COLORPLATE 12. Bacillary angiomatosis.

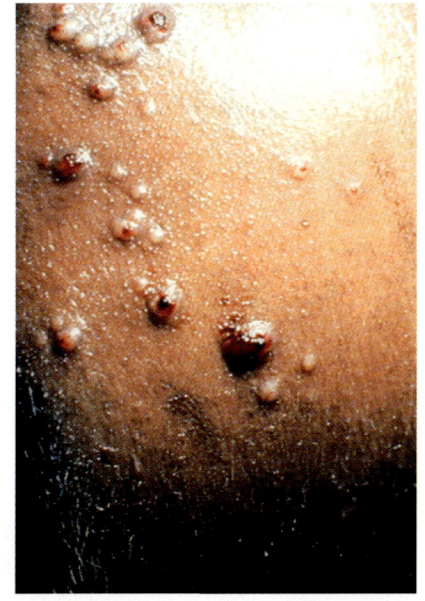

COLORPLATE 13. Cutaneous cryptococcosis.

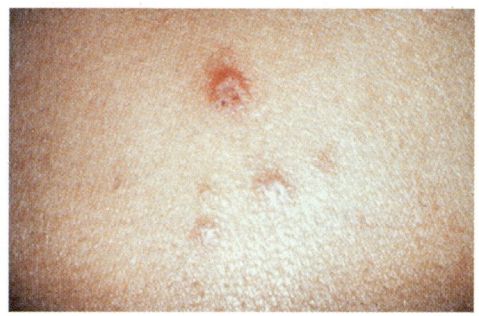

COLORPLATE 14. Histoplasmosis (skin).

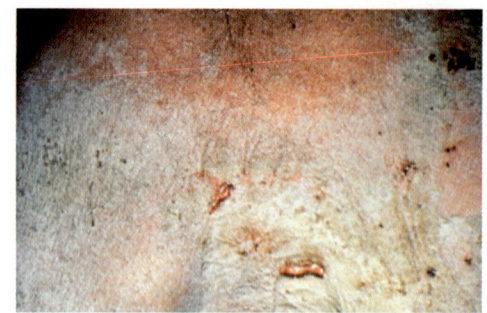

COLORPLATE 15. Crusted scabies.

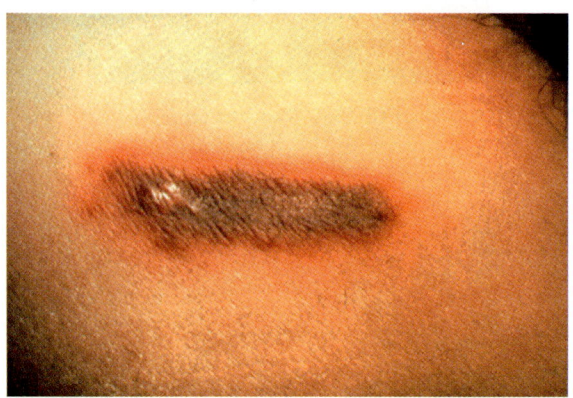

COLORPLATE 16. Kaposi's sarcoma.

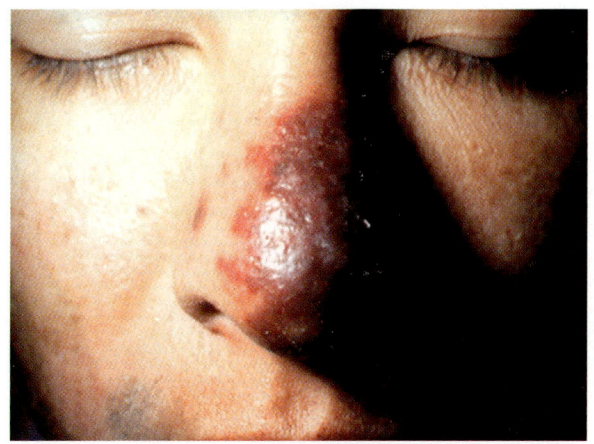

COLORPLATE 17. Kaposi's sarcoma.

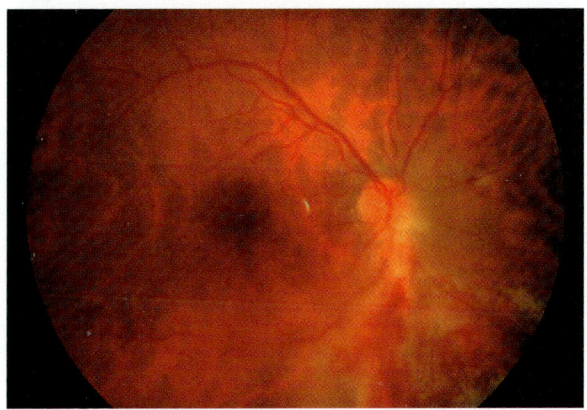

COLORPLATE 18. Cytomegalovirus retinitis.

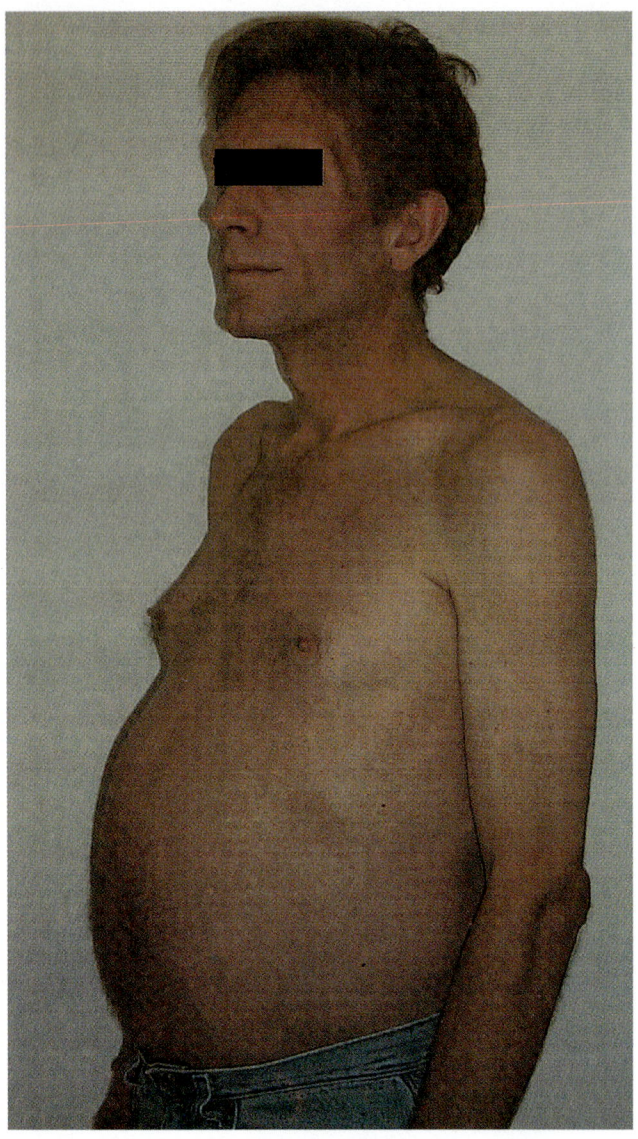

COLORPLATE 19. HIV-infected man with facial lipoatrophy, abdominal distension, and adipose tissue deposition in the breasts (lipomastia) associated with HAART.

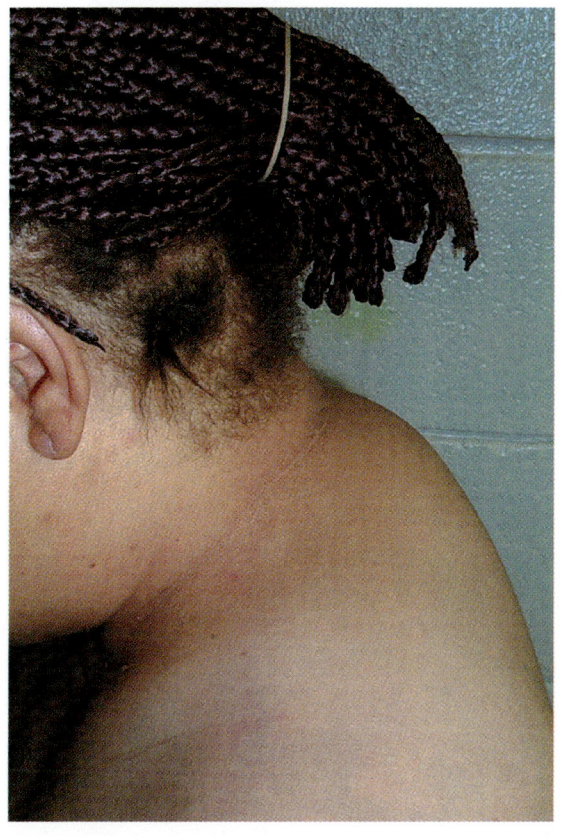

COLORPLATE 20. Dorsocervical adipose tissue deposition ("buffalo-hump") in an HIV-infected woman treated with HAART.

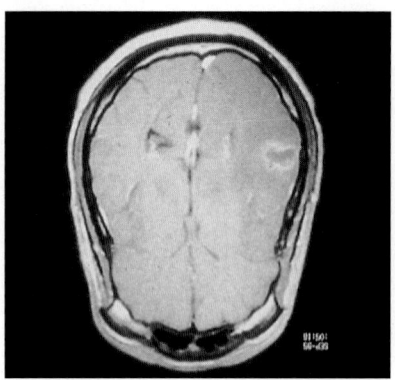

COLORPLATE 21. Magnetic resonance imaging scan of brain: toxoplasmosis.

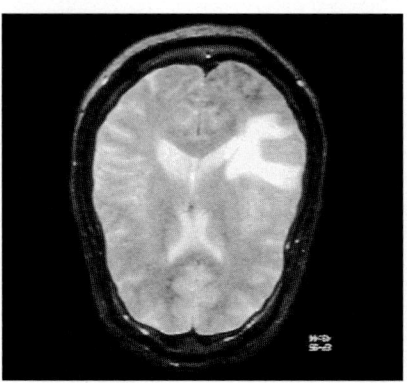

COLORPLATE 22. Magnetic resonance imaging scan of brain (T2-weighted image): toxoplasmosis with prominent white-matter edema.

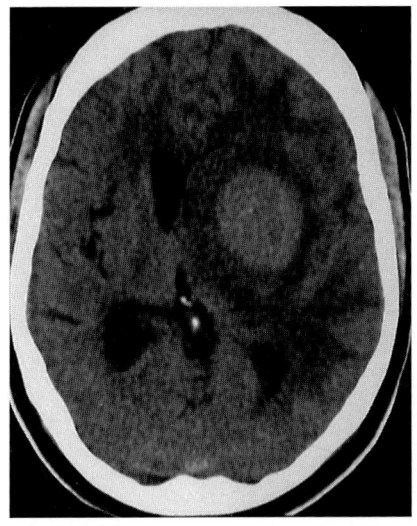

COLORPLATE 23. Computed tomography scan of brain: lymphoma. Note the marked mass effect.

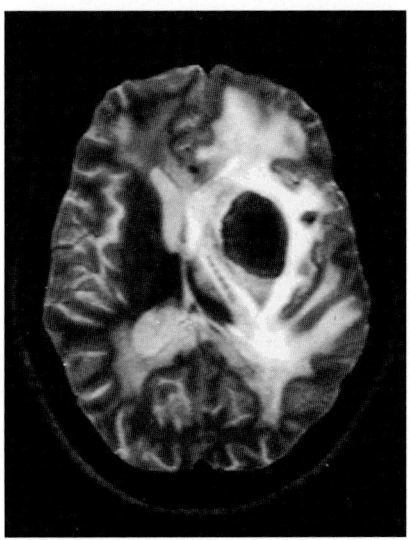

COLORPLATE 24. Magnetic resonance imaging scan of brain: lymphoma with massive edema.

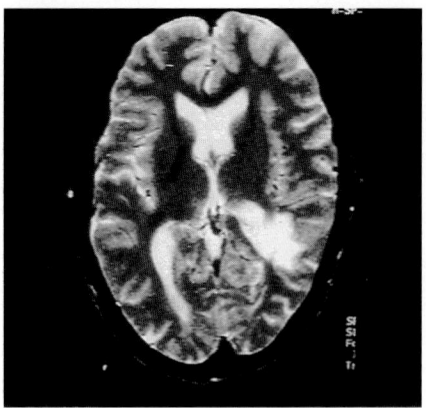

COLORPLATE 25. Magnetic resonance imaging scan of brain: progressive multifocal leukoencephalopathy with discrete white-matter parietal lesion.

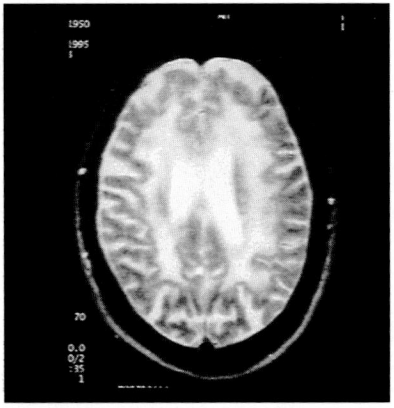

COLORPLATE 26. Magnetic resonance imaging scan of brain: human immunodeficiency virus encephalopathy with marked atrophy and diffuse white-matter changes.

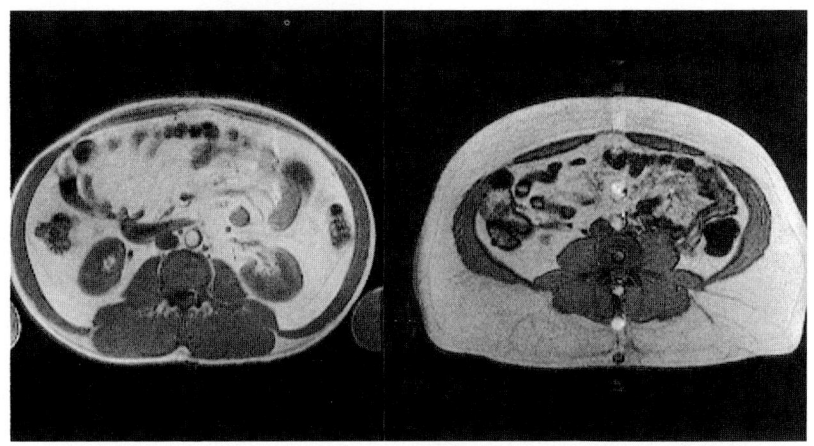

COLORPLATE 27. Proton magnetic resonance cross-sectional image of the abdomen at the level of the umbilicus in two men living with HIV and treated with HAART: A: Large intraabdominal adipose tissue depot, with small subcutaneous adipose tissue deposition. This pattern of adiposity has been associated with pro-atherogenic metabolic complications. B: Large subcutaneous adipose tissue depot, with small intraabdominal adipose tissue depot.

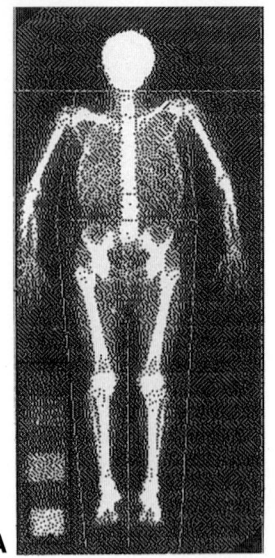

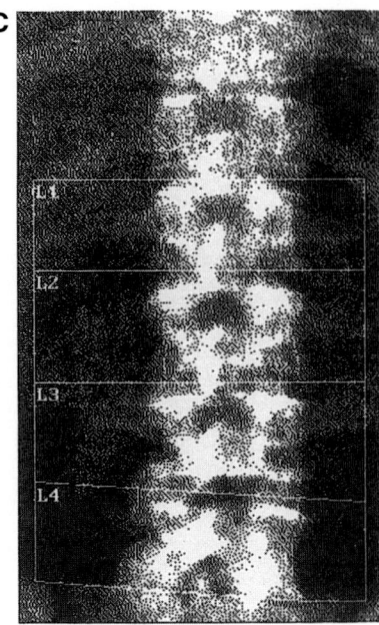

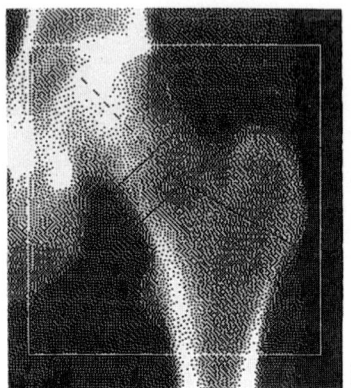

COLORPLATE 28. Dual-energy x-ray absorptiometer scans (DEXA) of an HIV-infected man. A: Whole-body image acquired in pencil-beam mode for measuring whole-body lean, bone, and adipose tissue masses. The white "cut-lines" denote regions of interest and are used to determine arm, leg, and trunk lean, bone, and adipose tissue masses. An indication of adipose tissue maldistribution can be derived from the ratio of truncal to appendicular adipose tissue masses. Bone mineral density is determined as the ratio of bone mineral mass to bone mineral area. B: DEXA scan of the proximal femur used to determine bone mineral density in the trochanter, femoral neck, and the region with the lowest bone mineral density (Ward's Triangle). C: DEXA scan of the anterior-posterior lumbar spine (L1–L4) used to determine bone mineral density of individual vertebrae.

be indicated in advanced disease. Patients with AIDS are not generally candidates for cardiac transplantation, given their immunosuppression status, although this may change with effective antiretroviral therapy.

E. Other cardiac abnormalities associated with HIV

  1. Primary pulmonary hypertension (PPH)

    a. Prevalence. Although pulmonary hypertension in HIV-infected patients is usually attributed to recurrent respiratory illnesses, there may be a subset of HIV+ patients at risk for developing PPH without any HIV-associated illnesses or known secondary causes of pulmonary hypertension with an incidence of 0.5% compared with an incidence of 0.02% in the general population.

    b. Features. Patients have dyspnea on exertion and may complain of chest pain. Patients may develop syncope and peripheral edema in advanced stages. Physical examination is significant for a prominent P_2, right-sided S_3, and tricuspid regurgitation.

    c. Diagnosis. Secondary causes of pulmonary hypertension such as thromboembolic disease, lung injury from recurrent respiratory illnesses, and connective tissue diseases must be excluded before a diagnosis of PPH is made. The chest radiograph is abnormal in 90%, depicting increase in size of pulmonary vasculature or attenuation of peripheral vessels. The ECG may reveal a right axis, right ventricular hypertrophy (RVH), or nonspecific T-wave changes. The ECHO reveals an enlarged right atrium, RVH with normal left ventricle, and tricuspid regurgitation. Pulmonary-function tests are usually nonspecific revealing a mild restrictive pattern with decreased diffusing capacity. Other studies that may be useful include V/Q scan, right-sided cardiac catheterization, pulmonary angiography, and lung biopsy.

    d. Therapy. Pulmonary vasodilatation is the only effective treatment for PPH. There is very little information regarding vasodilator therapy in patients with AIDS. However, the disease does appear to respond to epoprostenol in a way similar to that in non–HIV-infected patients with primary pulmonary hypertension. Patients should be given oxygen for hypoxemia and vasodilatory effects. Diuretics are recommended for management of peripheral edema. Calcium channel blockers should be initiated only under Swan–Ganz monitoring to ensure reduction of pulmonary pressures greater than systemic pressures. Patients should be given anticoagulants if not contraindicated, given the increased risk of mortality should a blood clot develop.

  2. Left ventricle dysfunction. Isolated LV dysfunction in the adult AIDS population is most likely the result of myocardial risk factors as seen in the general population. LV dysfunction attributable to cardiomyopathy or myocarditis is emerging as an important clinical manifestation in AIDS. Echocardiographic abnormalities are seen more frequently as the CD4+ count decreases. LV dysfunction may be more common and more clinically significant in the pediatric population. The origin of this remains unknown.

  3. Vascular lesions. A number of vascular lesions have been reported in AIDS, including arteriopathy, fibrocalcific arteriopathy, aneurysms, and vasculitis (Acierno. *J Am Coll Cardiol* 1989;13:1144–1154; see Chapter 18).

III. Secondary causes of cardiac disease

  A. Cardiac malignancies. Autopsy series report a 28% to 50% incidence of cardiac involvement in disseminated Kaposi's sarcoma. Lymphoma appears much less. Although focal involvement of the pericardium, epicardium, and subepicardial fat by Kaposi's occurs, few patients will have clinical cardiac disease (see Chapters 28 and 29 for therapy).

  B. Opportunistic infections. One-third to one-half of cardiac disease in AIDS can be attributed to opportunistic infections. These infections are often treatable, and rarely does death occur as a result of the cardiac aspect of the disease. The most common pathogens associated with cardiac involvement are *Toxoplasma gondii, Mycobacterium tuberculosis, Cryptococcus neoformans, Cytomegalovirus,* and atypical mycobacteria. Although the vast majority of patients with AIDS with either myocarditis or cardiomyopathy have a concomitant opportunistic infection, it is often difficult to attribute the cardiac disease to that pathogen. Aggressive therapy directed at the offending pathogen, especially in tuberculosis and cryptococcosis, can restore cardiac function to normal (refer to specific pathogen in Part III for therapy).

    C. Drugs. Several drugs used in the management of HIV-infected patients can contribute to cardiac dysfunction.

        1. Zidovudine has been implicated because of its known side effect of skeletal muscle myopathy. Pentamidine is associated with orthostatic hypotension and ventricular arrhythmias. Dapsone may induce methemoglobinemia, resulting in hypoxia. Eflorithine may cause conduction blocks. α-Interferon is associated with hypotension, hypertension, tachycardia, and congestive cardiomyopathy.

        2. The most common cardiotoxic drugs used in AIDS are the chemotherapeutic agents. Doxorubicin (Adriamycin) can cause mural thrombi. Doxorubicin induces myocarditis. Vinblastine is associated with an increased incidence of myocardial infarction, hypertension, and cerebral infarcts.

        3. Many other drugs not specific to management of HIV are associated with structural changes in the heart and peripheral vessels, as well as vasculitides; therefore, it is imperative to exclude a possible cardiotoxic agent as the cause of either myocarditis or cardiomyopathy in an HIV-infected patient.

        4. Another major class of cardiotoxic agents encountered in HIV are intravenous recreational drugs, especially cocaine. LV dysfunction has been reported in as many as 40% of intravenous cocaine users. Myocarditis is frequently seen in HIV-negative patients using intravenous cocaine.

        5. There have been anecdotal reports of myocardial infarction in HIV-positive patients receiving potent antiretroviral therapy. These have generally occurred in patients who also have hyperlipidemia on treatment, leading to speculation that they are causally linked. Further elucidation of this will require larger prospective studies that control for other cardiac risk factors.

IV. Summary. Although autopsy series have shown a large number of histopathologic abnormalities, clinical manifestations of cardiac disease have been observed in relatively small numbers. Signs and symptoms of cardiac disease have not been reported in primary HIV infection. Cardiac disease does appear to be more prevalent in AIDS patients than in HIV-positive non-AIDS patients, so an aggressive approach to exclude all treatable origins should be pursued. Advances in antiretroviral therapy have led to dramatically increased survival in patients with HIV infection. Patients are now living into a period of their life when cardiovascular disease becomes more prevalent. Many patients have additional risk factors for cardiovascular disease. Furthermore, hyperlipidemia is a complication of some antiretroviral drugs. Thus it is highly likely that we should see an increase of cardiac manifestations over the next decade as opportunistic infections are controlled and survival improves.

18. RHEUMATIC ASPECTS

The rheumatic manifestations of human immunodeficiency virus (HIV) infection, although relatively uncommon, may be a major source of morbidity to patients and an area of diagnostic and therapeutic challenge for the clinician. Unfortunately, during the complicated and prolonged natural course of HIV infection, rheumatic complaints such as arthralgia, arthritis, myalgia, and weakness often go unrecognized or unattended. Early recognition and treatment of such problems can often enhance quality of life. At times, rheumatic complications such as systemic vasculitis and other connective tissue diseases may dominate the clinical picture, and appropriate therapy can prolong life. Treatment of such complications of HIV infection generally requires the use of antiinflammatory drugs and at times the use of immunosuppressive agents, which require special considerations in the immunosuppressed host.

I. **Arthritis**
   A. **Reiter's syndrome and reactive arthritis**. Reiter's syndrome is an inflammatory form of arthritis found predominantly in young men and is believed to occur more often in those infected with HIV. Classic Reiter's syndrome includes an oligoarticular inflammatory arthritis, urethritis, conjunctivitis, and characteristic skin and mucous membrane lesions. Back pain and radiographic involvement of the sacroiliac joints are common. No features clearly distinguish between HIV-infected and other forms of Reiter's syndrome, although radiographic changes in the spine or other joints or both are extremely uncommon in HIV infection.
   B. **Reactive arthritis**. Reactive arthritis, or inflammatory arthritis of one or more joints associated with enteric or sexually transmitted infections, without the other features of classic Reiter's syndrome, is also well described in HIV infection. Infectious agents often associated with these syndromes include *Shigella flexneri, Campylobacter fetus, Yersinia enterocolitica,* and *Y. pseudotuberculosis*, although in many, no infectious origin is identified.
      1. **Conservative therapy**. Treatment should commence with conservative measures including nonsteroidal antiinflammatory drugs (NSAIDs). Agents such as indomethacin or even phenylbutazone may be more effective than other newer NSAIDs but should be reserved for refractory cases. Additional measures such as physiotherapy, rest, and adjunctive analgesics to control pain also are beneficial.
      2. **Aggressive therapy**. For the small percentage of patients with disease that is resistant to conservative treatment and highly disabling, more potent antiinflammatory agents may be needed to control joint symptoms to improve quality of life.
         a. The use of sulfasalazine has theoretic merits and appears no more toxic in this setting (Disla et al. *J Rheumatol* 1994;21:662).
         b. Early reports have suggested that low-dose methotrexate (7.5 to 15 mg per week) is associated with acceleration of immunosuppressive complications and thus should be avoided. More recent views of this issue have suggested that methotrexate may be used with an acceptable balance of risks to benefits if patients are given aggressive prophylaxis for opportunistic infections (Calabrese. *Rheum Dis Clin North Am* 1993;19:477) by adhering to the principles of immunosuppression (see Section III).
         c. Low-dose corticosteroids (prednisone, 5 to 10 mg per day) also may be useful in controlling inflammation without being highly immunosuppressive. A single inflamed joint can be injected with corticosteroids.

   d. There is no evidence that antiretroviral therapy is helpful for these forms of arthritis.
C. Psoriatic arthritis. In non–HIV-infected individuals with psoriasis, ~5% to 7% have psoriatic arthritis, whereas 32% of HIV-infected patients with psoriasis have arthritis. Those with psoriatic arthritis develop an asymmetric inflammatory arthritis similar to Reiter's syndrome and reactive arthritis, which rarely involves the spine. Curiously, patients with psoriatic arthritis may have one or more features of Reiter's syndrome and have been labeled by some as having undifferentiated spondyloarthropathy (Solomon et al. *Rheum Dis Clin North Am* 1991;17:43).

   Treatment of the underlying psoriasis is extremely important and may lead to remission of arthritis in selected patients (see Chapter 12).
D. Septic arthritis. Given the array of infectious disorders observed in the HIV-infected population, it is remarkable that septic involvement of joints and their surrounding tissues and bones is uncommon (Goldenberg. *Rheum Dis Clin North Am* 1991;17:149). Infections with bacterial pathogens such as *Staphylococcus aureus* and *Streptococcus* sp. are most frequently encountered in HIV-infected intravenous drug users. Rarely opportunistic pathogens, including fungi and mycobacterium, have been reported to cause infections of bones, joints, and surrounding tissues.

   1. It is vital that all episodes of unexplained acute or subacute inflammatory arthritis be considered infectious until proven otherwise. Wherever possible, synovial fluid should be obtained and examined, including Gram's stain of a centrifuged pellet and a joint-fluid leukocyte count, as well as be cultured for typical and opportunistic organisms.

   2. Treatment. Septic arthritis in the HIV-infected patient is given treatment similar to that of the non–HIV-infected case. The use of intravenous antimicrobials appropriate to each microbiologic situation is preferred as initial therapy. Maintenance of adequate drainage by repeated synovial aspiration, if necessary, is essential, and a decreasing leukocyte count in the fluid will reflect response to treatment. Rarely open surgical drainage may be required.

E. Miscellaneous arthritic conditions. Joint complaints caused by conditions other than those mentioned are quite common in HIV-infected individuals.

   1. Mono-, oligo-, and polyarticular joint pains, with or without associated swelling or limitation of motion, may occur throughout the clinical course and increase in incidence as the disease progresses. These generally are self-limiting and nonprogressive. Conservative treatment, similar to that outlined for Reiter's syndrome, is generally adequate to provide symptomatic control.

   2. One poorly understood condition particularly deserving of comment is the **"painful articular syndrome"** (Rynes. *Rheum Dis Clin North Am* 1991;17:79). Patients with this condition have acute, severe pain in one or more joints with or without periarticular or bone pain, lasting from a few hours to a few days. Synovial fluid has been reported to be noninflammatory and free of crystals. Treatment of the condition often requires narcotic analgesics until it spontaneously subsides. Relapses are rare. Recognition is clinically important because it is often mistaken for septic or crystal-induced disease (acute gout or pseudogout).

II. Connective tissue diseases
   A. Myopathy. Symptoms and signs of muscle disease, such as pain and weakness, are frequently observed in HIV infection. A broad spectrum of muscle problems has been recognized (Simpson et al. *Neurology* 1993;43:971), and these conditions can be conveniently separated into three groups: drug-induced, inflammatory, and noninflammatory disorders. Unfortunately, some patients may have muscle signs or symptoms that do not fit neatly into this classification.

   1. Drug-induced myopathies. Zidovudine is a common cause of myopathy associated pathologically with mitochondrial changes and encountered in 17% of patients undergoing long-term treatment.

a. **Diagnosis.** Clinical manifestations vary widely from asymptomatic elevation of muscle enzymes to a severe inflammatory myopathy with weakness and associated electromyographic (EMG) and histopathologic findings (Dalakas et al. *N Engl J Med* 1990;322:1098). A myopathy seen as a wasting syndrome, complicated by anorexia, nausea, and malaise, may also be associated with zidovudine therapy. Zidovudine myopathy is more frequently encountered at high doses and with advancing HIV infection.

b. **Treatment.** Fortunately, with the availability of alternative antiretroviral agents, merely switching from zidovudine to another drug may be adequate even for patients with severe symptoms. In patients with wasting caused by zidovudine, muscle strength and muscle enzymes may return to normal within 4 to 8 weeks after discontinuing therapy (Peters et al. *Q J Med* 1993;86:5). For patients in whom zidovudine therapy is essential, NSAIDs can be efficacious in alleviating myalgia, and if necessary, corticosteroids such as prednisone (in a dose of 0.5 mg per kg per day) may be of additional benefit.

2. **Inflammatory myopathy.** A myopathy clinically and pathologically indistinguishable from idiopathic polymyositis and not related to zidovudine therapy may arise in HIV-infected individuals.

a. **Diagnosis.** Progressive proximal weakness most prominent in the lower extremities is the usual presentation. Muscle enzymes (e.g., creatine kinase and aldolase) are increased, and EMG examination reveals an active, inflammatory myopathic process. Biopsy of involved muscle confirms an active necrotizing myopathy similar to idiopathic polymyositis. Myalgias, which may be severe, are experienced by about half of the patients.

b. **Treatment.** If the patient is taking zidovudine, the drug should be stopped because the condition may be difficult to distinguish from drug-induced disease. If the patient does not then improve, or is not taking zidovudine, the cautious use of immunosuppressives should be attempted, according to the principles of immunosuppression (see the following). Generally patients with HIV infection and inflammatory myopathy respond to much lower doses of corticosteroids than patients with idiopathic polymyositis. For patients with clinically significant weakness that compromises quality of life, initial therapy should be prednisone, in the range of 0.5 mg per kg per day, and this dose maintained until muscle enzymes and strength are normalized, generally for 4 to 8 weeks. The prednisone can then be tapered to the lowest possible dose needed to control symptoms.

3. **Noninflammatory myopathy.** Muscular weakness is the cardinal symptom of this type of myopathy and is also a feature of patients with wasting. Pathologically, there is a paucity of inflammatory changes in muscle and a variety of unusual ultrastructural changes. The presence of zidovudine therapy in such patients further complicates the clinical picture. There is no satisfying treatment for HIV-infected patients with noninflammatory myopathy complicated by wasting. Aggressive nutritional support is essential. The use of immunosuppressives should be avoided, given the advanced stage of immunodeficiency and debility in such patients. The role of other more specific therapies (i.e., human growth hormone, antitumor necrosis factor-based therapies, or anabolic steroids) is still unclear (see Chapter 39).

B. **Vasculitis.** A heterogeneous group of vascular inflammatory diseases has been reported in association with HIV infection (Calabrese. *Rheumatol Clin North Am* 1991;17:131). These conditions include a broad spectrum of disorders affecting different types, sizes, and distributions of blood vessels. Although it is unclear whether these two disorders (i.e., HIV and vasculitis) are pathologically related or merely coincidental in their occurrence, their co-occurrence often creates a serious therapeutic dilemma. Vasculitis, in the non–HIV-infected patient, can be life threatening when involving vital target organs [i.e., central nervous system (CNS), kidney, pulmonary organs]. Treatment frequently involves prolonged and high-intensity immunosuppression. Vasculitis should be at least considered in the differential diagnosis in a variety of settings including unexplained multisystem disease, unexplained myopathy or arthritis, unexplained ischemia of any organ, and in the presence of mononeuritis multiplex. It is most important in the diagnosis of systemic vasculitis to rule out mimicking conditions such as disseminated infections or malignancies, both of which are common in the HIV-infected patient and capable of producing many of the same clinical findings. Diagnosis requires both appropriate clinical features and biopsy evidence of the disease.

  1. **Specific diseases.** Vasculitis can be primary, as part of an autoimmune disorder, or it may be the result of a wide variety of conditions including infections, drug use, and malignancies. Several primary vasculitic syndromes have been reported in HIV, including polyarteritis nodosa with a particular propensity to involve peripheral nerves. A purely cutaneous leukocytoclastic vasculitis also has been reported. Finally a rare form of vasculitis that selectively targets the CNS also has been reported in HIV infection.
  2. **Management.** Management should include consultation with a physician experienced in the treatment of these disorders, and the principles of immunosuppression (see the following) should be applied. Immunosuppressive therapy is usually needed; its intensity should be individually tailored to the activity and distribution of target-organ involvement.
     a. **Corticosteroids** are the mainstay of the therapy in most forms of vasculitis and may be sufficient in mild cases, particularly those limited to skin. In more severe cases, high-dose therapy (1 mg per kg per day of prednisone) may be necessary for disease control.
     b. **Immunosuppressive agents,** such as cyclophosphamide, azathioprine, and methotrexate are routinely used in the non–HIV-infected patient with life-threatening vasculitis. For obvious reasons, these agents should be considered in only the rare case in which the morbidity and predicted mortality of the vasculitic disorder outweighs the clear risk of further exacerbating the underlying immunosuppressive state.
     c. **Immunoglobulin.** There are limited data supporting the use of intravenous immunoglobulin in patients with certain forms of vasculitis, and in particular, Kawasaki's disease. Such therapy would be particularly appealing in HIV-associated vasculitis because it is not associated with immunosuppressive side effects. There is no published experience with immunoglobulin therapy in HIV-associated vasculitis.
C. **Diffuse infiltrative lymphocytosis syndrome (DILS).** DILS is a unique illness of presumed autoimmune origin found in ~1% of patients with HIV infection. It is characterized by the presence of dryness of the eyes and mouth and often massive enlargement of the parotid glands. The histopathologic findings in the minor and major salivary glands are similar to those in Sjögren's syndrome, but the conditions differ in their underlying immunopathology and genetics (Itescu et al. *Ann Intern Med* 1990;112:3). The infiltrating lymphocytes are CD8 cells, which are often numerically expanded in both tissues and peripheral blood. A variety of extraglandular features have been observed in DILS, including lymphocytic interstitial pneumonitis, which occasionally can be life threatening, interstitial gastrointestinal and renal disease, and CNS disease, including bilateral seventh nerve palsies. Curiously, the natural history of patients with DILS includes the relatively slow progression of their underlying HIV infection but with a high frequency of the late development of high-grade lymphomas.
  1. **Diagnosis** is often suspected clinically with parotid gland enlargement and/or marked CD8 expansion in peripheral blood combined with a minor salivary gland biopsy demonstrating a CD8-predominant sialadenitis.

2. **Management** of DILS is determined by the severity of glandular and extraglandular features.

   a. For treatment of the parotid gland enlargement, which is frequently cystic and occasionally highly disfiguring, **antiretroviral therapy** has been associated with a major degree of clinical regression.

   b. Radiation therapy should generally be avoided because of concerns regarding malignant transformation.

   c. **Corticosteroids** will temporarily shrink enlarged glandular tissues, but swelling generally returns with tapering of the medication.

   d. For more serious and occasionally life-threatening forms of extraglandular involvement, high-dose corticosteroids (i.e., prednisone, 1 mg per kg per day) or even cytotoxic drugs (i.e., cyclophosphamide, chlorambucil, and others) may at times be necessary (Itescu. *Rheum Dis Clin North Am* 1991;17:99). As in the therapy of HIV-associated problems discussed previously, the clinician should follow the principles of immunosuppression (see the following).

III. **Principles of immunosuppression.** The use of immunosuppressive drugs in either chronic infection or a preexisting immunosuppressive state is clearly controversial and thus in HIV the issue is all the more complex. Immunosuppressive therapy in the HIV-infected patient should not be considered absolutely contraindicated out of fear of exacerbating the underlying immunosuppressive state for a number of reasons. First, it should be recognized that with corticosteroids, there is a major dose-response relation with immune-mediated toxicity. Prednisone at doses of <0.3 mg per kg per day is relatively safe and well tolerated. Second, there is a limited role for corticosteroids in the treatment of several infectious diseases or their complications or both, such as tuberculous meningitis or pericarditis, among others (McGowan et al. *J Infect Dis* 1992;165:1). Finally, emerging data support a role for modest immunosuppression for HIV infection and some associated complications, including oropharyngeal aphthae (see Chapter 20) and disseminated *Mycobacterium avium* infections (Andrieu et al. *J Infect Dis* 1995;171:523; Wormser et al. *Antimicrob Agents Chemother* 1994;38:2215). Collectively these observations suggest that, under certain circumstances, immunosuppressive therapy may be not only tolerated but also beneficial to the HIV-infected patient. Alternatively, there is clear evidence that long-term high-level immunosuppressive therapy (prednisone, ≥1 mg per kg per day) is associated with a marked increase in susceptibility to a variety of infections, including opportunistic pathogens. Thus the decision to use such therapy in the HIV-infected patient must be weighed carefully, keeping the following principles in mind:.

   A. **Risks and benefits** must be weighed individually. For example, if a patient with advanced HIV infection has prominent morbidity from weakness caused by polymyositis, and the use of corticosteroid therapy may lead to marked improvement in quality of life, then withholding such therapy merely because of the underlying HIV infection would not appear reasonable or ethical.

   B. **Adjunctive therapy** of the underlying HIV infection including **antimicrobial prophylaxis and antiretroviral therapy** should be individualized and aggressive. For example, if a patient with a CD4+ count of >300 cells/mm³ requires high-level immunosuppression for some indication, it would be reasonable to consider prophylaxis against *Pneumocystis carinii* pneumonia (PCP), in anticipation of the iatrogenic immunosuppression that will follow. This may be particularly true for a patient not receiving effective antiretroviral therapy. Established guidelines for antimicrobial prophylaxis by using CD4+ counts are based on predicted infectious complication rates in HIV-infected patients who have not had immunosuppressive treatment.

   C. A team approach is optimal in treating HIV-infected patients with life-threatening complications of autoimmune illnesses. Such a team would ideally include the primary HIV-treating physician and a physician with expertise in autoimmune diseases and the use of a variety of immunosuppressive therapies.

19. ENDOCRINE, METABOLIC, AND BODY COMPOSITION DISORDERS

Kevin Yarasheski, Donna Marin, Sheri Claxton, and William G. Powderly

Endocrine and metabolic disorders may complicate human immunodeficiency virus (HIV) infection in many ways. Endocrine and metabolic dysfunction may result from HIV-1 infection, opportunistic illnesses, or medications used to treat HIV infection and its complications. Infection with HIV and the antiviral medications used to treat HIV have been associated with several anthropomorphic and metabolic complications including: hyperglycemia, hypertriglyceridemia, hypercholesterolemia, central adiposity, peripheral lipoatrophy, muscle wasting, and osteopenia. Their similarity with diabetes mellitus, abdominal obesity, and pro-atherogenic processes have raised concern that these complications will increase the risk for cardiovascular disease in young and middle-age men and women infected with and treated for HIV. There is no clear, universally accepted and tested case definition for these syndromes. Some were noticed in patients treated with HIV-nucleoside analogue reverse transcriptase inhibitors (NRTIs). The recent availability of HIV-aspartyl protease inhibitors (PIs) and their use in combination with antiretroviral medications [i.e., highly active antiretroviral treatment (HAART)] appears to have increased the prevalence and severity of these complications. The cause(s) of the complications have not been delineated, although emphasis has focused on the use of antiviral medications. It is likely that the complications represent several different syndromes. For example, the combined presence of lipoatrophy and lipohypertrophy in the same patient has added confusion and doubt to the hypothesis that HAART-associated metabolic complications are due to a unique, singular pathogenesis. Potential contributors to the pathogenesis include: other chronic viral infections, rapid immune reconstitution associated with HAART, route of infection, chemical dependencies, advancing age, underlying genetic predispositions, nutrient/energy intake, physical inactivity, differences in antiviral pharmacokinetics among individuals, mitochondrial toxicity (especially with NRTIs), inhibition of hepatic cytochrome-P450 isozymes (especially with PI's) and alterations in liver metabolism, PI-induced inhibition of undiscovered cellular aspartyl proteases or dysregulation of other key biochemical pathways.

Patients' concerns are clear. The anthropomorphic changes add to the stigma and outward "AIDS-appearance." Some of the changes are disfiguring and physically uncomfortable. Some patients decide to delay or discontinue HAART based simply on the undesirable metabolic complications. Therefore an understanding of these changes is essential in managing HIV infection.

I. **Pancreatic dysfunction.** Endocrine and exocrine gland disorders have been associated with medications and opportunistic pathogens [cytomegalovirus (CMV) infection].

   A. **Hyperglycemia.** Both fasting hyperglycemia and diabetic ketoacidosis have been described in patients treated with **protease inhibitors**. Some developed diabetes within 2 weeks of initiation and some after 12 months of initiating HAART. Compelling evidence that PIs caused diabetes came from case studies where hyperglycemia was normalized after PIs were discontinued. When the same or a different PI was restarted after euglycemia was achieved, hyperglycemia often returned. Fasting hyperglycemia and hyperinsulinemia are characteristics of this metabolic syndrome. One prevalence study found diabetes in 7%, impaired glucose tolerance or fasting hyperglycemia in 27%, and insulin resistance with normal glucose tolerance in 18% of HIV-infected patients receiving PIs. It appears that insulin resistance non-insulin-dependent diabetes mellitus (NIDDM) rather than insulin deficiency insulin-dependent diabetes mellitus (IDDM) is the cause of HIV-protease inhibitor-associated hyperglycemia. **Drug-induced diabetes mellitus** has also been observed with **pentamidine** and **didanosine** (Vittecoq et al. *AIDS* 1994;8:1351), both of which can induce pancreatic injury. Zalcitabine, megestrol acetate, corticosteroids, famciclovir, or sulfonamides may be associated with hyperglycemia. **Ethionamide** and **isoniazid** may affect glycemic control in persons with diabetes mellitus.

1. **Signs/symptoms** of diabetes mellitus include polyuria, polydipsia, polyphagia, and cloudy vision. Acute complications include diabetic ketoacidosis, which may occur with severe pancreatic injury. Long-term complications of diabetes mellitus typically do not develop in the HIV-infected population.
2. **Diagnosis.** Increased fasting glucose levels and glycosuria.
3. **Management**
   a. **Dietary restrictions**, physical activity, **oral hypoglycemic agents**, or **insulin** therapy with monitoring of glucose and hemoglobin A_{1C} values. **Initial drug treatment of choice** is with a sulfonylurea agent such as glyburide, 5 to 10 mg p.o. b.i.d., or glypizide, 5 to 20 mg p.o. b.i.d. Insulin should be used in persons with prior diabetic ketoacidosis, because they usually lack sufficient insulin levels. Insulin should be given in divided doses with a mixture of regular and intermediate-acting insulin for optimal glucose control. The daily requirement of insulin for most persons is 35 to 50 U per day, although lower doses may be effective. Initial treatment is often begun in the hospital with dose adjustment based on maintaining glucose levels between 100 and 200 mg per dl.
   b. Optimal therapy for **protease inhibitor associated-hyperglycemia** and diabetes has not been determined.
      (1) Switching to a **protease-sparing regimen** often eliminates the problem.
      (2) Because **insulin resistance** is a usual feature of PI-associated diabetes mellitus, metformin and/or the thiazolidinediones (e.g., rosiglitazone and pioglitazone) have been suggested as optimal therapy. In one small study, metformin restored normoinsulinemia and reduced serum triglycerides and free-fatty acids in 21 HIV-infected patients (Saint-Marc et al. *AIDS* 1999; 13:1000).
   c. **Drugs** (such as pentamidine or didanosine) that cause pancreatic damage should be stopped.
B. **Hypoglycemia. Pentamidine** can cause hypoglycemia typically within 6 hours of infusion. Sweating, weakness, and confusion occur with hypoglycemia. Management includes slowing the rate of the pentamidine infusion, supplementing with 5% to 10% D/W i.v., or switching to another agent for treatment of PCP.
C. **Pancreatitis.** Pancreatic exocrine gland injury has been associated with CMV infection, *Mycobacterium avium* complex, and biliary tract involvement with Microsporidia or Cryptosporidia. Drugs associated with pancreatitis include didanosine, zalcitabine, stavudine, sulfonamides, metronidazole, tetracycline, famciclovir, and pentamidine. **Hypertriglyceridemia** (>1,000 mg per dl) is an important risk factor for pancreatitis, as is alcohol use.
   1. **Signs/symptoms.** Abdominal pain, nausea, vomiting, fever, tenderness, ileus, and decreased bowel sounds.
   2. **Diagnosis.** Increased amylase and lipase levels. In the absence of biliary tract disease, ethanol abuse, or a medication known to cause pancreatitis, a search for an opportunistic pathogen should be considered.
   3. It is recommended that patients taking **didanosine** (especially in combination with hydroxyurea) have regular monitoring of serum amylase and/or lipase. However, the utility of this in preventing pancreatitis is unknown.

        4. Management. Restriction of food and liquid intake with or without nasogastric drainage is the optimal approach to acute pancreatitis; Histamine$_2$-receptor antagonists (cimetidine or ranitidine), anitbiotics and analgesia may be needed. The agent responsible for pancreatitis, if drug-associated, should be stopped.

II. Dyslipidemias. Hypertriglyceridemia, hypercholesterolemia, and **insulin resistance** occur commonly in patients receiving protease-inhibitor based therapy, often accompanied by **adipose tissue maldistribution** (see below). Normal serum concentrations for triglycerides, total-, HDL-, LDL-cholesterol for the US population have been established (Table 1). In people living with HIV, fasting serum lipid concentrations should be monitored and compared to the published guidelines.

    A. Hypertriglyceridemia appears to be a complication of protease inhibitors, and occurs at varying rates with all drugs. It appears to be most commonly associated with ritonavir usage. Hyperinsulinemia may contribute to the hypertriglyceridemia syndrome.

        1. Elevated serum triglycerides increase the risk for **pancreatitis**. By themselves, elevated triglycerides are not a risk factor for **cardiovascular disease,** but, when combined with elevations in total- and LDL-cholesterol and a reduction in HDL-cholesterol, the cardiovascular disease risk escalates.

        2. In accordance with the American Heart Association guidelines, **modifying eating behavior** to reduce saturated fat and simple sugar intake, reducing alcohol consumption, and **increasing physical activity** should be considered first. However, it is unreasonable to believe that nutritional counseling and increased energy expenditure will normalize severe hypertriglyceridemia.

        3. Treatment with **gemfibrozil** reduced serum triglycerides in HIV-infected patients treated with PI-based HAART (Hewitt et al. *AIDS* 1999;13:868).

        4. Swithing to a protease sparing regimen can be considered.

    B. Hypercholesterolemia. Prior to HAART, HIV infection was associated with a decline in serum HDL-cholesterol levels, followed by a reduction in LDL cholesterol levels. Hypertriglyceridemia and increased VLDL levels marked the progression to AIDS. Decreased clearance rate and increased production rate of triglyceride-rich particles, was linked to hypertriglyceridemia and increased circulating concentrations of interferon-α. In the HAART-era, HDL-cholesterol levels are reduced, total- and LDL-cholesterol levels are increased, and concomitant severe hypertriglyceridemia is observed. Both the protease inhibitors and efavirenz have been associated with elevated cholesterol, but in the case of efavirenz, HDL levels often also rise.

        1. Dietary modification and exercise should be the initial approaches to hypercholesterolemia

        2. In cases of severe hypercholesterolemia, oral **lipid-lowering agents** may be used. The **HMG-CoA-reductase** inhibitors (e.g., pravastatin, and atorvastatin), along with the lipid-lowering fibric acid derivative **gemfibrozil** have been used to lower serum cholesterol and triglycerides in

Table 1. Serum lipids and risk for cardiovascular disease and pancreatitis

	Desirable		Borderline-high risk for CHD		High risk for CHD		High risk for pancreatitis	
	mg/dL	mM	mg/dL	mM	mg/dL	mM	mg/dL	mM
Total cholesterol	<200	<5.2	200–239	5.2–6.2	≥240	≥6.2	—	
LDL cholesterol	<130	<3.4	130–159	3.4–4.1	≥160	≥4.1	—	
HDL cholesterol	>60	>1.6	—		<35	<0.9	—	
Triglycerides	<200	<2.3	200–400	2.3–4.5	>400	>4.5	>1000	>11.3
Total/HDL	<5.0		5.0–6.0		>6.0		—	

HIV-infected patients with HAART-associated dyslipidemia (Henry et al. *Lancet* 1998;352:1031). Although HMG-CoA-reductase inhibitors are effective treatments for reducing total- and LDL-cholesterol levels and increasing HDL-cholesterol levels, these agents have severe toxicities (e.g., rhabdomyolysis and polymyositis). HMG-CoA-reductase inhibitors that are substrates for the liver CYP3A4 enzyme system should be used with caution with other drugs metabolized by this system. In particular, simvastatin and lovastatin are contraindicated in combination with protease inhibitors, especially ritonavir.

   3. **Switching to a protease-sparing regimen** may also be attempted in patients with severe hypercholesterolemia.

      a. **Short-term studies of switching to** nevirapine or **abacavir** have been associated with reduction in serum lipids (although body composition changes persist).

      b. Switching to efavirenz less consistently lowers serum lipids.

III. **Body Composition-Anthropomorphic Changes.** Prior to the current era, the most common change in body composition was loss of lean muscle tissue or wasting. With the advent of more effective antiretroviral therapy, changes in adipose tissue have assumed a greater importance.

   A. **Adipose Tissue Maldistribution**. Redistribution of fat is extremely common in patients receiving combination antiretroviral therapy. Although initially ascribed to protease inhibitors, it is increasingly apparent that the etiology is more complex and may involve both protease inhibitors and nucleosides acting through different pathogenetic pathways. Both fat accumulation and fat loss can occur and both can occur in the same patient.

      1. **Lipohypertrophy** is characterized by adipose tissue accumulation, most notably in the truncal region (Safrin et al. *AIDS* 1999;13:2493–2505). Adipose tissue accumulation may be localized as in central or abdominal obesity, dorsocervical adipose tissue deposition ("buffalo hump"), or symmetrical and asymmetrical breast enlargement in men and women (Schurmann et al. *AIDS* 1998;12:2232–2233). Adipose tissue deposition may be isolated as in the development of symptomatic (pain, tenderness) subcutaneous angiolipomas (Dank et al. *J Am Acad Dermatol* 2000; 42:129–131). These are uncommon benign tumors/lesions of normal karyotype that form within the subcutaneous adipose tissue. Estimates of lipohypertrophy are broad (1% to 56%). The physical appearance (phenotype) has been likened to Cushing's Syndrome, but the pituitary-adrenal hormone axis, adrenal function and cortisol metabolism appear normal (Lo et al. *Lancet* 1998;351:867–870; Miller et al. *Lancet* 1998;351: 871–875; Yanovski et al. *J Clin Endocrinol Metab* 1999;84:1925–1931). An association with PI-based HAART has been hypothesized, but lipohypertrophy has been reported in individuals who are not receiving a PI.

      2. **Lipoatrophy** refers to a decrease or absence of subcutaneous adipose tissue. In HIV, it is most notable in the face, arms, legs, and gluteal regions. Loss of facial adipose tissue gives a characteristic "gaunt" appearance, with sunken cheeks and zygomatic prominence resulting from the loss of preauricular adipose tissue. Reduced submandibular adipose tissue may accentuate the neck muscles. Subcutaneous lipoatrophy in the arms and legs makes the underlying vasculature and tendons more prominent: the former described as a "hypervascular appearance" or "venomegaly." Estimates of prevalence are broad (1% to 24%). Lipoatrophy has been reported in individuals naïve to PI therapy and has been linked to nucleoside use, especially stavudine. Some have suggested that lipoatrophy may be a mitochondrial toxicity of long-term nucleoside use. Combined lipoatrophy and lipohypertrophy has been denoted the "**lipodystrophy syndrome**."

      3. These syndromes are best **diagnosed** by using quantifiable measures.

         a. Direct measurement of the waist-hip ratio is the simplest approach, although the least accurate for formal investigation.

      b. Axial-proton **magnetic resonance imaging (MRI)** of the abdomen and thighs is perhaps the best method for measuring subcutaneous and intra-abdominal adipose tissue cross-sectional areas. A ratio of intra-abdominal-to-total abdominal adipose tissue area >0.40 may identify a syndrome (Miller et al. *Lancet* 1998;351:871–875), but an increase in this ratio over time is perhaps the best indicator. MRI can also distinguish between abdominal "bloating or distension" vs abdominal adiposity.

      c. **Dual-energy x-ray absorptiometry (DEXA),** which is simply soft tissue mass measured with a bone densitometer, has been used to quantify truncal and appendicular (arms and legs) adipose masses. A ratio of truncal-to-appendicular adipose mass of ≥0.9 in women (Grinspoon et al. *J Clin Endocrinol Metab* 1999;84:201–206) and ≥1.1 in men (St. Marc et al. *AIDS* 2000;14:37), may be adequate indicators of the syndrome. However, this ratio may be misleading because DEXA cannot discriminate between intra-abdominal and subcutaneous adiposity. The ratio may be artificially elevated in patients who possess both peripheral lipoatrophy and central adipose tissue deposition (Safrin et al. *AIDS* 1999;13:2493–2505). Both MRI and DEXA should be considered research tools at this time.

      d. The patients' or health care providers' **perception** of changes in body dimensions can factor into the diagnosis, but should be regarded as part of a constellation of symptoms that require confirmation with objective measures.

   4. Management of fat redistribution is difficult. Clinical trials of various strategies have been initiated.

      a. Changing antiretroviral therapy has not been associated with consistent reversals of fat redistribution. The only exception to this is preliminary evidence that lipoatrophy may be improved if stavudine is discontinued.

      b. Small studies of recombinant **human growth hormone** have shown some reversal of fat accumulation. It should be noted however, that growth hormone is lipolytic, and may accentuate lipoatrophy.

      c. Surgical treatment (liposuction, removal of localized adipose tissue accumulation) may be attempted but abnormal tissue often re-accumulates.

      d. Because fat redistribution is often accompanied by **insulin resistance and hyperlipidemias**, these should also be treated. Metoformin, 500 mg bid, may be considered in patients with insulin resistance and visceral adiposity (Hadigan et al. *JAMA* 2000;284:472).

B. HIV-associated wasting is a manifestation of advanced HIV infection and often results in profound weight loss, progressive loss in muscle mass, severe fatigue, and disfigurement, and in many cases, is associated with debilitating diarrhea. Wasting also may occur late in the course of AIDS and has been reported in 25% of patients during the last 6 months of life (Chan et al. *AIDS* 1995;9:1145). As with other complications of AIDS, the incidence and prevalence of wasting has declined dramatically with the advent of potent antiretroviral therapy.

   1. CDC case definition of wasting. "Wasting syndrome" was designated as an AIDS-defining condition by the Centers for Disease Control (CDC) and Prevention in 1987. The CDC case definition of the wasting syndrome is a weight loss of ≥10% in the presence of diarrhea or fever for >30 days that is not attributable to a concurrent condition other than HIV infection itself (*MMWR* 1987;36:3S). Weight loss in HIV infection is usually episodic. Rapid weight loss is typically associated with acute systemic infections, whereas more gradual weight loss occurs in individuals with malabsorptive disorders (Macallan et al. *Am J Clin Nutr* 1993;58:417). These individuals may have periods of weight stability and spontaneous weight gain, but their wasting is usually characterized by failure fully to regain weight lost. The anabolic potential to restore weight and lean tissue during HIV is present and demonstrated by episodes of spontaneous weight gain, increases in weight in response to enteral supplementation, a shift in protein turnover from net catabolism to net anabolism during feeding, and the ability to gain weight and lean body mass (LBM) in response to protein anabolic therapy. Thus wasting is not an inevitable consequence of HIV infection; rather it is another complication that can be managed and ultimately prevented.

2. **Evaluation of the patient with HIV-associated wasting**
   a. **Patterns of weight loss.** The most useful technique to diagnose and characterize wasting involves simple monitoring and plotting of weights (Grunfeld et al. *Am J Clin Nutr* 1993;58:317). Weights should be recorded on the same scales, which are routinely calibrated. Shoes and heavy clothing, which can contribute considerable variability, should be removed. Patients with unexplained rapid weight loss should be thoroughly evaluated for occult infection and malignancy. For patients with more gradual, progressive weight loss, a gastrointestinal evaluation may be more appropriate, although there is often overlap in causes of weight loss.
   b. **Dietary assessment.** A comprehensive dietary assessment should include dietary history and estimation of current energy intake, as well as identification of factors that might interfere with food intake.
   c. **Evaluation of diarrhea and malabsorption** (see also Chapter 14)
      (1) Identification of specific pathogens should begin with a workup of stool specimens for ova and parasites, cryptosporidia, microsporidia, acid fast bacteria, and *Clostridium difficile* toxin, as well as culture for routine bacterial pathogens. Blood cultures should be collected for *M. avium* and CMV. If these evaluations fail to identify a pathogen, an endoscopic workup should be considered.
      (2) **Malabsorption** may occur in the absence of diarrhea. Patients should be questioned about free-floating fat on the toilet water as evidence of fat malabsorption. Quantitative and semiquantitative diagnostic procedures can be used to detect and characterize malabsorption. These procedures include measurement of fecal fat content, d-xylose test (an index of carbohydrate malabsorption), presence of fecal α_1-antitrypsin (evidence of protein-losing enteropathy), and breath H_2 testing for evidence of lactose intolerance. Information about specific types of malabsorption can be useful in planning diets tailored to individual tolerances.

3. **Treatment. Aggressive management of HIV infection** is the key to prevention and management of wasting. However, because wasting now typically occurs in patients failing available antiretroviral therapy, additional measures may be needed.
   a. **Minimizing or interdicting weight loss.** Aggressive dietary counseling can in many cases create periods of weight stability and even weight gain. Dietary counseling by a registered dietitian can help to identify target energy intake and food choices to suit individual tastes, practices, and tolerances. Counseling should emphasize the importance of maintaining energy intake, even during periods when eating is not pleasurable or appetite is poor.
      (1) **Oral nutritional supplements** can increase net energy intake, despite some compensatory decrease in food consumption. Special formulations are sometimes better tolerated by individuals with HIV infection, but these are typically more costly. Thus, patients should be encouraged first to try the conventional, less expensive products before those targeted to specific conditions. The primary criteria for selection of a supplement include cost, palatability, and tolerability.
      (2) **Enteral nutrition.** Individuals with impaired upper gut function might be candidates for short-term nasogastric tube feed-

ing or, for longer periods, percutaneous endoscopic gastrostomy (PEG) or percutaneous endoscopic jejunostomy (PEJ). Standard or elemental enteral formulas should be used so that the cost of the nutrition is considerably less than for parenteral feeding.

(3) **Parenteral nutrition.** Central or peripheral parenteral nutrition may stabilize and maintain nutrition and hydration in patients with loss of gastrointestinal function. The costs and risks of superinfection associated with parenteral nutrition are greater than those for enteral therapies. In addition, increases in weight and body cell mass (BCM) were limited to HIV patients with malabsorptive disorders, whereas increases in weight in patients with systemic infections consisted exclusively of fat in one study (Kotler et al. *JPEN* 1990;14:454).

b. **Treatment of serious secondary infections and malignancies** is indicated in all cases if wasting is to be reversed.

c. **Treatment of diarrhea and malabsorption.** When possible, enteropathogens must be treated. In the absence of an identified origin or available therapy, a variety of nonspecific agents can effectively control diarrhea in many patients. These include antimotility agents (loperamide, diphenoxylate/atropine, and tincture of opium), luminal agents (cholestyramine), and hormonal therapy (octreotide). Patients should be encouraged to use these agents routinely, rather than simply for occasional relief. In addition, dietary modifications such as reduction in osmotic load, making alterations in fat content, or inclusion of soluble fibers may contribute to symptomatic management of diarrhea.

d. Symptomatic relief from **nausea and vomiting** can be obtained by use of antiemetic medications. Dietary modifications that can also provide relief include alterations in the timing, size, texture, temperature, and fat and sugar content of meals.

e. **Hypogonadism**. Because normal testosterone levels may be important in preserving and restoring LBM, replacement therapy should be administered to men with low testosterone. In fact, testosterone replacement in HIV-infected men who complained of sexual dysfunction resulted in modest increases in weight (Engleson et al. *J Acquir Immune Defic Syndr* 1996;11:510).

f. **Appetite stimulants**. Both megestrol acetate and dronabinol have been approved by the FDA for anorexia in individuals with HIV infection.

(1) **Megestrol acetate (Megace)** produced increases in energy intake, weight, and sense of well-being in two randomized, double-blind, placebo-controlled trials in individuals with HIV-associated weight loss of ~10% (Von Roenn et al. *Ann Intern Med* 1994;121:393; Oster et al. *Ann Intern Med* 1994;121:400). One study evaluated doses of megestrol acetate from 100 to 800 mg per day and demonstrated that weight and sense of well-being increased in a dose-dependent manner. In both studies, the increases in weight were predominantly or exclusively fat. However, treatment with megestrol acetate has been associated with marked decreases in serum testosterone, and less often, reversible adrenal insufficiency, usually on discontinuation of megestrol acetate (Leinung et al. *Ann Intern Med* 1995;122:843).

(2) **Dronabinol (Marinol)**, the active ingredient in marijuana, in a dose of 2.5 mg twice daily, increased self-reported appetite and mood, while decreasing nausea, in a multicentered, placebo-controlled trial in patients with HIV-associated wasting. However, no significant effect was demonstrated on body weight. The predominant side effects noted in both studies included euphoria, dizziness, thinking abnormalities, and somnolence.

g. Recombinant human growth hormone. In a double-blind, placebo-controlled, randomized trial, rhGH (0.1 mg per kg per day for 3 months) increased weight 1.6 kg and lean body mass 3.0 kg (by DEXA), and reduced adipose tissue mass 1.7 kg in men with HIV-associated wasting. Side effects of rhGH administration may limit its usefulness. They include arthralgia, myalgia, fluid retention, carpal tunnel compression, diarrhea, hyperglycemia, hyperinsulinemia, and hypertriglyceridemia. The latter side effects are most worrisome in the current era of HAART-associated impairments in lipid and glucose homeostasis. Growth hormone has been approved by the FDA for HIV-associated wasting in a dose of 6 mg per day for patients with weights >55 kg and lower doses for weights <55 kg. The cost of this recombinant agent limits its accessibility for many patients.

h. Pharmacologic use of anabolic steroids. The efficacy and safety of pharmacologic doses of testosterone and its derivatives have not been established in patients with HIV-associated wasting. These agents vary in the extent of their anabolic and androgenic properties and potential toxicities. Attention must be given to possible liver toxicity (especially peliosis hepatis and liver tumors), which is more likely with the 17-methyl substituted oral formulations.

IV. Metabolic disorders. Metabolic disorders are very common in advanced HIV disease. Typically these disorders are easily reversible. Table 2 indicates the most commonly observed metabolic derangements seen with medications often used in persons with HIV-1 infection.

Table 2. Medications that cause metabolic disorders

HYPOCALCEMIA	HYPOMAGNESEMIA
Didanosine	Amphotericin B
Foscarnet	Foscarnet
Ketoconazole	Aminoglycosides
Pentamidine	Cidofovir
HYPERCALCEMIA	HYPONATREMIA
Foscarnet	Amphotericin B
	Miconazole
HYPOGLYCEMIA	Vidarabine
Pentamidine	Pentamidine
	Trimethoprim
HYPERGLYCEMIA	
Didanosine	HYPERNATREMIA
Glucocorticoids	Amphotericin B
Pentamidine	Foscarnet
	Para-amino salicylic acid
HYPOKALEMIA	Penicillins
Aminoglycosides	Rifampin
Amphotericin B	
Didanosine	HYPOPHOSPHATEMIA
Foscarnet	Foscarnet
Penicillins	
Pentamidine	HYPERPHOSPHATEMIA
Cidofovir	Foscarnet
	Rifampin
HYPERKALEMIA	
Pentamidine	HYPERURICEMIA
Trimethoprim	Didanosine
	Ethambutol
	Pyrazinamide

A. Hyponatremia. Hyponatremia is usually classified by the volume status of the patient and is common in hospitalized persons with AIDS (Tang et al. *Am J Med* 1993;94:169). Causes other than the medications listed in Table 2 include diuretics, adrenal insufficiency, syndrome of inappropriate secretion of antidiuretic hormone (SIADH), excess free water consumption, fluid overload states (e.g., renal or heart failure), hyperglycemia, and renal losses. There are usually few symptoms unless hypotonic hyponatremia is present. Headaches, nausea, malaise, lethargy, cramps, delirium, psychosis, seizures, and coma may occur. Management is dependent on the underlying cause. Correction of hypotonic hyponatremia should not exceed 0.5 mEq per L per hour. The use of 3% saline is rarely indicated, as 0.9% saline is usually sufficient to correct the deficit.

B. Hypernatremia. Hypernatremia occurs only in hyperosmolar states. Common causes include dehydration and diabetes insipidus (DI). Diarrhea may be accompanied by hypernatremia. Clinical manifestations of hypernatremia include tremulousness, irritability, ataxia, spasticity, confusion, seizures, and coma. Correction of the fluid deficit should begin with isotonic saline if there is hypotension; otherwise, 0.45% saline is usually adequate. The volume deficit should be calculated to determine the required amount of fluid replacement with the following formula:

$$\text{Body water deficit (liters)} = [0.5 \times \text{current weight (kg)}$$

$$\times \{\text{plasma } [Na^+]/140) - 1\} \qquad (1)$$

C. Hyperkalemia. Renal failure, hypoaldosteronism, and medications are the leading causes of hyperkalemia. Clinical manifestations are uncommon unless the potassium increases to >6.5 mEq per L. Muscle weakness, paresthesias, areflexia, and ascending paralysis may occur. Cardiac manifestations are the most worrisome and include progression from bradycardia, heart block, asystole, and ventricular fibrillation. Peaked T waves and a shortened QT interval are the earliest signs on the electrocardiogram (ECG). **Treatment depends on the severity of the elevation of the potassium.** At potassium levels of 5.0 to 6.0 mEq per L without cardiac compromise, cation-exchange resins (sodium polystyrene sulfonate, 50 g) can be used to decrease the potassium level within 4 to 6 hours by 0.5 to 1.0 mEq per L. Higher potassium levels or serious manifestations require urgent treatment with glucose and insulin, sodium bicarbonate, and calcium. Hemodialysis may be necessary.

D. Hypokalemia. Renal and extrarenal losses are the most common causes in AIDS. Diarrheal illnesses (e.g., Cryptosporidiosis, wasting syndrome) and medications are the most important causes in HIV-1–infected patients. The signs and symptoms of hypokalemia are usually mild unless the potassium level decreases to <2.5 mEq per L. Malaise, fatigue, weakness, hyporeflexia, paresthesias, cramps, restless legs syndrome, paralysis, constipation, ileus, vomiting, and cardiac abnormalities (orthostatic hypotension, arrhythmias, and ECG changes) are the usual manifestations. For mild hypokalemia, oral potassium chloride, 10 to 40 mEq, may be given once or twice daily. Intravenous potassium may be necessary for severe manifestations or potassium levels <3.0 mEq per L. In HIV-1–infected patients, frequent monitoring of potassium levels is warranted when using amphotericin B or foscarnet. It is important to note that magnesium deficiency may cause persistent or refractory hypokalemia.

E. Calcium disorders (refer to Section III for manifestations and management recommendations) in general, are very uncommon in HIV-1–infected persons. Hypercalcemia occasionally occurs with granulomatous diseases (e.g., tuberculosis), lymphomas, and CMV infection (Zaloga et al. *Ann Intern Med* 1985;102:331). Hypocalcemia most commonly is associated with the use of medications listed in Table 2.

F. **Magnesium disorders**. Hypomagnesemia is a side effect of several medications used in the treatment of AIDS patients and occurs commonly in persons receiving prolonged courses of amphotericin B. The manifestations are similar to those seen with hypokalemia and hypocalcemia, which often accompany hypomagnesemia. Treatment of mild or chronic hypomagnesemia consists of magnesium oxide preparations providing 240 mg per day or twice daily of elemental magnesium p.o. Severe or symptomatic disease should be treated with 50% magnesium sulfate (4 mEq per mL), 2 to 4 mL i.v. over 15 minutes followed by an infusion over 3 to 7 days to replenish stores. Hypermagnesemia is not frequently encountered in patients with HIV-1 infection.

G. **Miscellaneous metabolic disorders**. Disorders of phosphate metabolism usually occur with treatment with medications (Table 2). Disorders of acid–base balance are usually the result of severe underlying illnesses. Amphotericin B, cidofovir, and aminoglycosides can cause renal tubular acidosis.

H. **Lactic acidosis** has been reported in HIV-1–infected patients usually accompanied by microvesicular steatosis of the liver. Virtually all such patients have received nucleoside analogs and cases have been reported with all NRTIs. More severe (fatal) cases have been reported in women.

   1. **Pathogenesis.** It is believed that nucleoside-associated mitochondrial toxicity leads to impaired oxidative phosphorylation and increased lactate. NRTI's are dideoxynucleosides that can potently inhibit mitochondrial DNA polymerase gamma activity, the only polymerase involved in replication of mitochondrial DNA. Inhibition of polymerase-gamma can impair the ability of mitochondria to provide ATP to the cell (especially muscle cells, hepatocytes, adipocytes) by inhibiting electron-transport and oxidative phosphorylation pathways. Tissues that transport and phosphorylate NRTIs, or rely heavily on mitochondrial oxidative phosphorylation for energy, or have slow mitochondrial DNA turnover rates (post-mitotic tissues) will accumulate the largest number of mitochondrial DNA impairments and potentially the greatest loss of function.

   2. **Diagnosis. Serum lactate** levels can be monitored. In a number of series, as many as 10% of patients taking chronic nucleosides had elevated serum lactates, usually without symptoms. Hyperlactatemia is defined as a lactate level above 2 mmol per L. If levels exceed 5 mmol per L, mortality is high.

   3. A syndrome of **nucleoside metabolic dysfunction** accompanied by lactic acidemia has recently been described and may represent another (earlier) manifestation of nucleoside-associated mitochondrial dysfunction. Symptoms include peripheral wasting, lipoatrophy, abdominal distension, weight loss, fatigue, nausea, abdominal pain. Biochemical evidence of liver dysfunction is common.

   4. **Management.** Early recognition is essential. Symptoms can include fatigue, nausea, abdominal pain, and shortness of breath.

      a. Immediate **cessation of nucleoside therapy** is necessary. It is unclear whether nucleosides can be resumed in the future.

      b. The role of supplemental therapy (dichloroacetate, coenzyme Q, thiamine, riboflavin, carnitine) to improve oxidative phosphorylation is unclear. There is anecdotal data only, and these agents have not be shown to be effective in other causes of metabolic acidosis.

V. **Disorders of the pituitary gland and hypothalamus**. These are uncommon in HIV-1 infection. *Toxoplasma gondii,* CMV, herpes simplex virus, varicella-zoster virus, *Mycobacterium tuberculosis, Cryptococcus neoformans, Pneumocystis carinii,* and lymphoma may affect the hypothalamus or pituitary gland (Sano et al. *Arch Pathol Lab Med* 1989;113:1066). Histopathologic abnormalities are observed more frequently than clinical disturbances. Headaches and visual disturbances (diplopia, visual field defects or decreased acuity) indicate mass effect from a lesion compressing the optic chiasm. MRI is the best test for detecting mass lesions of the pituitary gland or hypothalamus.

A. **Gonadotropin deficiency**. Hypogonadism is common in HIV-1 infection (see also Section V). Follicle-stimulating hormone (FSH) and luteinizing hormone (LH) levels can be normal. Hypogonadotropic hypogonadism [decreased production or release of gonadotropin-releasing hormone (GnRH)] is a common cause of sexual dysfunction in persons with AIDS (Croxson et al. *J Clin Endocrinol Metab* 1989;68:317).

   1. **Signs/symptoms**. Decreased libido, gynecomastia, impotence, or amenorrhea.
   2. **Diagnosis**. Low or normal levels of FSH or LH in response to GnRH stimulation (100 μg) suggest pituitary or hypothalamic disease. An MRI should be performed.
   3. **Management**. Therapy with hormone replacement should be individualized (see Section IX). Treatment of the underlying cause may not reverse hormonal abnormalities. Biopsy or surgical resection is rarely indicated.

B. **SIADH**. Although hyponatremia is not infrequent in HIV infection, SIADH is uncommon. SIADH has been associated with treatment of *Pneumocystis carinii* pneumonia (PCP) with pentamidine. SIADH is characterized by hypotonic hyponatremia with inappropriately increased urine sodium levels (>20 mEq per L). The diagnosis is made by fluid restriction with evaluation of the serum osmolality, urine osmolality, and sodium levels. Treatment includes water restriction, loop diuretics, and demeclocycline (150 to 300 mg p.o. b.i.d.).

C. **Diabetes insipidus**. DI is manifested by polyuria, polydipsia, dehydration, hypernatremia, and an increased serum osmolality. Nephrogenic DI has been reported in association with amphotericin B and foscarnet (Farese et al. *Ann Intern Med* 1990;112:955). The diagnosis is established by a water-deprivation test. Central DI responds to desmopressin (dDAVP), whereas nephrogenic DI does not. Amphotericin B–induced nephrogenic DI may respond to indomethacin (Hohler et al. *Clin Investig* 1994;72:769).

D. **Growth-hormone deficiency**. Growth failure is common in children with acquired immunodeficiency syndrome (AIDS); however, growth-hormone deficiency has rarely been reported in AIDS.

E. **Panhypopituitarism** has been reported in patients with extensive cerebral toxoplasmosis. Panhypopituitarism is manifested by signs and symptoms of multiorgan endocrine-gland failure. Diagnosis can be made by evaluating adrenal and thyroid gland function. **If target hormone levels are low, pituitary trophic hormone levels can be measured**. A cosyntropin (Cortrosyn) stimulation test is quite sensitive for secondary adrenal failure. An MRI should be performed. Therapy for thyroid and adrenal dysfunction is mandatory.

F. **Hyperprolactinemia**. Mild increase of serum prolactin levels in persons with advanced HIV disease is common but typically asymptomatic.

VI. **Thyroid function. Symptomatic thyroid disease is rare in persons with HIV infection**. However, abnormal thyroid-function studies are common in persons with chronic disease such as AIDS. The sick euthyroid syndrome with low free thyroxine (T_4) or triiodothyronine (T_3) levels or both is the most commonly observed problem. Kaposi's sarcoma, extrapulmonary *P. carinii* (Gallant et al. *Am J Med* 1988;84:303), and CMV infections have all been associated with thyroid gland disease. Typically, these infections cause thyroid gland masses or nodules without hormonal dysfunction.

A. **Signs/symptoms. Hypothyroidism** is manifested by cold intolerance, fatigue, somnolence, poor memory, constipation, menorrhagia, myalgias, and hoarseness. Signs include slow tendon-reflex relaxation, bradycardia, facial and periorbital edema, dry skin, and nonpitting edema (myxedema). **Hyperthyroidism** is manifested by heat intolerance, weight loss, weakness, palpitations, oligomenorrhea, frequent stools, and anxiety. Signs include brisk tendon reflexes, fine tremor, proximal weakness, stare, and lid lag.

B. Diagnosis. The plasma thyroid-stimulating hormone (TSH) level is the best initial diagnostic test for thyroid disorders.
  1. **Hypothyroidism.** A normal TSH value excludes primary hypothyroidism. An increased TSH level (>20 μU per mL) confirms the diagnosis of hypothyroidism. If plasma TSH is moderately increased (<20 μU per mL), the plasma T_4 index should be measured. If secondary hypothyroidism is suspected because of evidence of pituitary disease, the plasma T_4 index should be measured because TSH levels are usually within the reference range of normal.
  2. **Hyperthyroidism.** A plasma TSH level >0.1 μU per mL excludes clinical hyperthyroidism. If the plasma TSH is <0.1 μU per mL, then the plasma T_4 index and plasma T_3 levels should be measured to establish the diagnosis and determine the baseline therapy indicated.
C. Management. Therapy is not indicated for the euthyroid sick syndrome.
  1. **Hypothyroidism. Thyroxine is the drug of choice.** The usual replacement dosage is 75 to 150 μg per day p.o. Patients with hypothyroidism who take rifampin may need thyroxine dose adjustment because of increased levothyroxine clearance.
  2. **Hyperthyroidism.** Transient thyroiditis may require only symptomatic treatment with antiinflammatory medications (ibuprofen). Hyperthyroidism is treated with **radioactive iodine, thioanomides, or surgical therapy.** Consultation with an endocrinologist is useful in determining the most appropriate choice of therapy.
  3. **Thyroid gland mass.** The diagnosis of a thyroid gland mass or nodule is typically made by palpation. **Needle-aspiration biopsy** is the best method to evaluate for opportunistic pathogens. Kaposi's sarcoma, *P. carinii,* and CMV may all cause diffuse thyroid gland enlargement with or without thyroid gland dysfunction. Iodoquinal, sulfonamides, and *para*-aminosalicylic acid (PAS) may cause goiter.

VII. Parathyroid function
  A. Hyperparathyroidism is rarely associated with HIV infection and usually causes asymptomatic hypercalcemia. Symptoms do not usually occur until the calcium level increases to >12 mg per dL.
  B. Hypoparathyroidism. There are rare reports of hypoparathyroidism in AIDS (Lehmann et al. *Horm Res* 1994;42:295).
   1. **Signs/symptoms. Hypocalcemia** is the main problem. Manifestations include tetany, muscle cramps, paresthesias, or in more severe cases, confusion, lethargy, seizures, heart failure, or rarely, laryngospasm. Hypocalcemia can be a side effect of therapy.
   2. **Diagnosis.** Measurement of a low ionized calcium and serum parathyroid hormone (PTH) level in the absence of magnesium deficiency.
   3. **Management.** Short-term management consists of infusion of 10% calcium gluconate (90 mg elemental calcium per 10 mL), two ampules (20 mL) i.v. >10 minutes, followed by infusion of calcium gluconate in 500 mL 5% D/W (1 g per mL) at 0.5 to 2.0 mg per kg per hour for serious manifestations of hypocalcemia. Long-term management consists of calcium supplements (1 to 2 g of elemental calcium p.o. t.i.d. during acute phase and 0.5 to 1.0 g with meals t.i.d. thereafter) and vitamin D supplementation. Calcitriol in doses of 0.5 to 2.0 mg per day p.o. is usually sufficient. Dosing is usually started at 0.25 mg per day p.o. and increased over 2 to 4 weeks.

VIII. Adrenal function. Histopathologic abnormalities of the adrenal glands are commonly observed at autopsy, but clinical dysfunction is uncommon (Glasgow et al. *Am J Clin Pathol* 1985;84:594). *Histoplasma capsulatum*, CMV, *M. tuberculosis*, *M. avium* complex, *C. neoformans,* Kaposi's sarcoma, and medications (ketoconazole, rifampin, fluconazole, itraconazole, and megestrol acetate) may cause adrenal dysfunction.
  A. Adrenal insufficiency is the most common serious endocrine disorder, although it occurs in <5% of persons with AIDS.

1. **Signs/symptoms**. Weakness, fatigue, weight loss, anorexia, diarrhea, hypotension, hypovolemia, hyperpigmentation, hyponatremia, and hyperkalemia.
2. **Diagnosis** can be made by demonstrating low basal serum cortisol levels. A blunted response to the Cortrosyn stimulation test (administration of cosyntropin, 250 μg i.v., with baseline, 30-, and 60-minute measurements of serum cortisol levels) is diagnostic. The cortisol level should double its baseline value and is usually >20 μg per dl with normal adrenal function.
3. **Management. Adrenal crisis with hypotension should be treated immediately with hydrocortisone, 100 mg i.v. every 8 hours** and volume expansion with 0.9% saline. If the diagnosis has not been established, a single dose of dexamethasone, 10 mg i.v. should be given, and the cosyntropin (Cortrosyn) stimulation test performed. Maintenance therapy usually consists of prednisone, 5 mg p.o. every morning and 2.5 mg every evening. Fludrocortisone, 0.1 mg per day p.o. is usually added in persons with primary adrenal failure. Illnesses, injury, or surgery may all increase the need for steroid replacement.
   B. **Hypercortisolism.** Cushing's syndrome has rarely been reported in persons with HIV-1 infection. It has been reported in persons taking megestrol acetate. Rebound hypoadrenalism can occur when megestrol is stopped.
IX. **Hypogonadism is the most commonly observed endocrine disorder in HIV-1 infection** typically affecting persons with more advanced disease.
   A. **Testicular failure.** Testicular atrophy with fibrosis and low sperm counts is common. Testicular failure can result from opportunistic infections, HIV-1 infection, common sexually transmitted diseases, neoplasms, or medications (e.g., ketoconazole, megestrol acetate, antineoplastic drugs, corticosteroids, opiates, and antibiotics). Opportunistic pathogens reported to infect the testes include CMV, *T. gondii*, *H. capsulatum*, *M. avium* complex, and *M. tuberculosis*.
      1. **Signs/symptoms.** Decreased libido, gynecomastia, impotence, loss of muscle mass, infertility, and testicular atrophy.
      2. **Diagnosis.** The hallmark is a low serum testosterone level. Total and free testosterone levels are reduced. In primary testicular failure, the LH and FSH levels are increased. Testicular masses require biopsy for neoplasm or infection.
      3. **Management. Methyltestosterone**, 10 to 50 mg per day p.o., **testosterone** cypionate or enanthate 50 to 400 mg **i.m.** every 2 to 4 weeks, or **transdermal testosterone**, 6-mg patches applied to hairless area of the scrotum daily, are all effective.
   B. **Menstrual disorders/hypogonadism.** Approximately one-third of HIV-1–infected women have dysmenorrhea, oligomenorrhea, or amenorrhea although the role of HIV infection is unclear. Megestrol acetate and systemic azoles (i.e., ketoconazole) may cause menstrual disorders. Drugs that cause thrombocytopenia (e.g., chemotherapy or ganciclovir) may cause uterine bleeding.
      1. **Signs/symptoms.** Oligo- or amenorrhea, metromenorrhagia, cramps, fatigue, iron-deficiency anemia, vaginal dryness, hot flashes, flushing, and mood disorders.
      2. **Diagnosis and management.** There are no controlled trials on the optimal management of menstrual disorders or hypogonadism in women with HIV-1 infection. Standard approaches should be used.
         a. **Abnormal bleeding.** Evaluate for cervical or uterine abnormalities (tumors), use of hormonal therapy (i.e., birth control), pregnancy (serum β-HCG) thrombocytopenia, or prolonged bleeding time. Refer to a gynecologist for further evaluation and treatment.
         b. **Oligomenorrhea or amenorrhea.** Evaluate for use of hormonal therapy and pregnancy (serum β-HCG). Premature ovarian failure can be distinguished from hypogonadotropic hypogonadism by

measuring FSH, LH, and estradiol levels. In ovarian failure, the FSH and LH levels are high, whereas they are low or normal in hypothalamic or pituitary gland disease. Treatment with estrogens and progesterones (oral contraceptives) to regularize menstrual cycles may be considered.

  c. **Menopause.** Treatment with conjugated estrogens (Premarin), 0.625 mg per day p.o. often eliminates symptoms associated with menopause.

X. Bone Disorders.

  A. **Bone Demineralization.** Recent evidence suggests that osteopenia and osteoporosis of the lumbar spine (L_1–L_4) and proximal femur (hip) regions may occur as a complication of PI-based HAART (Tebas et al. *AIDS* 2000;14:F63). Hypogonadism or central adiposity does not appear to explain bone demineralization. Prior to HAART, only marginally lower spine BMD was noted in HIV+ men.

  B. **Avascular necrosis** has been reported in several case reports. The areas most often affected are the femoral and humeral heads, femoral condyles, proximal tibia, and some of the small bones in the hand and wrist. It may be limited to one site or involve multiple areas. If the hips are involved, bilateral disease is usual. In HIV+ individuals not receiving corticosteroid therapy, hypercoagulability and hyperlipidemia may influence the development of osteonecrosis. There is no clear relationship to antiretroviral therapy. Patients usually present with pain. Treatment usually requires joint replacement.

20. ORAL AND ENT PROBLEMS

The Mouth

The mouth is an important "window" to both the diagnosis and prognostic staging of human immunodeficiency virus (HIV) infection. In the absence of antimicrobial prophylaxis, almost all patients with acquired immunodeficiency syndrome (AIDS) will develop a characteristic oral lesion at some point in their clinical course, with oral candidiasis and hairy leukoplakia being most common. Prevalences of oral lesions in HIV-infected individuals have been reported to range from 15% to 100%; the higher figures reported in populations with advanced AIDS.

The finding of an oral lesion described in this chapter should raise the possibility in the mind of the treating physician of the presence of HIV infection in the patient, even when high-risk behavior for the infection has not been elicited. In a patient known to be infected with HIV, the presence of oral candidiasis or oral hairy leukoplakia is suggestive of significant immunosuppression and has prognostic significance for assessing the degree of clinical progression of the disease. In addition, these lesions are sometimes useful markers by which to judge the clinical response to the initiation or alteration of an anti-HIV therapeutic regimen. Kaposi's sarcoma and non-Hodgkin's lymphoma are two common neoplasms associated with HIV infection; they frequently are seen first in the mouth. Similarly, idiopathic aphthous ulcers and salivary gland disease, processes presumably caused by the HIV-induced derangement of the immune system, commonly manifest in the mouth.

I. Infections of the oral cavity

A. Fungal

1. **Candidiasis.** As noted, the presence of oral candidiasis in a patient may be an indicator of underlying HIV disease. In addition, it is associated with clinical progression of the HIV infection. However, other immunosuppressive illnesses (e.g., cancer, organ transplantation, or diabetes mellitus), old age, infancy, and the administration of antibiotics and immunosuppressive medications can predispose to the occurrence of oral candidiasis. Therefore, it is not a specific indicator of HIV infection. The diagnostic features of the different forms of oral candidiasis (erythematous candidiasis, pseudomembranous candidiasis, or angular cheilitis) and the treatment of this infection are reviewed in Chapter 24.

2. **Other fungal infections.** Patients with systemic fungal infections, such as histoplasmosis, cryptococcosis, and aspergillosis, may have oral lesions that may aid the diagnostic process. Refer to Chapter 24 for details of diagnosis and treatment.

B. Viral

1. **Oral hairy leukoplakia**

   a. **Description.** Hairy leukoplakia is a white corrugated lesion linked to **Epstein–Barr Virus (EBV)** that most commonly occurs bilaterally on the lateral surfaces of the tongue. From there, it may extend over to the ventral surface. Occasionally, it is found in other areas of the oropharyngeal mucosa. The presence of this lesion is highly suggestive of concurrent HIV infection, although it is occasionally found in organ-transplant recipients and other immunosuppressed individuals. There have been occasional reports of this lesion in seemingly immunocompetent persons. It is seen in 15% to 35% of HIV-infected persons, being more prevalent in those with advanced HIV

The author acknowledges the contribution of Jeffrey M. Jacobson to the previous edition of this chapter.

disease. Independent of CD4+ lymphocyte count, its presence has predictive value for the development of AIDS.

b. Diagnosis. The diagnosis usually can be made from clinical appearance. However, occasionally, a biopsy or cell scraping must be performed to distinguish it from candidiasis or other lesions. Histologic findings include a thickened epithelium, with acanthosis, hyperparakeratosis, and large vacuolated prickle cells. Some of these characteristic histologic features of hairy leukoplakia are occasionally present in other conditions, and the specific diagnosis is dependent on the demonstration of EBV in the sample by in situ hybridization, immunohistochemical staining, or electron microscopy.

c. Treatment. Hairy leukoplakia rarely needs to be treated. It has a fluctuating course and usually causes no symptoms. Effective antiretroviral and immune-restoration therapies have been reported to cause improvements in oral hairy leukoplakia (OHL) lesions. If treatment is necessary because of appearance or discomfort, acyclovir, 200 mg p.o. 5 times daily, is effective (Resnick et al. *JAMA* 1988; 259:384). Topical retinoids and podophyllin resin, 25% solution, are also effective. The topical retinoid, 0.05% solution, is applied to the lesion for 1 to 2 minutes daily for several days. The podophyllin resin, 25% solution, is applied 2 to 3 times in a 24-hour period. Wait 1 week to see the full effect of the treatment on healing. If complete resolution of the lesion has not occurred, the treatment may be repeated at that time. Recurrences are common with all these treatments.

2. Herpes simplex. This infection manifests as recurrent single or multiple intraoral ulcers or herpes labialis. The lesions occasionally enlarge and persist. The treatment of herpes simplex infections is described in Chapter 25.

3. Cytomegalovirus (CMV). This virus occasionally causes ulcerations of the oropharyngeal mucosa in patients with advanced HIV disease that may occur alone or as a manifestation of disseminated CMV infection. Because CMV can be shed in the saliva in the absence of disease, diagnosis is based on histologic evidence of CMV in the ulcer(s). The treatment is described in Chapter 25.

4. Varicella-zoster can manifest in the trigeminal dermatome. (See Chapter 25.)

5. Papillomavirus infection manifests in the mouth either as white or pink papillomaform warts that may be single or multiple, or as flat warts that resemble focal epithelial hyperplasia. The lesions are usually asymptomatic, but if they are bothersome, surgical or laser excision, cryotherapy, or electrocoagulation may be attempted. The warts frequently recur.

C. Bacterial

1. Periodontal infections. Although not a common problem, periodontal disease in the HIV-infected patient may become rapidly destructive and difficult to manage. The early involvement of adequately trained dentists is essential in the care of these infectious processes. Several lesions have been described, although their uniqueness to patients with HIV disease remains controversial. Similarly, the inter-relation of these entities is still poorly understood. It has not been firmly established whether the more severe forms of periodontitis are associated with more advanced HIV disease. As in non–HIV-infected patients, a mixture of anaerobic bacteria play the dominant role in these infections.

a. HIV gingivitis, or linear gingival erythema, consists of an erythematous band of inflammation along the marginal gingiva. This inflammation is unrelated to plaque and calculus formation, and unlike non-HIV chronic gingivitis, the regular removal of plaque does not improve the inflammation. A common clinical presentation is spontaneous gum bleeding. The treatment consists of irrigation of the affected area with 10% povidone–iodine solution followed by 0.12% chlorhexidine gluconate mouth rinses. Patients should rinse their mouths with chlorhexidine 3 times per day until healing is seen, and then twice daily as prophylactic therapy. Side effects are minimal but include taste disturbance, mucosal discomfort and desquamation, and staining of the teeth and tongue.

   b. **More aggressive necrosis and ulceration** of the periodontal tissues may occur. Such a process confined to the free gingival margin is referred to as **necrotizing ulcerative gingivitis**. Extension of the ulceration into the attached gingiva with exposure and destruction of bone is characteristic of **HIV periodontitis.** Tooth loosening and loss may result. Spread of this process to the adjacent oral mucosa or palate leads to a **necrotizing stomatitis.** All of these lesions may be accompanied by severe pain, fever, gingival bleeding, and foul breath. Treatment consists of irrigation with 10% povidone–iodine solution, debridement of necrotic gingival and bone tissue, removal of plaque and calculus, followed by the 0.12% chlorhexidine gluconate mouth-rinse regimen described previously. The more severe lesions require the administration of systemic antibiotics with antianaerobic bacteria activity. These include clindamycin, 450 mg p.o. 3 times a day; metronidazole, 250 mg p.o. 4 times a day; or amoxicillin/clavulanate, 250 mg p.o. 3 times a day; each for a 4- to 5-day course. Pain medication may be necessary. The patient should be followed up frequently to assess healing and the need for repeat debridements. The intervals will depend on the severity of the infection but should be at least every other day for the more aggressive lesions.

II. Neoplasms of the oral cavity
A. Kaposi's sarcoma
   1. **Background**. Kaposi's sarcoma was one of the first features to be associated with AIDS at the beginning of the epidemic, although cases have occurred in noninfected individuals. It is more common in homosexual men with HIV infection. The etiologic agent has now been identified as a virus in the herpes family, human herpesvirus 8 (HHV-8).
   2. **Clinical presentation**. The mouth is a common location for Kaposi's sarcoma. It is usually seen on the hard palate, but the gingiva and posterior pharynx also may be involved. Occasionally the tongue is a site. Lesions are usually red, blue, or violet and flat, raised, nodular, or bulky. Whereas the flat and smaller lesions may be asymptomatic, the bulkier ones may ulcerate and bleed. They may cause significant pain and, occasionally, swallowing problems. Biopsy should be performed to establish the diagnosis.
   3. **Treatment.** The treatment of Kaposi's sarcoma is discussed fully in Chapter 28. Oral lesions should probably be treated early to prevent progression to the more severe, bulkier forms. Excision of small lesions by either surgery, carbon dioxide laser, or cryotherapy may be attempted. Intralesion injections with chemotherapy (vinblastine, 0.1 mL, mixed with 0.1 mL saline); α-interferon, 3 to 5 million units 3 times per week; or a sclerosing agent (sodium tetradecyl sulfate, 3% solution, 0.2 mL per cm lesion up to 0:8 mL) are alternatives. These injections are painful and should be preceded by local anesthesia. Larger lesions should be treated with local radiation therapy (800 cGy or the equivalent in fractionated doses). Particularly troublesome disease may respond to systemic approaches (see Chapter 28).

B. Lymphoma. Non-Hodgkin's lymphoma associated with AIDS may manifest in the mouth as an ulcer, nodule, or diffuse swelling. Biopsy is essential for diagnosis. The treatment is described in Chapter 29.
C. Squamous cell carcinoma. Cases of oral squamous cell carcinoma in HIV-infected persons have been described, but it has not been firmly established that this cancer occurs at an increased frequency with HIV infection. An

unusual feature of HIV-associated oral squamous cell carcinoma is that it occurs at a younger age than reported in the general population. Most cases are in patients younger than 45 years. This is uncommon in non–HIV-infected individuals. Lesions may appear as either leukoplakia, erythroplakia, or ulceration. The most common locations are the posterior tongue, floor of the mouth, tonsillar fossa, and soft palate. The diagnosis is made by tissue biopsy. Treatment consists of surgery, radiation, or both, depending on the tumor stage and site of disease.

   D. Basal cell carcinoma. Reports of a number of cases of basal cell carcinomas in HIV-infected persons have led to an impression that there is an increased frequency of this lesion in those with HIV infection. The treatment is surgical excision.

III. Idiopathic oral aphthous ulcers

   A. Clinical presentation. Aphthous ulcers may manifest in the mouth as anything from self-limited pinpoint to progressively enlarging destructive lesions that can be single or multiple. They are frequently recurrent. Pain can be quite severe and interfere with eating. The larger destructive ulcers in particular are associated with advanced HIV disease, although oral and esophageal ulceration has been described in patients with acute HIV infection.

   B. Management. After a negative culture of the lesion for herpes simplex, the smaller ulcers may be observed for spontaneous clearing, and if that does not occur, empirically treated with a topical corticosteroid preparation (fluocinonide ointment, 0.05%, as a 50%/50% mixture with carboxymethylcellulose sodium in plasticized hydrocarbon gel to the lesions 4 to 6 times per day or dexamethasone elixir, 0.5 mg per 5 mL, mouth rinses, 1 to 2 tsp q.i.d.). Larger or persistent lesions should have biopsies to rule out infectious (herpes simplex, CMV) and neoplastic causes. It should be remembered that medications used by HIV-infected persons, such as dideoxycytidine (ddC), can cause oral ulcerations. A dental examination by an experienced practitioner should eliminate HIV-associated periodontitis as a possibility. **Thalidomide,** 200 mg per day p.o., given for 4 weeks, is the only medication proven effective for the larger lesion in a controlled study (Jacobson et al. *N Eng J Med* 1997;336:1487). Strict precautions should be taken to avoid exposure to thalidomide during pregnancy. Other adverse effects of thalidomide include excessive drowsiness, rash, constipation, and peripheral neuropathy. Alternatives include topical corticosteroid preparations and systemic corticosteroids (prednisone, 40 mg per day p.o.). Long-term suppressive therapy may be necessary to prevent recurrences. Patients should always be given maximally effective potent antiretroviral therapy, but the response of idiopathic ulcers to treatment of HIV has been inconsistent.

IV. HIV salivary gland disease

   A. Clinical features. HIV salivary gland disease is the Sjögren's syndrome–like manifestation of the diffuse infiltrative CD8 lymphocytosis syndrome (see also Chapter 18). Xerostomia, bilateral salivary gland enlargement (usually the parotids), or both occur. Xerophthalmia can be another feature. Salivary flow rates are reduced. Occasionally, lymphomas may develop. Other organs that may be involved with the lymphocytic infiltration include the lungs, liver, kidney, and stomach. The CD8 lymphocytosis syndrome is more common in children than adults. Patients with this syndrome rarely have opportunistic infections, and their prognosis is better than others with HIV disease. The cause is unknown.

   B. Management. The gland swelling may fluctuate in size but usually remains large. Fine-needle aspiration may be useful to reduce uncomfortable swelling. Saliva substitutes can be used. Fluoride treatments can reduce the danger of dental carries.

The Ear

I. External ear

   A. Seborrheic dermatitis is a very common problem in patients with AIDS. It usually involves the face and scalp, as well as other areas of the body, but occasionally the external ear is affected. Topical corticosteroid preparations can control the dermatitis, but recurrences are frequent. Low-potency steroid creams, hydrocortisone (1% to 2.5%) applied twice daily, may be tried first, but higher potency preparations, triamcinolone (0.1% applied twice daily), may become necessary for adequate control (see also Chapter 12). Desonide 0.05%–acetic acid, 2% otic solution, 3 to 4 drops into the ear 3 to 4 times per day, is also effective.

B. **Kaposi's sarcoma** can occur on the ear, usually the auricle, and less commonly the external auditory canal. If the canal, tympanic membrane, or middle ear is involved, hearing loss may result. Carbon dioxide laser treatment may be used for canal disease, but argon laser therapy is more sparing of tympanic membrane tissue, if this is involved. Middle ear involvement requires radiation therapy. (See Chapter 28.)

C. **Cellulitis** of the auricle may occur, particularly as a superinfection of a seborrheic dermatitis. The usual infecting organism is *Staphylococcus aureus* and is treated with dicloxacillin, 500 mg orally 4 times per day for 10 days.

D. **Otitis externa.** Mild otitis externa can be managed with ear drops containing antibiotics and steroids (corticosporin, four drops in the ear 3 to 4 times a day). A more aggressive malignant otitis externa with pain and ear drainage occasionally occurs in patients with AIDS. The organism is usually *Pseudomonas aeruginosa*, but Aspergillus has been reported. Systemic antipseudomonal (ceftazidime, piperacillin, ciprofloxacin with or without aminoglycoside) or antifungal (amphotericin B) therapy is required.

E. *Pneumocystis carinii and Mycobacterium tuberculosis* have been reported to cause tumorous lesions of the external auditory canal. Biopsy is essential for diagnosis. Treatment is the same as for these infections elsewhere in the body.

II. Middle ear

A. **Acute otitis media** occurs with greater frequency in children with HIV disease. Less commonly, HIV-infected adults can get this infection, usually as a complication of sinusitis or obstruction from nasopharyngeal neoplasms or lymphoid hyperplasia. The usual infecting organisms are *Streptococcus pneumoniae* and *Haemophilus influenzae*, as in the non–HIV-infected population. However, gram-negative bacteria and *S. aureus* are more common in HIV-infected individuals. Tympanocentesis may be necessary to identify more unusual or antibiotic-resistant organisms. Amoxicillin–clavulanate, 500 mg orally 3 times per day for 10 days, should be effective in most cases.

B. The occurrence of **serous otitis media** may require myringotomy and tube placement.

C. **Mastoiditis** is a rare complication. Surgical drainage should be performed if mastoid radiographs suggest coalescence of air spaces and abscess formation.

III. Inner ear

A. **Hearing loss.** Primarily high-frequency sensorineural hearing loss occurs in ~50% of patients with AIDS. The origin is probably central nervous system HIV infection, although this has not been firmly established. Other infectious, neoplastic, and medication causes should be excluded with serologic testing for syphilis, complete neurologic examination, lumbar puncture, brain imaging [computed tomography (CT) scan or magnetic resonance imaging (MRI)], and medication review. An audiogram and auditory brainstem response testing should be performed. Hearing aids should be prescribed as needed. Causes of conduction hearing loss include infections and neoplasms of the external ear canal and otitis media (see the preceding).

B. **Vertigo** usually occurs only as a component of multiple neurologic symptoms in AIDS dementia complex.

C. **Otosyphilis.** Eighth-nerve involvement with *Treponema pallidum* can be seen as fluctuating symptoms of hearing loss, tinnitus, vertigo, or a combination of these. A patient with positive serum treponemal serology and any of these symptoms should have a lumbar puncture performed for cerebrospinal fluid cell count, glucose, protein, and VDRL. However, the treatment should be aqueous penicillin G, 4 million units i.v. every 4 hours for 10 to 14 days, regardless of the lumbar-puncture results (see Chapter 27).

The Nose

I. **Kaposi's sarcoma.** The skin and mucous membranes of the nose are common sites for the appearance of Kaposi's sarcoma lesions. Although they are usually only a cosmetic problem in this area of the body, patients may complain of nasal obstruction, discharge, or epistaxis. If needed for symptomatic relief, laser therapy is effective for local lesions. More extensive disease may require radiotherapy or chemotherapy (see Chapter 28).

II. **Herpes simplex infection.** Large herpetic ulcerations may extend from the nasal vestibule onto the nasal and perinasal skin. For treatment, refer to Chapter 25.

III. **Seborrheic dermatitis.** This rash most commonly manifests in a bilateral "butterfly" distribution over the bridge of the nose and malar regions of the face. Treatment is with topical corticosteroid preparations (hydrocortisone, 1% to 2.5%, or triamcinolone, 0.1%, applied twice daily) as outlined in the External Ear section. Also effective is 2% sulfur/2% salicylic acid ointment applied twice daily.

IV. **Nasal obstruction.** A patient's complaint of nasal obstruction can be caused by sinusitis, allergic or viral rhinitis, adenoidal hypertrophy, Kaposi's sarcoma, or non-Hodgkin's lymphoma of the nasopharynx. CT scan or MRI should be performed to evaluate persistent complaints. A biopsy should be performed of mass lesions and asymmetric nasopharyngeal lymphoid hyperplasia to rule out a neoplasm. Nonmalignant adenoidal hypertrophy is usually homogeneous and symmetric. It is related to HIV infection in the same manner as is reactive lymphadenopathy elsewhere in the body. Surgical excision can be attempted for bothersome symptoms.

V. **Allergic rhinitis** is more common in HIV-infected persons. A similar approach as with non-HIV-infected patients should be taken to attempt to identify allergens to avoid. Steroid nasal inhalers (beclomethasone, 0.1%, 1 to 3 times daily) may help relieve symptoms (nasal obstruction and discharge and postnasal drip).

VI. **Epistaxis** may be caused by a neoplastic lesion (usually Kaposi's sarcoma), idiopathic thrombocytopenic purpura, or other origins unrelated to HIV infection. A defined bleeding point should be cauterized; otherwise, the nose should be packed.

VII. **Sinusitis** (see Chapter 26).

The Hypopharynx and Larynx

I. **Infection**

A. **Clinical presentation.** Symptoms of infection in the hypopharynx and larynx include dysphagia and odynophagia. Hoarseness may result from laryngeal involvement.

B. **Candida, herpes simplex, and CMV** can infect these regions. Lesions can usually be seen on indirect laryngoscopy. Ulcerative lesions are usually caused by herpes simplex. An empiric trial of acyclovir, 200 mg orally 5 times a day, may be initiated. If there is no response, direct laryngoscopy with biopsy and culture for herpes simplex should be performed. The histologic examination should include an evaluation for CMV. Culture for CMV is not useful because patients with AIDS may shed CMV in salivary secretions asymptomatically. See Chapters 24 and 25 for the treatment of Candida, herpes simplex, and CMV.

C. **Epiglottitis** has been described in HIV-infected patients. Signs and symptoms include fever, sore throat, odynophagia, and laryngeal tenderness. The diagnosis is made by indirect laryngoscopy or direct endoscopy. The patient should be hospitalized and observed for signs of evolving airway obstruction. Intubation should be immediate if endoscopy reveals significant airway compromise. Because the most common cause is *Hemophilus influenzae* and *Streptococcus pneumoniae* is the second, an intravenous antibiotic should be empirically started, e.g., cefuroxime, 1.5 g every 8 hours; ceftriaxone, 1 g every 12 hours; or ampicillin/sulbactam, 1 g every 6 hours. If the infection is not responding, repeated endoscopy with biopsy and culture should be considered.

II. **Idiopathic aphthous ulcers.** Occasionally aphthae involving these areas may occur. They can become quite large and destructive. Biopsy and herpes simplex culture should rule out other causes. Treatment is similar to that for oral aphthous ulcers.

III. **Lymphoid hyperplasia.** Hyperplasia of the tonsillar tissue at the base of the tongue may cause dysphagia and airway obstruction. Surgical removal is warranted for symptomatic relief and to rule out neoplasms such as Kaposi's sarcoma and non-Hodgkin's lymphoma, particularly if the enlargement is asymmetric.

IV. **Kaposi's sarcoma.** Lesions in this region may interfere with swallowing and breathing. Laryngeal involvement could cause hoarseness. Radiotherapy is effective. Prophylactic tracheotomy before the initiation of radiotherapy is indicated if the airway is endangered, as radiation may cause further swelling initially.

V. **Non-Hodgkin's lymphoma** is rare in this area in patients with AIDS.

The Neck

In addition to HIV lymphadenopathy and salivary gland disease, infections (tuberculosis, Mycobacterium avium complex infection, pneumocystosis, toxoplasmosis, cryptococcosis, histoplasmosis, coccidioidomycosis) and neoplasms (Kaposi's sarcoma, non-Hodgkin's lymphoma) can cause lymph node enlargement in the neck. If a neck mass is asymmetric or enlarging, a fine-needle biopsy is indicated to establish the diagnosis. Treatment issues are discussed in the relevant chapters.

21. HEMATOLOGIC PROBLEMS

I. Introduction

A. Abnormalities of the complete blood count are common in human immunodeficiency virus (HIV)-infected patients. Anemia and neutropenia frequently occur, and these findings generally correlate with the severity of the clinical disease. Lymphopenia occurs in most patients, reflecting a decline in the absolute number of $CD4^+$ T cells. Complete evaluation of the cellular elements of blood also involves a microscopic examination of the peripheral smear. Specific morphologic abnormalities (which may or may not be directly related to HIV infection) should be sought and may be important clues to the diagnosis.

B. Bone marrow samples are the result of an invasive procedure, and care should be taken in the proper handling of samples to ensure that all necessary diagnostic information is obtained during one procedure. Examination of the bone marrow should be considered in patients with fever, anemia, or pancytopenia. In contrast, the origin of isolated thrombocytopenia is rarely discovered on a bone marrow examination, so that this test is usually not helpful.

1. **An aspirate and biopsy** should be obtained on all samples and be evaluated by a hematologist or hematopathologist. If no aspirate is obtainable (i.e., "dry tap"), then touch preps of the core biopsy should be made.

2. **Suspicion of infection** in patients with unexplained fever or in cytopenic patients is frequently the reason for the bone marrow examination. A complete evaluation should always include fungal and mycobacterial cultures. Histologic staining for fungal and mycobacterial organisms also should be prepared because this is a rapid method of diagnosis when compared with blood or bone marrow culture. Disseminated fungal infections are typically diagnosed on a stained bone marrow sample. The presence of granulomas in the bone marrow frequently correlates with the presence of opportunistic infections, but their absence does not eliminate this possibility. Bacterial and viral cultures should also be considered but may not add to the diagnostic sensitivity compared with cultures of the blood or buffy coat.

3. **Special testing** of bone marrow samples for the evaluation of malignancy should be used judiciously because the initial diagnosis of Hodgkin's disease or non-Hodgkin's lymphoma (NHL) is not usually made on a bone marrow exam. **Flow cytometry** is most helpful for the phenotypic evaluation of blasts or for the establishment of clonality and immunotyping of NHL in the bone marrow. In the absence of histologic evidence of NHL in the bone marrow, flow cytometry rarely establishes the diagnosis. **Cytogenetic and molecular diagnostic studies** are helpful in the characterization of malignancy such as NHL but are rarely useful in the absence of a known diagnosis.

4. **Dysplasia of the hematopoietic cells** is a frequent bone marrow finding in HIV-infected patients. These findings resemble those found in primary myelodysplastic disorders. Striking dysplasia of the erythroid, myeloid, and megakaryocytic lines may be present. Whether these findings represent direct retroviral infection of hematopoietic cells remains uncertain. Additional bone marrow findings include lymphoid aggregates, increased numbers of plasma cells or eosinophils, and fibrosis.

The author acknowledges the contribution of Morey A. Blinder to the previous edition of this chapter.

Unlike primary myelodysplasia, evolution to acute myeloid leukemia in this setting is rare.

II. Disorders of red blood cells

A. Anemia is common in HIV-infected individuals and is related to the decline in the $CD4^+$ count. The anemia associated with HIV infection is normocellular and normochromic, and the reticulocyte count is inappropriately low. In addition to a direct consequence of HIV infection, other causes of anemia should be considered. **Treatment-induced effects on erythropoiesis** that lead to anemia are common with antiretroviral and other antimicrobial therapy (see Section VI).

1. ***Mycobacterium avium complex* (MAC)** infections are frequently associated with severe anemia, and this may occur in the absence of other cytopenias. This diagnosis should be considered in patients with new-onset or worsening anemia. The presence of anemia is a negative predictor for survival in MAC-infected patients. The treatment of MAC is described in Chapter 24.

2. **Parvovirus B19** should be considered in HIV-infected patients with transfusion-dependent anemia and a low reticulocyte count. The levels of antiparvovirus antibodies, which develop in immunocompetent patients and provide long-term immunity, are typically not increased in HIV-infected patients. The diagnosis is suggested by finding severe erythroid hypoplasia with giant pronormoblasts in the bone marrow and can be confirmed by identification of viral DNA sequences in the serum. Treatment with immunoglobulin [intravenous immunoglobulin (IVIG), 0.4 g per kg per day i.v. for 5 to 10 days] typically results in erythropoietic recovery. Relapses have occurred between 2 and 6 months and may be successfully managed with intermittent IVIG at an empiric maintenance dose of 0.4 g per kg per day i.v. given every 4 weeks (Frickhofen et al. *Ann Intern Med* 1990;113:926).

3. **Autoimmune hemolytic anemia (AIHA)** occurs infrequently in HIV-infected patients. When it occurs, ineffective erythropoiesis related to the underlying HIV infection may cause a low reticulocyte count and mask the diagnosis. Treatment with glucocorticoids (e.g., prednisone, 1 mg per kg per day p.o.) is generally recommended for initial therapy. The majority of patients will also respond to splenectomy. The use of antiretroviral therapy in this setting is unproven. In contrast to the uncommonly diagnosed AIHA, the direct antiglobulin (direct Coombs) test is frequently positive in HIV-infected patients. In most cases, this is because of deposition of immune complexes on the red blood cell (RBC) membrane and is not the principal cause of anemia.

B. Low levels of vitamin B_{12} are a frequent finding in HIV-infected patients. Anti-intrinsic factor antibodies, indicative of pernicious anemia, are not detected. The Schilling test to identify vitamin B_{12} malabsorption may be abnormal in patients with either normal or subnormal levels and is generally not helpful in this setting. The use of ZDV correlates with low vitamin B_{12} levels. Because ZDV directly causes a macrocytic anemia, an effect of low vitamin B_{12} on hematologic parameters (e.g., mean cellular volume) is uncertain. Low levels of vitamin B_{12} are associated with more advanced HIV disease and gastrointestinal symptoms. Therapy with vitamin B_{12} supplementation is of unproven value (Paltiel et al. *Am J Hematol* 1995;49:318).

III. Leukopenia includes both lymphopenia and neutropenia (granulocytopenia). Most patients with advanced disease have leukopenia.

A. Lymphopenia is a direct effect of HIV infection and worsens over time. All lymphocyte subsets decline in patients with acquired immunodeficiency syndrome (AIDS). A low $CD4^+$ count is an important marker for the development of opportunistic infections. Effective treatment with antiretroviral therapy will stabilize or improve the lymphopenia.

B. Neutropenia worsens as the $CD4^+$ count declines. Neutropenic patients with AIDS are at risk for bacterial infections similar to patients with neutropenia and cancer. The causes of neutropenia are complex but include direct and indirect effects on bone marrow myelopoiesis, as well as treatment-related neutropenia (see Section VI). Morphologic abnormalities of neutrophils, including hyposegmentation of the nuclear lobes, prominent cytoplasmic granulation, and Howell–Jolly bodies, are common.

1. **Treatment.** The use of granulocytic growth factors has a significant role in the management of HIV-infected patients by increasing the neutrophil count within several days. After stopping therapy, the effect reverses in ~48 hours. These agents are generally safe and effective, but their exact role and optimal dosages are not well defined. Lower doses, including alternate-day or less frequent intermittent dosing, may be considered. The dose should be modified to maintain the neutrophil count at ≥1,000 per μl (Miles. *Curr Opin Hematol* 1995;2:227).

   a. **Granulocyte colony-stimulating factor (G-CSF**; Filgrastim, 1 to 5 μg per kg per day s.c.; available as 300- and 480-μg vials) is effective in increasing the neutrophil count in patients with AIDS and in those receiving myelosuppressive therapy. At this dose, toxicity is uncommon. Patients receiving myelosuppressive agents such as ZDV or cancer chemotherapeutic agents generally require daily dosing.

   b. **Granulocyte-macrophage CSF (GM-CSF;** Sargramostim, ~2 μg per kg per day s.c.; available as 250- and 500-μg vials) has been shown to improve the neutrophil count in patients with advanced AIDS, in patients taking ganciclovir, and in those receiving other myelosuppressive agents. Toxicity, including fatigue, myalgias, and asthenia, worsens with long-term administration. Although both agents are similar in increasing neutrophil counts, the better tolerance profile of G-CSF and the theoretic risk of retroviral stimulation of GM-CSF make G-CSF the favored agent. There has been some renewed interest in GM-CSF as an immunomodulatory agent in the management of HIV but this remains investigational.

IV. **Thrombocytopenia** frequently occurs in HIV-infected patients at some point in their disease. Evaluation should include review of the blood smear to rule out spurious effects, and consideration should also be given to secondary causes of thrombocytopenia, such as disseminated intravascular coagulation (DIC) or treatment-related toxicity. In many cases, a cause other than HIV-related thrombocytopenia will not be found.

A. **HIV-related thrombocytopenia** occurs in ~5% of asymptomatic seropositive individuals and in as many as 40% of patients at some time during their disease. Only a small number of patients will have platelet counts ≤50,000 per μl. In HIV-infected asymptomatic persons, thrombocytopenia is not a prognostic factor for the development of AIDS.

   1. **The mechanism** of HIV-related thrombocytopenia differs from that in patients with immune thrombocytopenic purpura (ITP) who are not infected with HIV. In HIV-infected individuals, platelet survival is decreased by about one half compared with that in nonthrombocytopenic HIV-infected patients. By comparison, platelet survival is much shorter in seronegative patients with ITP. An immunologic mechanism (either antiplatelet antibodies or immune complex deposition on the platelet surface) appears to account for the impaired platelet survival. Furthermore, platelet production also is decreased in HIV-related thrombocytopenia, which may be the result of HIV infection of megakaryocytes.

   2. **Treatment** of thrombocytopenia should be initiated in patients with a platelet count ≤20,000 per μl and considered in patients with a platelet count ≤50,000 per μl. Because spontaneous improvement of the platelet count may occur in some patients, and others have mild thrombocytopenia (50,000 to 150,000 per μl), treatment need not be initiated in all patients. Because of the underlying bleeding disorder, treatment of thrombocytopenia in patients with hemophilia requires a more aggressive approach (see Section V.A.2).

        a. Immunoglobulin, given as 0.4 g per kg per day i.v. for 5 days or 1 g per kg per day i.v. for 2 days, has an initial response rate of ~75% but results in few sustained responses. **Anti-Rh(D) immune globulin** (WinRho SD, 25 to 50 μg per kg i.v.) may be considered in place of IVIG in patients who are Rh positive and who have an intact spleen (Oksenhendler et al. *Blood* 1988;71:1499). The response rates appear similar to those with IVIG, and the cost is less. Toxicity from Anti-Rh (D) immune globulin includes hemolysis leading to a decline in hemoglobin of ≤2 g per dl in ~10% of patients.

        b. Zidovudine (300 mg b.i.d P.O.) also will result in an increase in platelet count by ~50,000 per μl in about one half of HIV-infected patients (Oksenhendler et al. *Ann Intern Med* 1989;110:365). The mechanism by which ZDV improves the thrombocytopenia may be unrelated to the antiretroviral action. Platelet production is enhanced by ZDV so that replacing ZDV with another antiretroviral agent may cause a subsequent decrease in platelet count. In general, attempts should be made to maintain ZDV in combination regimens.

        c. Prednisone (1 mg per kg per day p.o.) has a response rate of 50% to 70%, and some patients will remain in a sustained remission after therapy. Concern over the immunosuppressive and systemic toxicity has tempered the enthusiasm for this drug in HIV-infected patients with thrombocytopenia.

    3. Resistant or relapsed disease

        a. Splenectomy results in a complete response rate in ~70% of patients and is associated with minimal perioperative morbidity. Sustained remissions occur in most patients (Oksenhendler et al. *Blood* 1993; 82:29). Splenectomy does not appear to alter the progression of HIV infection to clinical AIDS. Pneumococcal vaccine, 0.5 mL i.m., should be administered before the anticipated splenectomy.

        b. Interferon-α (3 X 10[6] units s.c. 3 times per week for 4 weeks) has been used in ZDV-resistant patients and results in an improvement of platelet count to ≥ 50,000 per μL in ~67% of patients (Marroni et al. *Ann Intern Med* 1994;121:423). Fever, malaise, and chilling are commonly observed with this agent.

B. Thrombotic thrombocytopenic purpura (TTP) has been described in both asymptomatic and symptomatic HIV-infected patients. Persons with HIV infection appear to be at an increased risk for TTP compared with those without.

    1. The diagnosis is characterized by a pentad of findings including fever, neurologic changes, renal insufficiency, hemolytic anemia, and thrombocytopenia. Most patients do not demonstrate all of the features of the disease. The peripheral blood smear shows characteristic schistocytes, and the serum lactate dehydrogenase (LDH) is increased in almost all patients. No specific laboratory test is available to confirm the diagnosis of TTP.

    2. Treatment is similar in both HIV-positive and -negative patients. Untreated, the disease is almost always fatal. The usual approach to initial therapy includes daily plasma exchange, which should be started as soon as possible and continued until the platelet count has normalized (Rock et al. *N Engl J Med* 1991;325:393). Additional initial therapy has typically included a glucocorticoid (e.g., prednisone, 1 to 2 mg per kg per day p.o. or equivalent), but this is of uncertain benefit. The role of platelet inhibitors (e.g., aspirin, 325 mg per day p.o., or dextran-70, 500 mL per 12 hours i.v.) is also unproven. Complete response rates are seen after ~1 week of therapy and occur in ~80% of HIV-positive or -negative patients (Thompson et al. *Blood* 1992;80:1890). In patients who do not achieve an initial complete response or in patients who relapse, splenectomy should be considered. Additional therapy including plasma exchange by using cryosupernatant plasma or treatment with vincristine (2 mg i.v. push on day 1, followed by 1 mg i.v. push on days 4, 7, and 10) has been used successfully in HIV-negative patients.

V. Disorders of coagulation

A. Patients with hemophilia A or B who received clotting factor concentrates before 1986 have a high incidence of HIV infection caused by product contamination. HIV-related disease has become the leading cause of death in patients with hemophilia in the United States. Progression to AIDS in hemophiliacs seems to occur at a slower rate than that in other groups of HIV-infected patients.

  1. **Factor VIII–replacement therapy** should be guided by a hematologist experienced in the use of these products. All currently available products are treated with one of various virucidal methods, and all available data suggest that the transmission risk of HIV and hepatitis B and C has been eliminated. Bleeding episodes in asymptomatic HIV-infected hemophiliacs should be treated with either plasma-derived high-purity factor VIII or with a recombinant factor VIII product. These preparations may slow the decline of the CD4$^+$ count compared with factor VIII concentrates of an intermediate purity. In severe hemophilia A patients with previously diagnosed high-responder inhibitors, the development of HIV infection may result in the loss of alloantibody and improvement or elimination of the inhibitor effect. When necessary, this allows for rechallenge with factor VIII concentrates in many of these patients (Bray et al. *Am J Hematol* 1993;42:375). **Factor IX–replacement** therapy for hemophilia B should be with a plasma-derived high-purity product.

  2. **HIV-related thrombocytopenia** poses an additional hemostatic challenge to hemophiliacs. Bleeding risk, including intracranial bleeding, is high, so treatment should be initiated in patients with a platelet count ≤50,000 per μl. Immunoglobulin (0.8 to 1.0 g per kg i.v. monthly) and ZDV (200 mg p.o. every 6 hours) have resulted in a sustained response in the platelet count (Ragni et al. *Blood* 1990;75:1267). Splenectomy has also benefitted hemophiliacs with HIV-related thrombocytopenia.

  3. **Treatment of HIV infection and AIDS complications in hemophiliacs** generally reflects treatment of other populations of HIV-infected patients.

B. Lupus anticoagulants and anticardiolipin antibodies are commonly observed in HIV-infected patients. A lupus anticoagulant should be suspected in patients without a bleeding history who develop an increased activated partial thromboplastin time (aPTT) that does not correct after an equal mixing with normal pooled plasma. The dilute Russell's viper venom time (dRVV) and platelet-neutralization test should be measured to confirm the diagnosis. Lupus anticoagulants predispose to bleeding only when there is a prolongation of the prothrombin time (PT) or thrombocytopenia. Occasionally lupus anticoagulants result in thrombosis, which should be treated with conventional anticoagulant therapy. Anticardiolipin antibodies, detected by an immunoassay, occur in HIV infection but do not correlate with a decline in the CD4$^+$ count or the development of AIDS or thrombocytopenia.

C. Protein S deficiency has been described in HIV-infected patients. The mechanism is unclear. About 5% of these patients develop thrombosis requiring anticoagulation.

VI. Hematologic toxicity is frequently observed and is a common dose-limiting effect of HIV-related therapy. Because the clinical experience with many of these agents is limited, other idiosyncratic or uncommon reactions may not have been identified. Bone marrow toxicity from combination chemotherapy is anticipated and may be severe, so that these agents should be administered by medical oncologists.

A. Drug-induced bone marrow suppression

  1. **Dideoxynucleoside agents. Zidovudine** induces a macrocytic anemia in all patients and can be used as a crude marker for patient com-

pliance. In patients who either require red cell transfusions or have a hematocrit <30%, consideration should be given to stimulation of erythropoiesis. **Erythropoietin** (100 to 200 U per kg s.c. 3 times a week) improves the hematocrit in patients with an endogenous erythropoietin level of <500 mU per mL. Transfusion requirements are decreased by about one half, and ~40% of patients become transfusion independent. No hematologic benefit occurs if the serum erythropoietin level is >500 mU per mL (Henry et al. *Ann Intern Med* 1992;117:739). Dose-related leukopenia responsive to G-CSF or GM-CSF also occurs. Idiosyncratic pancytopenia, occurring within 4 to 6 weeks of starting ZDV, also may occur. **Zalcitabine (ddC) and lamivudine** can cause leukopenia and thrombocytopenia at high doses.

   2. **Antimicrobial agents** including ganciclovir, pentamidine, and amphotericin B are frequently associated with dose-related bone marrow suppression, and these medications should be used with caution in patients with cytopenia. Idiosyncratic aplastic anemia may be caused by sulfonamide-containing antibiotics, requiring discontinuation of the offending agent.

B. **Drug-induced oxidative hemolysis** may result from sulfa-containing agents (e.g., dapsone, sulfamethoxazole, or sulfadoxine) and some antimalarials (primaquine). Typical findings on the peripheral smear, including bite cells and blister cells, as well as the identification of Heinz bodies by special stain, may aid in the diagnosis. Although agents such as dapsone usually cause a low level of hemolysis, glucose-6-phosphate dehydrogenase (G6PD) deficiency is a frequent finding when hemolysis is severe.

C. **Megaloblastic anemia** caused by a cellular deficiency in folic acid may be caused by trimethoprim and is more likely to occur in patients receiving a high dose or in those treated for the long term. Treatment with folinic acid (leucovorin), 15 mg p.o. every 6 hours for 2 days, has been used to restore normal hematopoiesis. Folic acid supplementation will not correct trimethoprim-induced hematotoxicity.

D. **Thrombotic thrombocytopenic purpura** has been associated with valciclovir, and this agent is not recommended for long-term use in HIV-infected patients.

E. **Effects on anticoagulation.** Care should be taken in all patients receiving warfarin because its activity is commonly affected by other medications. Protease inhibitors, non-nucleoside reverse transcriptase inhibitors, and azole antifungals are known to potentiate the effect of warfarin, which leads to a prolongation of the INR (international normalized ratio) and increased risk of bleeding.

VII. **Transfusion therapy and HIV infections.** Between 1982 and 1991, ~2% of the 222,000 AIDS cases reported to the Centers for Disease Control (CDC) were thought to be associated with transfusion. Almost all of the cases were from infections before blood screening for HIV antibodies.

A. **Screening of all blood products** for HIV began in 1985. In addition to laboratory screening, currently used strategies such as a questionnaire appear to be successful in deferring high-risk donors so that ~1:10,000 donors are seropositive for HIV. Recent estimates of HIV transmission risk are ~1 in 500,000 donations of screened blood (Lackritz et al. *N Engl J Med* 1995;333: 1721). The primary risk appears to be donation while in the seronegative window period occurring between the onset of infection and the development of detectable antibody. With current HIV-testing methods (using p24 antigen detection as well as antibody screening), the infectious window is estimated to be ~15 to 30 days. Additional strategies to decrease this window period are ongoing. It is estimated that there continue to be a very small number of transfusion-related AIDS cases in the United States per year.

B. **Directed donations** of blood and blood components have increased dramatically with the onset of the HIV epidemic. In general, individuals who are directed donors have a similar incidence of viral infection to that of the overall population, so that these individuals should be evaluated and their blood tested in the same manner as for anonymous donors. An additional risk to patients who receive directed donor blood products from a human leukocyte antigen (HLA)-identical donor is transfusion-associated graft-versus-host disease. Because this disease is frequently fatal, blood donated from first-degree relatives should be irradiated to avoid this complication.

C. **Viral inactivation of blood products.** Numerous approaches to the removal of pathogens including HIV are ongoing. At present, RBC transfusions, platelet concentrates, and fresh frozen plasma are screened for HIV antibody but are not virally inactivated. All plasma-derived products for the treatment of hemophilia and all preparations of IVIG undergo one of several available viral-inactivation procedures, which has eliminated the risk of transfusion-associated HIV infection. However, both hepatitis A and parvovirus B19 outbreaks have been reported with the solvent-detergent virucidal technique of factor VIII preparations, and hepatitis C transmission has been associated with several brands of IVIG. Although the transmission risks are small, no product derived from human blood can be guaranteed to be free of infectious agents, especially against viruses that are still unknown.

22. PROTOZOAN INFECTIONS

I. *Pneumocystis carinii*

A. Diagnosis. Although *Pneumocystis carinii* is genetically linked to the fungi, it is susceptible to antiprotozoal therapy, and antifungal therapy is not effective against *P. carinii* organisms. *P. carinii* cannot be cultured in the laboratory. No antigen or antibody assays can be used for diagnosis. Definitive diagnosis of infection depends on the morphologic demonstration of *P. carinii* organisms in biological samples, such as expectorated sputum, bronchoalveolar lavage fluid, or lung biopsy tissue.

   1. Sputum induction for diagnosis of *P. carinii* pneumonia (PCP) requires a dedicated effort, and many centers have been unable to attain a high sensitivity.

   2. Bronchoscopy is the diagnostic procedure of choice; bronchoalveolar lavage is reported to have >90% sensitivity for PCP. With the large array of possible pulmonary pathogens, bronchoscopy also provides a method for the diagnosis of bacterial, mycobacterial, viral, fungal, and neoplastic lung diseases that may be in the differential diagnosis for people immunosuppressed by human immunodeficiency virus (HIV) infection (see Chapter 1).

B. The clinical presentation of PCP is nonspecific. Dyspnea, nonproductive cough, and fever are common symptoms. The duration of symptoms before diagnosis is often several weeks. Lung examination may be normal or may demonstrate diffuse or localized crackles. Most commonly, the chest radiograph shows diffuse interstitial infiltrates. However, localized disease (especially upper-lobe infiltrates) and normal chest radiographs may occur. Arterial blood gas (ABG) results usually show some hypoxemia with an increased alveolar-to-arterial oxygen difference ($D_{A-a}O_2$).

C. Severity of illness

   1. Calculation of $D_{A-a}O_2$. For a room-air ABG at sea level, the $D_{A-a}O_2$ is calculated by the formula

   $$D_{A-a}O_2 = [150 - (PCO_2/0.8)] - PO_2$$

   where the PCO_2 and PO_2 are taken from the room-air ABG.

   2. Mild disease is classified as a PO_2 >70 mm Hg on a room-air blood gas and a $D_{A-a}O_2$ <35 mm Hg.

   3. Moderate disease is defined as a PO_2 <70 mm Hg with a $D_{A-a}O_2$ of 35 to 45 mm Hg on a room-air ABG.

   4. Severe disease is defined as a $D_{A-a}O_2$ of >45 mm Hg on a room-air ABG.

D. Therapy

   1. General principles of therapy apply to mild, moderate, and severe disease. Available medications and recommended doses are shown in Table 1. **Trimethoprim–sulfamethoxazole** is considered the best therapy from an efficacy and cost standpoint for all levels of disease severity. Therapy generally continues for 3 weeks based on early observations that patients with HIV infection tended to improve more slowly and have more relapses than did other immunosuppressed patients; 3 weeks of therapy may result in better long-term results. However, for selected patients such as those with mild disease, receiving ~2 weeks of therapy may be sufficient. For instance, patients who are otherwise doing well but

The author acknowledges the contribution of Michael N. Dohn and Peter T. Frame to the previous edition of this chapter.

Table 22-1 Therapy for *Pneumocystis carinii* pneumonia

Drug	Dosage	Formulations
Trimethoprim–sulfamethoxazole	15 mg/kg/d based on the trimethoprim component and administered in divided doses every 8 h	Intravenous. Double-strength oral tablets with 160 mg trimethoprim and 800 mg sulfamethoxazole
Pentamidine isethionate	4 mg/kg once daily	Intravenous (may also be administered by intramuscular injection, although this is not generally recommended)
Trimetrexate with leucovorin	Trimetrexate: 45 mg/m^2 body surface area; leucovorin: 20 mg/m^2 body surface area. Dose may be doubled to 40 mg/m^2 if hematologic toxicity occurs. Leucovorin should be continued for 3 days after trimetrexate is discontinued	Intravenous trimetrexate. Oral leucovorin tablets: 5, 10, 15, and 25 mg
Dapsone and trimethoprim	Dapsone: 100 mg/d; trimethoprim: 20 mg/kg/d administered in divided doses every 6 h	Oral tablets: dapsone, 50 and 100 mg; trimethoprim, 100 and 200 mg
Clindamycin and primaquine	Clindamycin: 300–450 mg every 6 h; primaquine: 30 mg base once daily	Intravenous clindamycin, also oral capsules, 150 and 300 mg; primaquine, oral tablets, 15 mg of base/tablet
Atovaquone	750 mg (5 mL) twice daily with food	Oral suspension: 750 mg/5 mL
Adjunctive corticosteroids		
Prednisone	40 mg twice daily for 5 days, then 20 mg twice daily for 5 days, then 20 mg once daily until therapy is complete. No taper from the 20-mg daily dose is necessary	Oral tablets of various sizes. Equivalent doses of parenteral corticosteroid preparations may be substituted

have a dose-limiting drug toxicity after completing 2 weeks of therapy for PCP may not need additional therapy. **Prophylaxis for recurrent *P. carinii* disease is indicated for all patients completing therapy** and should be started promptly after the end of treatment for the acute episode.

2. **Mild disease** in most patients may be treated with oral therapy in an outpatient setting. Medications with oral formulations are most appropriate for mild disease. Close follow-up is indicated. Approximately half of the patients with mild disease will have transient worsening of their hypoxemia or symptoms during the first 4 days after therapy starts. Because of this early deterioration, judgments concerning the effectiveness of treatment may be difficult during the first week of therapy. By the end of 1 week of treatment, a patient's clinical condition should be at least as good as that at the time of therapy initiation. Adjunctive corticosteroids are not indicated for patients with mild disease; these patients should have a ~95% survival with anti-Pneumocystis therapy alone.

3. **Moderate and severe disease** are treated similarly. Initial oral therapy may be appropriate for patients with moderate disease who have few or mild symptoms. Generally oral therapy is not recommended for severe disease. **All patients should receive adjunctive corticosteroids.** Patients requiring supplemental oxygen and other supportive therapy should be hospitalized initially. Improvement to the point that supplemental oxygen is no longer necessary is a practical marker of when a patient may be ready for hospital discharge.

4. **Adjunctive corticosteroids** are indicated for all patients with moderate or severe PCP (*N Engl J Med* 1990;323:1500) (Table 1). Corticosteroids mitigate the early clinical deterioration observed after treatment starts and decrease the overall morbidity and mortality for patients with moderate and severe disease. Steroids must be started as the anti-Pneumocystis therapy begins; a delay in initiating adjunctive corticosteroids decreases their effectiveness.

5. Recent molecular studies have demonstrated mutations in the Pneumocystis carinii dihydropteroate synthase gene in patients receiving long term trimethoprim-sulfamethoxazole prophylaxis (Helweg et al. *Lancet* 1999;354:1347). These enzymes are involved in folate biosynthesis and are targets for the sulfa component of trimethoprim-sulfamethoxazole. Furthermore, patients with these mutations who developed PCP fared poorly, compared to patients whose organisms had no mutations. This raises the possibility of **drug resistance** to trimethoprim-sulfamethoxazole among patients who are on long-term prophylaxis. Patients in this situation who develop PCP should receive an alternative treatment, e.g., pentamidine for severe disease or atovaquone or clindamycin-primaquine for mild disease.

E. **Management during treatment**
   1. **Monitoring patients on therapy** can be variably scheduled to fit the circumstances. Follow-up of outpatients twice weekly while they receive therapy allows the early recognition of therapeutic failures and drug toxicities, as well as poor compliance with therapy. For improving patients with reliable compliance, single weekly visits during the second and third weeks of therapy may be sufficient.
   2. **Monitoring response to therapy** is accomplished by tracking oxygenation and symptoms.
      a. **Repeated ABGs** should be performed on any patients for whom there is a doubt about oxygenation status.
      b. **Chest radiographs** can demonstrate worsening disease if infiltrates increase; however, as improvement in the chest radiograph may lag behind clinical improvement, they are less useful in monitoring the improving patient.

3. **Early deterioration in oxygenation** occurs in about half of the patients treated for acute PCP over the first 3 or 4 days after therapy begins.
   a. Adjunctive steroid therapy generally eliminates this early deterioration for patients with **moderate and severe disease**. In patients with moderate and severe disease who continue to worsen with therapy after 5 to 7 days in spite of steroid use, consideration should be given to the possibility that this case is a therapeutic failure.
   b. Patients with **mild disease** do not receive adjunctive steroid therapy, and evaluation of treatment efficacy is problematic during the first week of therapy. Despite early deterioration, the vast majority of patients with mild disease (>90%) are treated successfully. By the end of 1 week to 10 days of therapy, patients with early deterioration should be no worse than they were when anti-Pneumocystis therapy began. If oxygenation or symptoms are not at least as good as when therapy was started, then consideration must be given to the possibility that the patient has a therapeutic failure.
4. **Therapeutic failure** occurs when there is deterioration or no improvement in clinical status with anti-Pneumocystis therapy. Therapy should be changed for patients for whom therapy is failing. Consideration should be given to whether a patient receiving oral therapy may have had malabsorption or compliance problems contributing to the therapeutic failure and to whether intravenous therapy may be a better alternative. As noted, patients who have developed PCP while receiving PCP prophylaxis may have acquired resistant infection and should receive an alternative agent. Patients who have therapeutic failure with their first drug have an increased rate of failure with subsequent drugs and a higher mortality risk for this episode of PCP.
5. **Drug reactions and toxicity** during treatment for *P. carinii* infection are common among HIV-infected patients. Depending on the particular therapy, specific toxicity monitoring is indicated.
   a. **Trimethoprim–sulfamethoxazole**. The incidence of dose-limiting allergic reactions with rash is ~50%. Systemic reactions including fever are not uncommon. Most reactions resolve with discontinuation of the drug and symptomatic treatment. Trimethoprim–sulfamethoxazole suppresses bone marrow, and periodic monitoring of complete blood counts (CBCs) is prudent. Blood urea nitrogen/creatinine (BUN/Cr) monitoring also is recommended. Trimethoprim–sulfamethoxazole is well absorbed after an oral dose; checking levels is generally not helpful unless malabsorption is suspected.
   b. **Pentamidine**. Intravenous pentamidine has many toxic effects. Most toxicities occur later in therapy as the cumulative dose increases.
      (1) However, acute hypoglycemia related to the pentamidine infusion may occur at any time. All symptomatic patients should be evaluated for hypoglycemia, and all patients monitored for hypoglycemia with blood glucose determinations 60 to 90 minutes after the infusion.
      (2) Pentamidine is nephrotoxic, and regular determinations of BUN concentration, Cr, magnesium, calcium, and phosphorus levels are indicated. Magnesium, calcium, and phosphorus should be replaced as necessary. Other nephrotoxic drugs should be avoided.
      (3) Hepatic chemistry profile may be monitored for hepatotoxicity.
      (4) Prompt evaluation for pancreatitis should be performed in patients with new abdominal pain or hypoglycemia.
      (5) Prolongation of the QT interval with ventricular arrhythmias may occur and may be related to abnormal levels of magnesium, calcium, and phosphorus. A baseline electrocardiogram (ECG) should be performed and the QT interval monitored by at least twice-weekly ECGs.

5

      c. Trimetrexate with leucovorin. Bone marrow suppression is the major toxicity, especially thrombocytopenia, and monitoring is performed with CBCs. The leucovorin dose may be doubled as the initial step to counteract toxicity. If the bone marrow suppression persists, then trimetrexate should be stopped and the leucovorin **continued** for an additional 3 days.

      d. Dapsone and trimethoprim. Hemolytic anemia may occur in individuals with glucose-6-phosphate dehydrogenase (G6PD) deficiency; assessment of pretreatment levels in populations at high risk for G6PD deficiency (African-Americans) may avoid a hemolytic episode. However, G6PD deficiency is unusual even in high-risk groups in the United States, and waiting for the results of a G6PD assay will delay initiation of treatment for *P. carinii*. Many clinicians start therapy and monitor closely for hemolytic anemia in high-risk groups. This combination may be bone marrow suppressive for any patient, and monitoring the CBC is indicated.

      e. Clindamycin and primaquine. Allergic reactions are reported. Typically a mild rash with fever develops 7 to 10 days after initiation of therapy. Many patients can continue therapy with symptomatic treatment. Bone marrow suppression may occur, and CBC monitoring is useful. Possible hepatotoxicity and nephrotoxicity may be evaluated in the third week of therapy with BUN/creatinine and hepatic chemistry profile.

      f. Atovaquone has a very low toxicity profile. The major problem with atovaquone is poor enteric absorption and consequent treatment failure. Hepatic chemistry profiles are sometimes recommended, but the occurrence of hepatotoxicity is unusual.

F. Prophylaxis (see also Chapter 4) is recommended for anyone with a previous episode of acute PCP and generally begins within 2 weeks after short-term therapy ends. Other indications for prophylaxis in an individual with HIV infection include a CD4+ lymphocyte count of <200 cells per µl, oral candidiasis, or persistent fevers and the initiation of chemotherapy for malignancy.

    1. Trimethoprim–sulfamethoxazole is the agent of choice (Table 2). Dapsone and atovaquone are alternatives for patients intolerant of trimethoprim–sulfamethoxazole. Aerosolized pentamidine is also active as prophylaxis but is less effective in patients with CD4+ lymphocyte count of <100 cells per µl.

    2. Primary prophylaxis can be discontinued in patients whose CD4+ lymphocyte counts rise to values >200 cells per µl while receiving **potent antiretroviral therapy**. Patients who have rises in CD4+ cell counts but whose viral replication is not completely suppressed should be monitored closely as immunological improvement may not be sustained; prophylaxis should be restarted if the CD4+ lymphocyte count falls again below

Table 22-2 Prophylaxis for *Pneumocystis carinii* pneumonia

Drug	Dosages
Trimethoprim–sulfamethoxazole	One double-strength tablet daily; one single-strength tablet daily; one double-strength tablet 3 times weekly
Dapsone	100 mg tablet daily
Atovaquone	750 mg twice daily or 1500 mg daily
Aerosol pentamidine	300 mg via nebulizer every 4 weeks; 150 mg via nebulizer every 2 weeks

200 cells per µL. There is less information about the safety of stopping secondary prophylaxis (i.e., for those who have had an episode of PCP); however, it is reasonable to consider stopping prophylaxis in such patients if they have sustained increases of CD4+ counts >200 cells per µL, with continued suppression of viral replication.

II. **Toxoplasmosis**
   A. **Latent *Toxoplasma gondii* infection in asymptomatic HIV patients**
      1. **Epidemiology.** Human infection by the obligate intracellular protozoan, *Toxoplasma gondii* (TG), is common, with 10% to 40% of American adults and up to 90% of adults in some other countries showing serologic evidence of infection. Seroprevalence in American HIV-infected patients ranges from 15% to 40% (Luft et al. *Clin Infect Dis* 1992;15:211). Wild and domestic cats are the definitive hosts for *T. gondii*, and all other mammals, including humans, are secondary hosts. Toxoplasma reproduces sexually in the cat gut, from which large numbers of oocysts are shed. Oocysts mature in the soil, becoming infectious after 5 to 7 days. Herbivorous, omnivorous, and carnivorous mammals, including humans, ingest infectious oocysts in soil or food contaminated with soil.
      2. During **primary infection**, asexual Toxoplasma tachyzoites are widely disseminated to cells in all tissues of the secondary host, especially muscle, brain, eye, and lymphatic tissue. Normal humoral and cellular immune responses induce intracellular and extracellular killing of the tachyzoites. Most humans are asymptomatic or have undiagnosed mild febrile syndromes during acute infection.
      3. **Latent infection** with tissue cysts is common after acute infection, and bradyzoites in the tissue cysts can remain viable for years. Latent infection has two important implications:
         a. **Meat** of any secondary host may contain viable *T. gondii*. Tissue cysts are present in up to 25% of commercially available lamb and pork. They are less common in beef. Eating meat containing tissue cysts is probably the most common route of infection for humans. (Vegetarians can acquire toxoplasmosis by ingesting oocysts from soil or food contaminated with soil.) Most primary human infections apparently occur during childhood.
         b. **Reactivation** of disease can occur during immune deficiency, in transplant patients, and in immune-suppressed oncology patients, as well as in HIV-infected patients. Reactivation of *T. gondii* tissue cysts is the most common pathogenesis of disease in patients with acquired immunodeficiency syndrome (AIDS).
      4. **Toxoplasma serology**. Primary infection with TG leads to a host immune response, which includes the development of immunoglobulin M (IgM) and then IgG antibodies. A number of tests detect Toxoplasma antibodies; the Immune Fluorescent Antibody (IFA) test is the most widely available. After an acute infection, the IgG antibody titer increases to very high dilutions and remains easily detectable for the life of the patient. Quantitation of IgG antibody titer gives little information as to when the primary infection occurred. Because most AIDS-associated toxoplasmosis is the result of reactivation of a latent infection, nearly all AIDS patients with toxoplasmosis have IgG antibody. For this reason, **HIV-infected patients should be screened for the presence of Toxoplasma IgG antibody with the IFA test.** Absence of IgG antibody indicates a low risk of developing toxoplasmosis if there is no further exposure to the organism. Conversely, the presence of a positive Toxoplasma IFA test identifies an HIV-infected patient with a lifetime risk of up to 45% for developing symptomatic toxoplasmosis. Some physicians recommend repeated IFA testing yearly to detect patients who may acquire TG infection after an initial negative screening test. Antibody testing is best done early in the course of HIV infection, when antibody production is less likely to be impaired. Because most local clinical

laboratories send the test to a reference lab, there is usually a delay in obtaining results. Therefore the presence or absence of prior TG infection should be part of the information obtained during the initial evaluation of any HIV-infected patient (see Chapter 4).

5. **Infection prevention**

   a. Most Toxoplasma infection is acquired from poorly cooked meat. Bringing the internal temperature of meat to 150°F (just barely pink) is an important recommendation for all HIV-infected patients. This practice also will prevent infection with *Salmonella* and other enteric pathogens. Hand washing after handling raw meat and careful washing of fresh vegetables also are important.

   b. Direct exposure to cats does not present a risk for Toxoplasma infection. Mature cats that do not go outside and do not eat uncooked meat are at little risk of acquiring the organism. In addition, the freshly excreted oocyst in cat feces is not infectious because it requires several days to mature in the soil. If litter boxes are changed daily, preferably by someone who is not HIV positive, there is little risk from keeping cats as pets.

6. **Primary prophylaxis** for toxoplasmosis is appropriate in HIV-infected patients who have Toxoplasma antibody and CD4+ counts <100/mm³. **Trimethoprim–sulfamethoxazole**, one double-strength (DS) tablet daily, has been shown to reduce the incidence of toxoplasmosis. **Dapsone**, 100 to 350 mg total weekly dose, with **pyrimethamine**, 50 to 100 mg total weekly dose, and **folinic acid**, 10 to 25 mg weekly dose, is also effective. Dapsone alone is ineffective. For patients who must receive aerosolized pentamidine for PCP prophylaxis, there is no available TG prophylaxis of known efficacy. **Atovaquone** is being studied as a prophylactic agent but has not yet been shown to be effective when used in this manner. Although there is less information on stopping prophylaxis for toxoplasmosis in patients on **potent antiretroviral therapy**, the same principles that apply to PCP prophylaxis can be used here also.

B. **Toxoplasma encephalitis (TE)** occurs by reactivation of latent tissue cysts in the brain or as a brain manifestation of disseminated toxoplasmosis. Dissemination through the bloodstream occurs when a latent focus of Toxoplasma becomes reactivated. Because Toxoplasma can be isolated from the blood in up to 50% of patients with encephalitis and because brain lesions are most often multiple, it is likely that TE is most frequently a manifestation of disseminated toxoplasmosis.

   1. **Diagnosis**

      a. **Clinical features.** Encephalitis is the most common manifestation of toxoplasmosis in AIDS. CD4+ counts almost always are <100 and usually <50. The most common clinical features of TE are those associated with an intracranial mass lesion. More than half of the patients have severe **headache, focal neurologic deficit, fever**, or **confusion**. Altered consciousness, ranging from **somnolence to coma**, may be present. **Seizures or abnormal behavior** also may be present alone or in association with other findings. The onset of the illness can be acute, subacute, or chronic, and there may be no focal neurologic signs. Thus, the presentation can be nonspecific, with only a disorder of consciousness or behavior. TE should be included in the differential diagnosis of any HIV-infected patient with marked immune deficiency and nonspecific central nervous system (CNS) complaints, with or without fever.

      b. **Brain imaging**. HIV-infected patients in whom toxoplasmosis is being considered should undergo a brain **magnetic resonance imaging (MRI) scan with gadolinium** contrast or **computed tomography (CT) scan with double contrast** (Levy et al. *J Acquir Immune Defic Syndr* 1990;3:461). The absence of lesions on one of these scans makes toxoplasmosis unlikely. Most patients with cerebral toxoplasmosis have multiple space-occupying lesions throughout the brain substance, especially in the region of the basal ganglia. Lesions can occur in the brain stem and cerebellum as well; thus, MRI is the preferred scan if it is available and the patient can tolerate the procedure. MRI also provides additional information about possible white-matter disease, aiding in other neurologic diagnoses in this population (see Chapter 13). Characteristic lesions on MRI scan with gadolinium contrast have a central hypodense region, surrounded by a contrast enhancing rim on the T_2-weighted image. The lesions are often surrounded by a surprisingly large area of edema. Similar contrast-enhancing lesions with central necrosis and surrounding edema are seen on the contrast CT scan. Because noncontrast CT scanning is often performed in the emergency setting to rule out CNS bleeding, a follow-up contrast study should be performed in patients whose differential diagnosis includes TE. The brain lesion in AIDS patients most often confused with toxoplasmosis is that of a CNS lymphoma, which more often is seen as a single lesion, tends to be periventricular or intraventricular, and can be differentiated by its ability to take up thallium (see Chapter 29).

c. **Other diagnostic tests for the evaluation of suspected TE**

   (1) The serum Toxoplasma IgG **IFA** is positive in >95% of TE cases, which indicates a previous infection. Patients without antibody are unlikely to have toxoplasmosis. On rare occasion, the IFA is negative because of the remoteness of the primary infection, because of an extended period of immune suppression with impaired IgG production, or because the patient has recently acquired primary TG infection.

   (2) Routine tests done on **cerebrospinal fluid** (CSF) do not provide additional useful information for the diagnosis of toxoplasmosis. CSF pressure may be elevated, and nonspecific protein and cellular changes may be present. Lumbar puncture should be performed only if it is necessary to evaluate the patient for other conditions.

   (3) **Polymerase chain reaction (PCR) and culture.** Toxoplasma PCR performed on a peripheral blood or CSF sample can establish the diagnosis of TE with certainty. When performed in a laboratory with proper PCR controls, a positive test on a peripheral blood or CSF specimen establishes the diagnosis of active toxoplasmosis, making brain biopsy unnecessary except in cases in which a comorbid CNS condition is suspected. Since false negative TG PCR tests occur in 80% of blood and up to 50% of CSF specimens, a negative PCR result does not exclude TE. The Toxoplasma PCR most often will be used as a confirmatory test after a treatment trial has already begun. *T. gondii* can be **cultured from blood, CSF, or biopsy** specimen in many cases, by using tissue culture or mouse injection. However, only a few medical centers have this capability.

   (4) **Brain biopsy.** A definitive diagnosis of TE requires histologic examination of a brain biopsy. Although brain biopsy in "silent" areas of the brain has relatively low morbidity, some lesions are not easily accessible without risk. In addition, demonstration of tachyzoites in stained sections of brain is difficult, and a negative brain biopsy does not exclude toxoplasmosis. Therefore, brain biopsy is usually reserved for patients with atypical lesions on brain imaging, patients with negative TG antibody, and patients who have failed to respond to a treatment trial.

d. **Treatment response as a diagnostic test**. If the clinical and radiologic features are consistent with toxoplasmosis and the patient has a positive serum IFA, empiric therapy for toxoplasmosis as a diagnostic test is appropriate with careful follow-up. Most patients with TE begin responding to therapy within 1 week, and **90% will show a clinical response within 2 weeks.** CNS lymphomas sometimes show a ring-enhancing pattern on contrast imaging, and occasionally toxoplasmosis is accompanied by a second intracranial diagnosis. In patients who respond clinically to this treatment strategy, a follow-up MRI or CT scan should be performed to document regression of the lesions, which usually occurs within 3 weeks. Smaller lesions often completely resolve after 6 to 8 weeks, but larger lesions may not completely resolve, leaving a residual abnormality on the scan. It is important to obtain a follow-up imaging study after clinical resolution or stabilization of findings to exclude coexisting diagnoses and to establish a new baseline picture.

   e. The **differential diagnosis** of toxoplasmosis most commonly includes cryptococcal meningitis, with or without a cryptococcal abscess (see Chapter 24) or CNS lymphoma (see Chapter 29) or both. Less likely are nocardiosis and other brain abscesses (see Chapter 26). Herpesvirus encephalitis [cytomegalovirus (CMV), herpes simplex virus (HSV), or varicella-zoster virus (VZV)] usually does not have the characteristic discrete lesions of TE, and progressive multifocal leukoencephalopathy (PML) is a diffuse white-matter disease without mass effect (see Chapter 13). HIV encephalopathy is characterized by loss of brain substance, primarily from the white matter, without mass effect or enhancement (see Chapter 13).

2. Treatment

   a. Antimicrobials

      (1) The treatment of choice is **sulfadiazine**, 25 mg per kg p.o. every 6 hours, to a maximum 8 g per day, plus **pyrimethamine**, 200 mg during the first 24 hours, followed by 50 to 75 mg per day, and **folinic acid**, 10 mg per day, to protect the bone marrow from the megaloblastic effect of pyrimethamine (Dannemann et al. *Ann Intern Med* 1992;116:33). Treatment should continue for 4 to 6 weeks, until the lesions have resolved or stabilized at a reduced size. When the response to treatment is considered satisfactory, the dose of sulfadiazine can be reduced to 2 g per day, and the three drugs are then continued indefinitely as suppressive therapy, because relapse can occur in up to 80% of patients who have recovered from an episode of toxoplasmosis. Neither sulfadiazine nor pyrimethamine is available in parenteral form. More than half of patients with AIDS will have adverse reactions to this treatment combination. Sulfadiazine can cause allergic reactions of rash and fever and occasionally bullous erythema multiforme (Stevens–Johnson syndrome). Less commonly, nephrolithiasis, interstitial nephritis, toxic hepatitis, and toxic encephalopathy can occur. Pyrimethamine also causes rash and interferes with folate metabolism, with bone-marrow toxicity being its most common side effect. The addition of folinic acid reduces this effect. All three drugs can be associated with nausea and vomiting. Drug compliance can also be a problem, because this regimen requires ~10 pills per day in patients who are ill and require other medications as well.

      (2) Clindamycin, 600 mg i.v. every 6 hours, combined with the same doses of **pyrimethamine** and **folinic acid** described previously, is as effective as sulfadiazine for the short-term treatment of toxoplasmosis (Dannemann et al. *Ann Intern Med* 1992;116:33; Luft et al. *N Engl J Med* 1993;321:995). Clindamycin in high doses causes nausea, vomiting, and diarrhea, and is associated with the induction of *Clostridium difficile* colitis. Fever or rash or both occur in equal frequency with the sulfadiazine-containing regimen.

(3) Other drugs. Several other drug regimens have been reported to be effective for toxoplasmosis in small uncontrolled studies.

    (a) The anti-*Pneumocystis* drug, **atovaquone**, has been used to treat toxoplasmosis with some success, If used, the better-absorbed liquid formulation of atovaquone, 750 mg twice daily, should be given in combination with **pyrimethamine** and **folinic acid**. There are no large comparisons of this combination with the first-choice regimens of pyrimethamine plus sulfadiazine or clindamycin, and it should be considered a third-choice alternative.

    (b) **Trimethoprim–sulfamethoxazole** in PCP doses, as well as **azithromycin**, have been used to treat toxoplasmosis, with success rates inferior to sulfadiazine–pyrimethamine.

  b. Adjunctive therapies. The mass lesions of TE with surrounding edema can be associated with stupor or coma and may lead to intracranial herniation. Although the use of steroids in infectious processes is controversial, in patients with brain-stem dysfunction suggesting incipient transtentorial herniation, **dexamethasone** can be given in an initial dose of 10 mg i.v., followed by 4 mg every 6 hours. Steroids should be tapered slowly over several weeks, after the initial improvement has occurred. Oral dosing can be substituted when the patient has improved enough to take dexamethasone by mouth. The use of steroids may **confound the interpretation of response** to treatment as a diagnostic test, however. Because the reduction of edema around any lesion may give temporary improvement, careful follow-up with contrast-imaging studies is necessary to document that the improvement is a result of the response of the encephalitis to specific therapy rather than the nonspecific effect of dexamethasone. In addition, steroids are lympholytic and thus can effect a temporary response of CNS lymphoma.

  c. Long-term suppression. Relapse of TE is common in patients with AIDS. Up to 80% of patients who are successfully treated for toxoplasmosis will have relapses after therapy is discontinued. Therefore treatment is considered to be life-long. After the patient has responded clinically and radiographically, the dose of **sulfadiazine** may be reduced to 500 mg every 6 hours. The **pyrimethamine** and **folinic acid** should be continued at the same dose used in acute treatment. Long-term **clindamycin** or **atovaquone** for suppressive therapy have not been extensively studied. If a patient responds to either of these second-line therapies, the same doses used in acute treatment should be used for chronic suppression. Reducing the dose of clindamycin after a response to therapy with clindamycin/pyrimethamine has been associated with a higher relapse rate. Pyrimethamine alone has been shown to be ineffective for long-term suppression of TE. All patients should receive **potent antiretroviral therapy**. If this successfully suppresses viral replication, and raises CD4+ cell counts, it may be possible to discontinue treatment for toxoplasmosis.

C. Other clinical syndromes cause by *Toxoplasma gondii* in patients with AIDS

  1. Interstitial pneumonitis. An interstitial pneumonia indistinguishable from PCP can be caused by TG, usually as a component of disseminated disease. Cough, shortness of breath, and a reticulonodular radiograph pattern are the most common features. Diagnosis is made by pathologic examination of lung tissue or bronchoalveolar lavage fluid, and the treatment is the same as that for TE.

  2. Chorioretinitis. During the systemic dissemination of the primary infection, tissue cysts can develop in the choroid. Reactivation of these cysts causes chorioretinitis, with eye pain, photophobia, and visual loss.

Examination of the eye often reveals vitreal inflammation. If the retina can be visualized, multiple necrotizing nodular white infiltrates are seen. Unlike CMV retinitis, vasculitis is not present. Most patients with AIDS in whom chorioretinitis is diagnosed also have encephalitis, and the treatment is the same.

III. Cryptosporidiosis

A. Clinical features and diagnosis. *Cryptosporidium parvum* is a ubiquitous protozoan parasite of humans and other mammals, especially cattle, which infects the columnar epithelium of the small intestine, causing severe diarrhea and malabsorption. In patients with severe immune deficiency, diarrhea can be chronic and severe enough to require continuous intravenous hydration. Patients with chronic cryptosporidiosis often have severe malnutrition and weight loss, and survival is shortened compared with that in similar patients without cryptosporidiosis. Extension to the **biliary tree** is associated with obstructive jaundice, and chronic productive cough occurs with infection of the **respiratory mucosa**. A modified **acid-fast stain** of a stool specimen is the usual method of diagnosis. This test often is not included in a routine "ova and parasite" stool examination and must be ordered separately.

B. Treatment. The disease is self-limited in normal hosts and in HIV-positive patients with some immune function (generally CD4$^+$ counts >150 to 200).

   1. Diphenoxylate/atropine, loperamide, and **tincture of opium** are partially effective in controlling the symptoms of acute infection and are often used heavily and continuously by patients with AIDS.

   2. The nonabsorbed aminoglycoside **paromomycin,** 2 to 4 g per day in divided doses, is the most frequently prescribed specific therapy for cryptosporidiosis in patients with unremitting diarrhea. Anecdotal reports and small trials suggest that some cases of chronic cryptosporidiosis may improve with this therapy (Fichtenbaum et al. *Clin Infect Dis* 1993;16: 298). However, a recent multicentered placebo-controlled trial showed that paromomycin was ineffective for treating cryptosporidiosis.

   3. No other antiprotozoan agent has been shown to be effective treatment for cryptosporidiosis. Spontaneous remission can occur in patients whose immune function improves with **successful antiretroviral suppression**. Therefore, all patients should receive maximally effective potent antiretroviral treatment.

   4. Some patients require **bowel rest and hyperalimentation** to obtain symptomatic relief and maintain nutrition. Intravenous **octreotide** has been reported to give temporary relief of symptoms, but in most cases, the response to this very expensive therapy is of short duration.

C. Prevention. *Cryptosporidium parvum* is transmitted most often by contaminated drinking water. Unfortunately, standard municipal water treatment does not always eliminate *Cryptosporidium*. Some have recommended that patients with severe immune deficiency drink **bottled or boiled water**. No regulations control the source or processing of bottled water, however, so that it cannot be considered totally safe. Careful **washing, peeling, or cooking of fruits and vegetables** can reduce the risk of acquiring the infection from agricultural sources, and **avoidance of fecal–oral transmission** is important because *C. parvum* is mature and infectious in stool.

IV. Isosporiasis.
Isospora belli is a protozoan parasite common in tropical and subtropical climates that can cause chronic diarrheal disease with malabsorption in immune-compromised patients. Infection in patients living in the United States is uncommon. HIV-infected patients from Mexico, Central America, the Caribbean, and Africa are at the greatest risk for this infection. Transmission is by fecally contaminated food, but human-to-human transmission is not a problem. Diagnosis is made with **acid-fast examination of stool specimens. Trimethoprim–sulfamethoxazole,** two double-strength tablets twice daily for 2 to 4 weeks, is effective therapy in adult patients. **Pyrimethamine,** 25 mg 3 times daily, and **folinic acid**, 5 mg per day, is an alternative for patients intolerant of sulfa drugs. Chronic suppression with one DS tablet of trimethoprim–

sulfamethoxazole or 25 mg pyrimethamine and 5 mg folinic acid is recommended after short-term therapy for patients with CD4+ counts <200. **Potent antiretroviral therapy** should be initiated if possible.

V. Microsporidiosis. Hundreds of species of protozoan parasites are designated microsporidia. Several species have been associated with human disease, although in some instances, the causal relation has not been firmly established. Diagnosis is usually made by pathologic examination of tissue specimens, for example, endoscopic biopsies of small-bowel mucosa, lung biopsies, or autopsies. *Enterocytozoon bieneusi* has been associated with chronic diarrhea and sometimes malabsorption in HIV-infected patients with severe immune deficiency. However, asymptomatic patients also have been found to harbor these organisms, so the causal nature of the association is not always clear. Other than **symptomatic therapy** for diarrhea, there is **no known specific treatment** for *E. bieneusi*, although a number of agents have been tried. Two other organisms, *Septata intestinalis* and *Encephalitozoon* sp., have been histologically demonstrated in endothelium and blood vessels of the lung, kidney, and gallbladder in a few patients with AIDS. **Albendazole,** 400 mg b.i.d., has appeared effective in a few reported cases of infection with these species of microsporidium. The drug is not effective for *E. bieneusi*, however. **Potent antiretroviral therapy** should be initiated if possible.

23. MYCOBACTERIAL INFECTIONS

I. **Tuberculosis (TB)**
   A. **Epidemiology and risk factors.** TB is caused by *Mycobacterium tuberculosis*, a slowly growing, aerobic, non–pigment-producing acid-fast bacillus. TB is probably the most common opportunistic infection worldwide in persons infected with human immunodeficiency virus (HIV). A disproportionate number of new cases of TB are diagnosed in persons coinfected with HIV. In 1992, among United States–born persons with TB between the ages of 30 and 39 years, 35% of men and 20% of women were coinfected with HIV (Onorato et al. *J Infect Dis* 1992;165:87). Demographic groups at high risk for TB and HIV overlap and embody those who are homeless, housed in institutions, injection drug users, or located in urban areas where TB rates are high. In urban areas where coinfection with TB and HIV is more common among high-risk demographic groups, there is also an increased risk of acquisition of multiple-drug-resistant TB (MDRTB), particularly among individuals previously treated with antimycobacterial drugs. In 1994, 8% of TB isolates recovered from patients in the United States were resistant to at least isoniazid, and 2.2% were resistant to at least isoniazid and rifampin (*MMWR* 1995;44:387). Development of MDRTB has been associated with poor adherence to therapy, failure to recognize drug resistance leading to a delay in initiation of appropriate treatment or use of ineffective treatment regimens, and failure to institute appropriate infection-control measures in institutions (Edlin et al. *N Engl J Med* 1992;326:1514).
      1. **Immunosuppression** related to HIV enhances the risk of acquiring new TB infection and developing active disease after infection or reactivation; reinfection with a second strain can occur during or after completion of antimycobacterial therapy (Small et al. *N Engl J Med* 1993;328:1137). *M. tuberculosis* is a virulent pathogen capable of causing disease at any stage of HIV infection, although the median CD4$^+$ cell count reported for HIV-infected patients with TB ranges from 150 to 300 cells/μl (Hopewell. *Clin Infect Dis* 1992;15:540). After exposure to TB, HIV-infected individuals are more likely to become infected. Active TB develops in a greater proportion of those coinfected with HIV, 30% to 40% compared with 5%, and at accelerated rates, 8% to 10% per year compared with 5% to 10% over a lifetime, than in immunologically healthy persons without HIV infection (Selwyn et al. *N Engl J Med* 1989;320:545).
   B. **Clinical manifestations of TB** in persons coinfected with HIV are in part dependent on the underlying degree of HIV-related immunosuppression. Earlier in HIV disease, when CD4$^+$ cell counts remain >200 to 250 cells per μL, the most common clinical presentation of TB is that of reactivation pulmonary disease characterized by productive cough, fever, night sweats, weight loss, and occasionally pleuritic chest pain, hemoptysis, or dyspnea. Chest radiographs typically demonstrate upper lobe cavitation; other radiographic findings may include pleural effusion, mediastinal lymphadenopathy, single or multiple pulmonary nodules, or in the instance of "miliary" TB, diffuse reticulonodular infiltration with tiny nodules the size of millet seeds.
      1. **Extrapulmonary TB** occurs more frequently in HIV-infected patients, regardless of HIV disease stage, than in the immunocompetent individual but is seen most frequently in those with advanced immunosuppression, as reflected by **CD4$^+$ counts of <200 cells per μL.** The sites most frequently involved are the **central nervous system** (tuberculous menin-

The author acknowledges the contribution of Constance A. Benson to the previous edition of this chapter.

gitis), the **reticuloendothelial system** (lymph nodes, spleen, liver, bone marrow), or **bone** (vertebral bodies). Tuberculous meningitis may be seen with fever, headache, mental-status changes, or focal neurologic deficits. Lymphoreticular disease may be seen with fever, lymphadenopathy, hepatomegaly, splenomegaly, or various cytopenias. Vertebral involvement may be characterized by fever and back pain. Virtually any other organ can be infected during hematogenous dissemination, and other less common sites of extrapulmonary involvement include the pericardium, skin, gastrointestinal tract, peritoneum, reproductive organs, and kidneys. Symptoms are often nonspecific constitutional symptoms of fever, night sweats, and weight loss but may also reflect the organ system(s) involved.

2. One other **atypical manifestation** of TB in HIV-infected patients is **primary progressive lung disease,** characterized by the acute or subacute onset of fever, cough, dyspnea, and hypoxemia accompanied by lobar consolidation or patchy alveolar or interstitial infiltrates. The latter are often bilateral. Symptoms and signs may be difficult clinically to distinguish from other progressive pulmonary opportunistic infections. Primary progressive disease most often follows recent acquisition of a new infection occurring in an individual with advanced immunosuppression.

3. **Clinical manifestations of MDRTB** among patients with HIV infection do not appear to differ substantially from those associated with drug-susceptible disease, with the possible exception that MDRTB may progress more rapidly, may follow a more aggressive course with more frequent extrapulmonary manifestations, and **may be associated with a higher TB-attributable mortality rate** than drug-susceptible disease. These features, however, may also depend in part on the degree of underlying immunosuppression of the host and the early recognition and initiation of appropriate therapy. Epidemiologic and clinical features that increase the suspicion of MDRTB include the following.

   a. A history of prior **irregular or incomplete antituberculous treatment.**

   b. Exposure in a setting where MDRTB is known to have been transmitted or in a geographic area where MDRTB is common.

   c. **Persistently positive sputum smears or cultures** or progression of radiographic abnormalities or symptoms despite initiation of appropriate multiple drug therapy.

4. Unusual clinical manifestations have also been described in patients receiving **potent antiretroviral therapy.** In the first few months after starting antiretroviral therapy, patients may experience apparent worsening with increased fever, pleural effusions, enlarging lymph nodes (especially mediastinal) (Narita et al. *Am Rev Respir Dis* 1998;158:157). Cerebritis has also been described. This paradoxical worsening is probably immune-mediated, does not imply failure of anti-TB treatment, and may respond to corticosteroids.

C. **The diagnosis of TB** requires several elements, including the epidemiologic and exposure **history**, the recognition of a constellation of **signs and symptoms**, potentially supported by a positive **tuberculin skin test** or a positive **acid-fast bacillus (AFB) smear** of infected secretions or tissue, ancillary **radiographic studies**, and the **recovery of** *M. tuberculosis* **in culture** from respiratory tract secretions, blood, or other body fluids or tissue samples. Blood cultures may be positive in as many as 26% to 42% of HIV-infected patients with TB (Shafer et al. *Am Rev Respir Dis* 1989;140:1611).

1. **The yield of sputum AFB smears** in HIV-infected patients is likely a function of the clinical syndrome and the degree of underlying immunosuppression. HIV-infected persons with active cavitary pulmonary TB are probably as likely to have positive sputum AFB smears as are non–HIV-infected persons with a similar disease presentation. The sensitivity of sputum AFB smears in patients with AIDS may be lower for those with more advanced immunosuppression who have atypical pulmonary dis-

ease or with extrapulmonary TB, especially if nonfluorescent stains are used. It is also likely that a lower burden of microorganisms is responsible for the development of active disease in this highly susceptible population. The smaller number of organisms may result in a lower yield for AFB smears as immunosuppression progresses.

2. **Rapid isolation and species identification** of TB organisms is the cornerstone of diagnosis; all initial isolates and isolates recovered from persons for whom therapy fails or who relapse after completion of therapy should undergo **drug susceptibility testing.** The latter is key to the **appropriate modification of initial drug regimens to assure adequate therapy.** Most clinical laboratories currently use a combination of radiometric detection systems and DNA probes for culture and identification, which substantially reduces the time to recovery and identification from an average of 8 to 12 weeks (with conventional culture methods) to 3 to 4 weeks. The use of radiometric methods for susceptibility testing further reduces the time for acquiring these data. Newer diagnostic techniques using polymerase chain reaction assays for detection and luciferase enzyme-based luminescence systems for rapid drug-susceptibility testing may further reduce these times.

D. **Therapy**

1. **General guidelines**. Successful treatment requires use of an adequate number of active antituberculous drugs for a prolonged duration. Treatment should be guided by antimycobacterial drug-susceptibility testing. All initial isolates and isolates recovered from those who relapse or for whom therapy fails should be tested for susceptibility to antituberculous drugs. Initial treatment should include multiple drugs while awaiting susceptibility-testing results, and subsequent treatment regimens should be modified based on those results. Use of a single drug for treatment or the addition of a single drug to a failing regimen should not be done. Assuring adherence to therapy is key; directly observed (DOT) or supervised therapy, which can be facilitated by using intermittent dosing regimens, is recommended for all patients but particularly for those with HIV infection or with MDRTB.

2. **Impact of antiretroviral therapy** (Havlir et al. *N Engl J Med* 1999; 340:367). Most regimens for TB include **a rifamycin** (rifampin or rifabutin) which are potent inducers of the hepatic cytochrome P450 system. HIV protease inhibitors are metabolized by this enzyme system. Some protease inhibitors and non-nucleoside reverse transcriptase inhibitors (NNRTIs) also inhibit P450 enzymes. Administration of rifampin with a protease inhibitor may decrease levels of the protease inhibitor and elevate rifampin levels. Rifabutin has the same effect though it induces the P450 system to a lesser degree; limited studies have demonstrated that it is possible to administer rifabutin with indinavir, nelfinavir, and probably amprenavir and maintain acceptable levels of both drugs although adjustments may be necessary in the dosing. Ritonavir can be given with rifabutin; the recommended dosage is rifabutin 150 mg every other day (*MMWR* 2000;49:185). NNRTIs also interact with rifampin. Efavirenz, nevirapine, and delavirdine levels are lowered with rifampin coadministration; rifampin levels are unchanged by NNRTI use. Rifabutin-plus-nevirapine or rifabutin plus efavirenz appear safe to use; however, the combination of rifabutin plus delavirdine is contraindicated.

3. **Treatment regimens** depend on whether patients are being treated with concomitant protease inhibitors or NNRTIs (*MMWR* 1998;47 (RR-20):1). In general, antiretroviral therapy should be delayed in patients if possible (e.g., in patients at higher CD4+ counts).

   a. **Initial therapy for uncomplicated TB in whom potent antiretroviral therapy is not started should include at least four drugs:** isoniazid, rifampin, pyrazinamide, and either ethambutol or streptomycin. Adult doses and common adverse reactions are summarized in Table 1. These agents should be continued for the first

Table 1. First- and second-line antimycobacterial drugs recommended for initial treatment of tuberculosis among HIV-infected individuals

Drug	Average adult dose[a]	Common adverse reactions
FIRST-LINE ANTIMYCOBACTERIAL DRUGS		
Isoniazid	300 mg/d (900 mg 2×/wk)	Hepatotoxicity (risk increases with age >35 yr), peripheral neuropathy
Rifampin	600 mg/d (600 mg 2×/wk)	Nausea, vomiting, diarrhea, rash, hepatitis, red-orange discoloration of body fluids, neutropenia, thrombocytopenia
Pyrazinamide	15–30 mg/kg/d (50–70 mg/kg 2×/wk). Max, 2 g/d (max, 4 g 2×/wk)	Nausea, vomiting, abdominal pain, hepatotoxicity, hyperuricemia, gout (rare)
Ethambutol	15–25 mg/kg/d (50 mg/kg 2×/wk)	Nausea, vomiting, abdominal pain, hepatotoxicity, optic neuritis, peripheral neuropathy (rare), hyperuricemia
Streptomycin	15 mg/kg/d (25–30 mg/kg 2×/wk). Max, 1 g/d (max 1.5 g 2×/wk)	Ototoxicity (vestibular and cochlear), nephrotoxicity
SECOND-LINE ANTIMYCOBACTERIAL DRUGS		
Kanamycin, amikacin, capreomycin	15 mg/kg/d (max, 1 g/d)	Ototoxicity (vestibular and cochlear), nephrotoxicity
Ethionamide	0.5–1 g/d	Anorexia, rash, metallic taste, peripheral neuropathy, nausea, vomiting, thrombocytopenia, visual changes (rare)
Cycloserine	250 mg-1 g/d	Rash, headache, hepatotoxicity, neurologic dysfunction, cerebellar ataxia
Para-aminosalicylic acid	4–12 g/d	Anemia, nausea, vomiting, diarrhea, hepatitis, rash, jaundice, leukopenia, thrombocytopenia

HIV, human immunodeficiency virus.
[a]2×/wk, twice weekly option; requires daily therapy with four drugs for the first 2 weeks and then four drugs given twice weekly as directly observed therapy (DOT) for 6 weeks, and subsequently, for drug-susceptible isolates, with isoniazid and rifampin twice weekly (DOT) for 16 weeks. Three times weekly DOT regimens for the full course of therapy is a third option. From *MMWR* 1993: 42:3, with permission.

2 months of therapy. For **drug-susceptible isolates**, isoniazid and rifampin should then be continued for an additional 4 months. It is currently recommended that HIV-infected patients with TB should be treated for a **minimum of 6 months.** Controlled clinical trials in this patient population suggest that with adequate DOT, the response is similar, and a 6-month course of therapy is equally effective for both HIV-seropositive and HIV-seronegative persons with uncomplicated TB (Kassim et al. *AIDS* 1995;9:1185). Much or all of the therapy can be given in intermittent dosing regimens to facilitate DOT. Treatment for extrapulmonary TB is the same as that for pulmonary disease, except for children with disseminated TB, bone or joint TB, or tuberculous meningitis, for whom 12 months of therapy is recommended (Bass et al. *Am J Respir Crit Care Med* 1994;149:1359). Mortality does appear to be higher among HIV-infected patients with TB; however, the higher mortality seen in many studies appears to reflect other opportunistic infections or HIV-related complications and may not be excess mortality directly attributable to TB.

   b. In HIV-infected patients with TB for whom **initiation of a potent antiretroviral therapy is indicated** or who are **already on a successful antiretroviral regimen** which contains a protease inhibitor or NNRTI, two options have been suggested.

   (1) A 6-month anti-TB regimen with **rifabutin** (150 mg qd if used with indinavir, nelfinavir, or amprenavir; 300 mg qd in other combinations) in place of rifampin.

   (2) A 9-month **streptomycin-containing** anti-TB regimen in place of a 6-month rifamycin-based anti-TB regimen.

   c. Initial treatment for those suspected of having **MDRTB** should include **at least five or six drugs delivered by DOT**; the choice of which drugs should be based on the susceptibilities of the source strain or of the strain(s) prevailing in the community, if known (*MMWR* 1993;42:1). If this information is unavailable, isoniazid, rifampin, pyrazinamide, ethambutol, and streptomycin (with or without a fluoroquinolone such as ofloxacin or ciprofloxacin) should be used and the regimen modified once drug susceptibilities are known. Persons being retreated should receive **at least three new drugs not previously administered.** The outcome may be better with the use of at least three drugs to which the isolate is susceptible in the treatment of those with MDRTB (Iseman. *N Engl J Med* 1993;329:784). A number of the second-line (Table 1) or other nonconventional antituberculous agents may be necessary, and consultation with an expert knowledgeable in the treatment of TB is indicated. The duration of therapy for MDRTB should be at least 18 to 24 months or 12 months beyond sputum-culture conversion.

   4. Monitoring of treatment. Patients should be followed up at least monthly with repeated sputum smear and culture, when applicable, radiographic testing, and laboratory and clinical assessment for adverse reactions. AFB seen on smears should decrease and clinical and radiographic improvement should be evident within 8 weeks of treatment; if negative cultures are not obtained by the end of 2 months of treatment, TB isolates should be retested for drug susceptibility, and the therapeutic regimen should be reevaluated.

E. Screening and prevention. The most useful screening methods for detection of TB infection are an appropriate **clinical and epidemiologic history and tuberculin skin testing.** As the proportion of HIV-infected individuals who are anergic varies inversely with the degree of immunosuppression, those who are HIV-seropositive should be tuberculin skin tested as early in their disease course as possible. The need for repeated tuberculin skin testing should be determined by the likelihood of continued or repeated exposure to infectious cases of TB (*MMWR* 1995;44:19). The **Mantoux** or intradermal method using **5 tuberculin unit strength purified protein derivative**

(PPD) is the recommended method; a PPD is considered **positive when ≥5 mm of induration develops.** HIV-positive patients may have a false negative PPD test because HIV infection causes anergy to cutaneous antigens. However because it is not predictive in identifying patients at higher risk for TB, **anergy testing is not recommended** for the evaluation of tuberculosis risk in patients with HIV infection (*MMWR* 1997;46:1).

1. **Chemoprophylaxis.** All HIV-infected individuals with a positive PPD (or a history of a positive PPD who have not previously received prophylaxis) should receive chemoprophylaxis regardless of age. Those who have been recently exposed to a known infectious case of TB should receive chemoprophylaxis regardless of PPD response. Prophylaxis may be considered for anergic HIV-infected persons if they are at high risk for development of TB although this has not been shown to be useful. High-risk populations include immigrants from areas where TB is highly endemic, injection drug users, homeless persons, or persons housed in correctional facilities, homeless shelters, or hospitals or clinics where recent outbreaks of TB have occurred.

   a. **Active tuberculosis** should be ruled out prior to starting chemoprophylaxis by performing a clinical examination and a chest X-ray.

   b. **Isoniazid,** 300 mg per day, is the chemoprophylactic drug of choice for those thought to be infected with drug-susceptible strains of *M. tuberculosis*. Higher doses administered by DOT twice weekly is an alternative regimen (Bass et al. *Am J Respir Crit Care Med* 1994; 149:1359). Isoniazid should be administered with pyridoxine, 25 to 50 mg per day, to prevent neuropathy. The recommended duration of isoniazid prophylaxis is currently 12 months.

   c. **Shorter courses of chemoprophylaxis** combining rifampin 600 mg per day and pyrazinamide 20 mg per kg daily for 2 months have been shown in HIV positive patients to protect against TB at rates equivalent to isoniazid (Gordin et al. *JAMA* 2000;283:1445). These may be considered in particular in situations where adherence may be an issue.

2. **Chemoprophylaxis for MDRTB.** The most effective chemoprophylaxis for those who may have been exposed to or infected with MDRTB is unknown. Suggested regimens include daily pyrazinamide and ethambutol or pyrazinamide and a fluoroquinolone such as ofloxacin or ciprofloxacin (Bass et al. *Am J Respir Crit Care Med* 1994;149:1359). Some experts have recommended chemoprophylaxis with multiple-drug regimens similar to those used for treatment, with the choice of drugs based on the known susceptibilities of the exposure strain(s).

3. **Bacille Calmette-Guérin (BCG)** vaccination is contraindicated in individuals with HIV infection, as disseminated disease caused by BCG strains may result.

4. **Infection-control procedures** are important adjuncts in the prevention of TB. These encompass early initiation of effective respiratory isolation procedures, including housing patients in a single room equipped with six or more air exchanges per hour, negative pressure with respect to the hallways, and ventilated to the outside; early recognition of disease with initiation of appropriate antituberculous therapy; use of appropriate personal protective devices or masks; barrier precautions for cough-inducing procedures; and screening and identification of exposed patients and health care workers. More aggressive engineering controls may be necessary in high-risk settings.

II. *Mycobacterium avium* **complex (MAC) disease**
   A. **Epidemiology and risk factors.** MAC disease is among the most common opportunistic infections in persons with AIDS in the United States and other developed countries, with an incidence ranging from 18% to 43% in the absence of chemoprophylaxis or effective antiretroviral treatment (Nightingale et al. *J Infect Dis* 1992;165:1082–1085). The MAC consists of *M. avium*, *M. intracellulare*, and some strains not classified as either; the organisms are

slowly growing, nonphotochromogens, although some strains may produce a yellow pigment that increases with light exposure. More than 95% of infections attributable to MAC in patients with AIDS are caused by *M. avium*, with serovars 1, 4, and 8 predominating in the United States (Benson. *Clin Infect Dis* 1994;18:S218). The organisms are ubiquitous in the environment, found in soil, water, and a variety of animals and foods, and are thought to be acquired through inhalation or ingestion (Horsburgh. *Am Rev Respir Dis* 1989;139:4). The risk of developing disseminated MAC disease is greatest for those who have CD4+ lymphocyte counts <50 cells per µl and who have had a prior opportunistic infection; the estimated yearly rate of occurrence of disseminated MAC in this patient population is 12% to 24% in the absence of chemoprophylaxis (Chaisson et al. *Am Rev Respir Dis* 1992;146:285; Nightingale. *J Infect Dis* 1992;165:1082). Demographic features, geographic location, gender, and risk factors for HIV transmission do not appear to influence the risk of developing disseminated MAC disease. Colonization of the respiratory or gastrointestinal tract with MAC in persons with advanced immunosuppression is uncommon; however, when present, it is associated with an increased risk of developing MAC bacteremia with a positive predictive value of ~60% (Chin et al. *J Infect Dis* 1994;169:289; Haulick et al. *J Infect Dis* 1993; 168:1045). Epidemiologic studies in HIV-infected patients have shown an association between daily showers or occupational exposure to water and a decreased risk of developing MAC bacteremia and between exposure to MAC-contaminated potable water supplies in hospitals and an increased risk of developing MAC bacteremia (Horsburgh et al. *J Infect Dis* 1994;170:362; von Reyn et al. *Lancet* 1994;343:1137). Despite these findings, epidemiologic data are insufficiently convincing to allow specific recommendations regarding avoidance of environmental exposure to MAC.

B. **Clinical manifestations.** Most patients with AIDS and MAC disease have disseminated multiorgan involvement.

1. The most frequently described **symptoms** are fever, night sweats, weight loss, wasting, fatigue, diarrhea, and abdominal pain.

2. The most frequently identified **laboratory abnormalities** include anemia and an elevated alkaline phosphatase. Anemia is often severe (Hct, <30) or out of proportion to that expected from other underlying conditions or related to medications such as zidovudine, and is thought to be related to suppression of erythropoiesis by a MAC-induced soluble factor (Gascon et al. *Am J Med* 1993;94:41). Abnormalities of liver chemistries other than alkaline phosphatase also may be seen in the presence of infiltrative MAC disease of the hepatic parenchyma or biliary tract.

3. **Common physical findings** include hepatomegaly or splenomegaly. Intraabdominal lymphadenopathy may be demonstrated by radiographic imaging procedures. Peripheral lymphadenopathy is uncommon.

4. **Less common localized manifestations** of MAC disease include pneumonitis, pericarditis, osteomyelitis, skin lesions, soft-tissue abscesses, or central nervous system lesions. Other symptoms, signs, and laboratory abnormalities may reflect these local sites of involvement. Localized infection, especially lymphadenitis, is also seen in patients who develop MAC while on **antiretroviral therapy** (Phillips et al. *J Acquir Immunodef Synd* 1999;20:122).

5. **Asymptomatic or transient MAC bacteremia** can occur in a small proportion of individuals with advanced HIV disease; the majority of such patients eventually developed recurrent or sustained bacteremia accompanied by symptoms (Kemper et al. *J Infect Dis* 1994;170:157).

C. **The diagnosis** of disseminated MAC disease is generally based on **recovery of MAC in culture** of blood or bone marrow. Recovery of MAC from other normally sterile body fluids or tissue, such as cerebrospinal fluid or tissue-biopsy samples, accompanied by systemic symptoms, provides presumptive evidence of disseminated disease (although if only a local or single normally sterile site is culture positive and other sites are culture negative, some patients may truly have local disease). The most rapid and highest-yield technique for culture of MAC combines radiometric detection in liquid media with DNA-probe species identification.

1. **A positive AFB smear** of blood, tissue, or secretions is nonspecific, and until culture and species identification data are available, the finding of AFB in specimens should be interpreted as indicative of *M. tuberculosis* infection.

2. **Susceptibility testing for MAC** has not yet been standardized and is not routinely recommended as a guide to initial therapy for MAC disease. Clinical trials in patients with AIDS have demonstrated a correlation between pretreatment susceptibility test results and microbiologic and clinical response only for clarithromycin, azithromycin and rifabutin (Heifets et al. *Antimicrob Agents Chemother* 1993;37:2364; Chaisson et al. *Ann Intern Med* 1994;121:905). Testing isolates for susceptibility to the macrolides may be clinically useful for patients for whom chemoprophylaxis with a macrolide fails or who fail to respond to or relapse after initial therapy. Quantitative colony counts to determine the amount of bacteria in blood are most useful in clinical trials when determining the relative activity of treatment regimens; **routine quantitative monitoring of blood cultures is not recommended.**

D. **Treatment**

1. **General guidelines.** Patients with AIDS and disseminated MAC disease have reduced survival compared with those who do not have disseminated MAC disease; appropriate treatment improves survival (Ives et al. *AIDS* 1995;9:261). Antimicrobial agents with anti-MAC activity include clarithromycin, azithromycin, rifabutin, newer rifamycins (rifapentine, KRM-1648), ethambutol, ciprofloxacin, amikacin, and liposome-encapsulated gentamicin (Table 2). Clarithromycin, azithromycin, and ethambutol have been demonstrated most consistently to have single-drug activity in clinical trials. Patients with AIDS and MAC bacteremia or disseminated MAC disease should be treated with a **multiple-drug regimen** consisting of **two or more drugs** known to be active against MAC to delay or **prevent the emergence of resistance** (Masur. *N Engl J Med* 1993;329:898). Most patients require 2 to 8 weeks of treatment before a substantial reduction in clinical symptoms can be demonstrated.

2. **Treatment regimens. Oral clarithromycin**, 500 mg twice daily, or azithromycin, 500 to 1000 mg per day, form the cornerstone of multiple-drug regimens for the treatment of MAC disease. **Ethambutol, 15 mg per kg per day,** has been widely recommended as a second drug, based on its singular activity. The role of rifabutin, 300 mg qd, as a third agent is less certain. Conflicting data are available from prospective randomized trials with evidence for improved survival with three drugs in one large study, and no difference when rifabutin is added to a clarithromycin/ethambutol regimen in another. It is clear, however, that initiation of potent antiretroviral therapy dramatically improves outcome. As noted earlier, the use of rifamycins is complicated in patients taking protease inhibitors and NNRTIs. The decision to add rifabutin should take into account clinical considerations of toxicity, **drug interactions, and underlying disease conditions.**

3. **Drug interactions** have particular impact in the treatment of MAC disease in this patient population. Clarithromycin, when combined with rifabutin, may be associated with a 77% increase in rifabutin concentrations. Fluconazole increases rifabutin concentrations by 80% when the two drugs are combined (Narang et al. *N Engl J Med* 1994;330:1316). These two interactions have been associated with an increased risk of developing rifabutin-associated uveitis when the drugs are combined (*MMWR* 1994;43:658). This risk is substantially reduced when rifabutin doses do not exceed 300 mg per day. Clarithromycin interacts with terfenadine and astemizole, accelerating the risk of dysrhythmia. Significant interactions between the rifamycins and protease inhibitors also have been reported. Concomitant use of rifampin and the protease inhibitors

Table 2. Antimycobacterial drugs suggested for treatment of *Mycobacterium avium* complex (MAC) disease in patients with AIDS

Drug	Adult dose	Common adverse reactions
Amikacin	10–15 mg/kg/d	Ototoxicity (cochlear and vestibular), nephrotoxicity
Azithromycin	500–1,000 mg/d	Diarrhea, nausea, vomiting, abdominal pain, rash, elevated liver transaminases
Ciprofloxacin	500–750 mg b.i.d.	Nausea, vomiting, abdominal pain, diarrhea, rash, insomnia, tremors, mental-status changes
Clarithromycin	500 mg b.i.d.[a]	Nausea, vomiting, abdominal pain, diarrhea, dysgeusia, rash, elevated liver transaminases, hearing loss, possible mania
Ethambutol	15 mg/kg/d	Nausea, vomiting, abdominal pain, diarrhea, hepatitis, optic neuritis, peripheral neuropathy (rare)
Rifabutin	300–450 mg/d[b]	Nausea, vomiting, abdominal pain, diarrhea, rash, uveitis, brown–orange discoloration of body fluids, neutropenia, arthralgia, myositis, increased liver transaminase levels
Rifampin	600 mg/d	Nausea, vomiting, diarrhea, rash, hepatitis, red–orange discoloration of body fluids, neutropenia, thrombocytopenia

[a] Clarithromycin, 500 mg b.i.d., is the dose approved by the U.S. Food and Drug Administration for prophylaxis and treatment of *Mycobacterium avium* complex (MAC) disease.
[b] Rifabutin, 300 mg/d, is the dose approved by the U.S. Food and Drug Administration for prophylaxis of MAC disease. Dose must be adjusted when used with protease inhibitors.
From Korvick JA, Benson CA. Advances in the treatment and prophylaxis of *Mycobacterium avium* complex in individuals infected with human immunodeficiency virus. In: Korvick JA, Benson CA, eds. *Mycobacterium avium complex infection: progress in research and treatment.* New York: Marcel Dekker, 1996, with permission.

is contraindicated, as is the concomitant use of rifabutin and delavirdine. If rifabutin is used in conjunction with indinavir, nelfinavir, or amprenavir, a dose of 150 mg qd should be used.

   4. **Duration of therapy.** Antimycobacterial therapy should be continued for the lifetime of the individual to prevent relapse unless effective antiretroviral therapy is given to improve immune function. If the CD4+ count rises to sustained levels >100 cells/mm³ with potent antiretroviral therapy, small studies suggest that treatment for MAC can be discontinued after 6 to 12 months.

   5. **Salvage therapy.** Prospective clinical trials suggest that a substantial proportion of patients with disseminated MAC disease will **relapse** with therapy. Reasons for relapse are several, including poor **adherence to therapy**, inadequate **absorption** of or intolerance to drugs, and development of **drug resistance.** The most appropriate management for patients who relapse after an initial clinical or microbiologic response depends in part on the reason for the relapse. Many experts recommend testing relapse isolates for susceptibility to macrolides, altering therapy based on the results, and adding at least two new drugs not previously used to the therapeutic regimen.

   6. **Adjunctive immunomodulator therapy with interferon-γ** resulted in a reduction in clinical symptoms in a small number of non–HIV-infected

patients with MAC disease for whom antimycobacterial therapy alone was failing; its role in salvage treatment for patients with HIV and MAC has not been established (Holland et al. *N Engl J Med* 1994;330:1348). Adjunctive therapy with **glucocorticoids** resulted in a similar response in a small number of HIV-infected individuals (Wormser et al. *Antimicrob Agents Chemother* 1994;38:2215). Preliminary results of a small study of azithromycin combined with **granulocyte–macrophage colony-stimulating** factor showed that the latter enhanced monocyte function and intracellular killing of MAC. Larger prospective clinical trials of immunomodulator therapy have not been completed, and such approaches remain **investigational**. Results from ongoing clinical trials must be awaited to define the most appropriate treatment for those who relapse or for whom initial treatment fails.

E. **Chemoprophylaxis** is recommended for HIV-infected individuals who have CD4+ cell counts of <50 cells per μL, particularly those who have had a prior opportunistic infection (*MMWR* 1999;48(No. RR-10)).

  1. **Chemoprophylaxis regimens. Rifabutin**, 300 mg per day, decreases the incidence of MAC disease by ~50%, may prolong MAC-free survival, and is not associated with emergence of resistance (Nightingale et al. *N Engl J Med* 1993;329:828; Chaisson et al. *AIDS* 1997;11:311). **Clarithromycin**, 500 mg twice daily, decreases the incidence of MAC disease by 69%, prolongs MAC-free survival, and is associated with emergence of resistance to clarithromycin in 58% of those for whom chemoprophylaxis fails with this agent (Pierce et al. *N Engl J Med* 1996;335:384). **Azithromycin**, 1,200 mg per week, decreases the incidence of MAC disease by 59% compared with placebo. Due to their greater efficacy, **azithromycin or clarithromycin are the recommended drugs for prophylaxis**. Rifabutin is an alternative for those who cannot take azithromycin or clarithromycin. Combining a macrolide with rifabutin is not recommended.

  2. Primary prophylaxis can be discontinued in patients whose CD4+ lymphocyte counts rise to values >100 cells per μL while receiving **potent antiretroviral therapy**. Patients who have rises in CD4+ cell counts but whose viral replication is not completely suppressed should be monitored closely as immunological improvement may not be sustained; prophylaxis should be restarted if the CD4+ lymphocyte count falls again below 100 cells per μl. There is less information about the safety of stopping secondary prophylaxis (i.e., for those who have had an episode of MAC); however, it is reasonable to consider stopping therapy in such patients if they have sustained increases of CD4+ counts >100 cells per μl, with continued suppression of viral replication.

III. **Other mycobacterial infections**

  A. *Mycobacterium kansasii* is a photochromogenic, slowly growing, AFB that causes disease more commonly in HIV-infected patients from the southwestern and midwestern United States and in those who use injectable drugs (Bamberger et al. *Clin Infect Dis* 1994;18:395).

  1. The presenting **clinical manifestations** are often those of cavitary pulmonary disease clinically indistinguishable from that caused by *M. tuberculosis*, although disease caused by this relatively less virulent pathogen may occur in individuals with more advanced stages of immunosuppression, and as such, may be associated with atypical radiographic manifestations including lower lobe, interstitial, nodular, or diffuse pulmonary infiltrates. As with TB in this patient population, extrapulmonary disease may occur concomitant with or overshadow pulmonary infection and most commonly involves the gastrointestinal tract, resulting in abdominal pain, organomegaly, intraabdominal lymphadenopathy, diarrhea, or weight loss. Disseminated disease caused by *M. kansasii* also occurs and mimics the manifestations of MAC disease.

  2. The **diagnosis** rests on recovery of the organism in culture from sputum, blood, bone marrow, or other normally sterile body fluid or tissue

with a compatible clinical syndrome. No skin-testing antigens are available to assist in screening for the presence of infection.

3. **Treatment** consists of a combination of isoniazid (300 mg per day), rifampin (600 mg per day), and ethambutol (15 mg per kg per day) for 12 months' duration. Longer courses of therapy may result in lower relapse rates. The use of isoniazid remains somewhat controversial as the organism is nearly uniformly resistant to this drug *in vitro*; however, relapse and emergence of resistance have been reported in patients treated with two-drug combinations of rifampin and ethambutol or isoniazid and rifampin; therefore most experts recommend treatment with all three drugs. A number of the sulfonamides and clarithromycin also have *in vitro* activity and may be useful additional drugs in some settings.

B. A variety of **other mycobacteria** occasionally cause disease in patients with HIV infection. The organisms and their most frequently recognized clinical syndromes are summarized in Table 3. In general, treatment of infections

Table 3. Other nontuberculous mycobacterial infections: associated clinical manifestations in patients with AIDS and drugs with potential activity in treatment regimens

Mycobacterial species	Clinical manifestations	Drugs with potential activity
M. bovis	Cavitary pneumonia; disseminated multiorgan disease (may be seen after BCG vaccination)	Isoniazid, rifampin, ethambutol, streptomycin (uniformly resistant to pyrazinamide)
M. chelonae	Skin, soft tissue, bone and joint; chronic inflammation and sinus tract formation is common	Amikacin, doxycycline, erythromycin, imipenem, tobramycin (all variable activity)
M. fortuitum	Cutaneous lesions, soft tissue, bone, disseminated multi-organ disease	Amikacin, cefoxitin, fluoro-quinolones, sulfonamides, doxycycline, clarithromycin
M. genovense	Disseminated multiorgan infection similar to MAC disease; molecular techniques may be necessary for species identification	Unknown (clarithromycin, ethambutol, amikacin, rifamycins, ciprofloxacin have been used in treatment regimens)
M. hemophilum	Cutaneous lesions, bone and joint, disseminated disease, grows optimally at 32°C and requires iron-containing media	Isoniazid, rifampin, ethambutol, clarithromycin, minocycline, doxycycline, ciprofloxacin, amikacin
M. marinum	Cutaneous lesions; bone, usually associated with water exposure	Rifampin, ethambutol, tetracyclines, trimethoprim–sulfamethoxazole
M. scrofulaceum	Cervical lymphadenitis; disseminated disease (rare)	Surgical excision usually the treatment of choice; isoniazid, rifampin, streptomycin, cycloserine, clarithromycin, sulfonamides
M. xenopi	Pulmonary nodules or diffuse reticulonodular infiltrates	Isoniazid, rifampin, ethambutol, streptomycin

AIDS, acquired immunodeficiency syndrome; BCG, bacille Calmette-Guérin; MAC, *Mycobacterium avium* complex.

caused by the nontuberculous mycobacteria require multiple-drug regimens to prevent or delay the development of resistance. Although susceptibility testing for the nontuberculous mycobacteria is not standardized, individualized therapy may be necessary based on the results. However, studies demonstrating a clear correlation between *in vitro* susceptibility and clinical and microbiologic response to therapy are for the most part lacking, particularly for HIV-infected patient populations. As therapy may be distinctly different depending on the species causing the infection, a culture-confirmed microbiologic diagnosis is of paramount importance.

24. MANAGEMENT OF MYCOSES

Mucosal candidiasis and systemic mycoses are major causes of illness in patients with acquired immunodeficiency syndrome (AIDS). Thrush occurs in nearly all patients, and systemic mycoses in 10% to 20% as the CD4$^+$ count decreases to < 200 per µl. Cryptococcal meningitis is the most common life-threatening mycosis in the United States and other endemic mycoses have regional importance in different areas of the world.

I. **Candidiasis**
 A. **Clinical features**. Candida generally causes mucosal disease: cutaneous, oropharyngeal, vulvovaginal, and esophageal. Systemic invasive Candida infection is rare except in patients with long-term indwelling intravenous catheters or those with neutropenia.
  1. **Oropharyngeal candidiasis**. Symptoms of oropharyngeal candidiasis include burning pain, altered taste sensation, and difficulty swallowing liquids and solids. However, many patients are asymptomatic. The oral manifestations of candidiasis have been classified into four distinct categories.
   a. Pseudomembranous candidiasis (**thrush**), characterized by the occurrence of painless, white spots on the tongue, gums, buccal membranes, or throat. These plaques are easily removable.
   b. Acute **atrophic candidiasis** (erythematous), which occurs as red patches affecting the tongue, buccal membranes, and gums.
   c. Chronic atrophic candidiasis (e.g., **angular cheilitis**), which is seen as painful white or red fissuring at the corners of the mouth.
   d. Chronic hyperplastic candidiasis (**leukoplakia**): chronic, discrete lesions that vary in size and appearance and cannot be scraped away.
  2. **Vaginal candidiasis** generally is seen as a creamy white abnormal vaginal discharge. Symptoms include vaginal or vulvar pruritus, burning pain, and dyspareunia. On examination, the vagina may appear erythematous, and pseudomembranous plaques are often seen.
  3. Patients with **esophageal candidiasis** generally have odynophagia or dysphagia.
 B. **Diagnosis.** Both thrush and vaginal candidiasis are diagnosed by direct examination. Demonstration of fungal organisms by stains may be needed to distinguish oral candidiasis from hairy leukoplakia. Fungal culture from the oropharynx is not helpful because Candida species are normal mouth flora. Candida esophagitis is diagnosed presumptively if dysphagia or odynophagia are present with thrush; antifungal therapy without endoscopy is appropriate. Endoscopy should be performed if dysphagia persists despite 7 to 10 days of presumptive therapy (Porro et al. *Am J Gastroenterol* 1989;84:143–146).
 C. **Treatment**. Treatment is effective in most cases, but recurrence is common (>60%).
  1. **Initial management**
   a. Initial episodes of oral **candidiasis** respond to either topical therapy with clotrimazole troches, 10 mg dissolved slowly in the mouth 5 times per day, or nystatin, 100,000 units as swish and swallow 3 to 4 times per day. Systemic therapy with ketoconazole (200 mg/day p.o. for 7 to 14 days), fluconazole (100 mg per day p.o. for 7 to 14 days), or itraconazole 200 mg per day (oral solution) p.o. for 7 to 14 days is also effective but more costly. Systemic therapy often is required for patients with multiple recurrences. A hierarchical approach beginning with clotrimazole and advancing to ketoconazole and then other oral azoles is less expensive and may reduce the incidence of fluconazole-refractory infection.

      b. Candida vaginitis responds to local therapy with miconazole or clotrimazole vaginal cream or suppositories, 100 mg intravaginally at bedtime for 7 days or 200 mg at bedtime for 3 days. The response may be better with longer regimens or a higher total dose. Nystatin vaginal suppositories, 100,000 units at bedtime for 14 days, are also effective. In patients who do not respond to topical therapy, ketoconazole, 200 mg per day p.o., or fluconazole, 100 mg per day p.o. for 5 to 10 days may be effective.

      c. Candida esophagitis is more serious and should be treated with fluconazole (200 mg per day p.o. for 14 to 28 days). Although itraconazole capsules are less effective than fluconazole, an oral solution of itraconazole, 200 mg/day swish and swallow for 14 to 28 days, is effective.

   2. Fluconazole-refractory disease is most likely to be seen in patients with advanced human immunodeficiency virus (HIV) disease (CD4$^+$ counts <50) who have received extensive prior courses of fluconazole (as therapy or prophylaxis). Failure of fluconazole, 200 mg per day, occurs in 5% of cases and is usually associated with organisms with high *in vitro* minimal inhibitory concentrations (MICs) to fluconazole. Response may occur to higher doses of fluconazole (400 to 800 mg per day p.o.) or oral solutions of itraconazole (200 mg per day p.o.) or amphotericin B (500 mg, q.i.d.) as a swish and swallow, 5-fluorocytosine, 500 mg t.i.d., or parenteral amphotericin B (0.3 to 0.5 mg per kg per day i.v.) (Fichtenbaum et al. *Clin Infect Dis* 1998;26:556). Response to treatment typically is slow (1 to 4 weeks) in patients with extensive disease.

   3. Suppressive therapy. Frequent relapses off therapy (i.e., occurring every 1 or 2 months), Candida esophagitis, or fluconazole-refractory infection may be indications to continue treatment to prevent recurrence. In general, fluconazole, 100 to 200 mg qd is the most commonly used suppressive therapy. Liberal use of suppressive therapy may be a factor in the selection of resistant organisms.

   4. Candidemia is usually a nosocomial infection and commonly is catheter related. Such infections may clear spontaneously with removal of the catheter and modification of other risk factors (e.g., discontinuation of antibiotics). Treatment is recommended for most patients. In patients without evidence of dissemination, a brief course of as little as 200 mg amphotericin B may be adequate, provided that fungemia resolves promptly with removal of the catheter. Other patients should receive therapy for disseminated disease with amphotericin B, 0.5 mg per kg per day, with a 0.5- to 1.5-g total dose. Fluconazole, 400 to 800 mg i.v. or p.o., is an alternative.

   5. Effect of potent antiretroviral therapy. As with other opportunistic infections, the incidence of mucosal and esophageal candidiasis has decreased significantly. In addition, oropharyngeal candidiasis clears rapidly in patients receiving protease inhibitor-based treatment

II. Cryptococcosis. Meningitis is the most common manifestation, but pneumonia, retinitis, skin disease, and dissemination to multiple organs may occur (Powderly. *Clin Infect Dis* 1993;17:837). Intracranial hypertension is a common complication of meningitis and may cause blindness or death (Denning et al. *Am J Med* 1991;91:267).

  A. Clinical features

   1. The most common manifestation is a subacute **meningitis** or **meningoencephalitis** with fever, malaise, and headache. Patients are usually symptomatic for 2 to 4 weeks before presentation. Some patients also have symptoms compatible with encephalopathy, such as lethargy, altered mentation, personality changes, and memory loss.

   2. Symptoms of **pulmonary cryptococcosis** may be the initial manifestation of disease, with fever, cough, dyspnea, and hypoxemia. Chest radiographs typically show bilateral alveolar or interstitial pneumoni-

tis, although focal or nodular patterns, pleural effusions, and lymph-adenopathy have been described. All such patients should be evaluated for meningitis.
3. Several types of **skin lesions** occur, including papules, nodules, and ulcers. The most common skin lesion resembles molluscum contagiosum.
4. In occasional patients, all cultures are negative, but **serum crypto-coccal antigen is positive.** Such patients should be assumed to have systemic infection and treated accordingly.
B. **Diagnosis.** Rapid diagnosis may be established by cryptococcal antigen detection in serum or cerebrospinal fluid (CSF), each positive in ~95% of cases. **Lumbar puncture** should be performed to confirm the diagnosis of meningitis in patients with cryptococcal infection identified in other tissues. An **opening pressure should always be measured** when a lumbar puncture is performed on patients with suspected cryptococcal meningitis. India-ink stain of CSF is positive in 75% of cases. Cultures may be positive from blood, alveolar lavage fluid, or other sites of dissemination.
C. **Treatment.** Aggressive treatment has improved the outcome of cryptococcal meningitis, but chronic suppression is essential to prevent recurrence.
1. **Induction treatment.** A regimen of amphotericin B, 0:7 mg per kg per day for 2 weeks, followed by fluconazole for 8 weeks is associated with a mortality rate of ~5% in clinical trials (van der Horst et al. *N Engl J Med* 1997;337:15). Fluconazole (200 to 400 mg per day p.o.) is the preferred choice for oral therapy once patients improve. Itraconazole, 400 mg per day can be used for patients who cannot tolerate fluconazole. Addition of 5-flucytosine (25 mg per kg p.o. q.i.d.) appears not to improve mortality but is associated with an improved outcome (more rapid sterilization of the CSF) and may have long-term benefits such as a lower risk of relapse. The use of 5-flucytosine as therapy is not associated with significant additional toxicity when given for a short period of treatment. Newer liposomal preparations of amphotericin B (AmBisome) may be more tolerable and appear to be as effective in initial clinical trials.
2. **Management of intracranial hypertension.** Aggressive management of intracranial hypertension is essential (Graybill et al. *Clin Infect Dis* 2000;30:47). Repeated removal of CSF (~25 mL) is appropriate in patients with opening pressures >180 mm H_2O who are lethargic or confused or have cranial nerve palsies, visual impairment, or symptoms of severe headache or vomiting, and in all patients with markedly elevated pressures (>350 mm). The role of corticosteroids in reducing pressure in cryptococcal meningitis is unproven; if used, they should be used cautiously because they further impair host defense. Lumbar drains or ventriculoperitoneal shunting may be tried if other therapies have failed.
3. **Oral induction regimens.** The combination 5-flucytosine (37.5 mg per kg p.o. q.i.d.) and fluconazole (400 mg per day p.o. for 6 weeks), followed by fluconazole (400 mg per day p.o.) alone, has been evaluated and was effective in 63% of patients with cryptococcal meningitis (Larsen et al. *Clin Infect Dis* 1994;19:741). Patients with mild symptoms may be candidates for such oral therapy.
4. **Prognostic factors.** The most important predictor of early mortality is the mental status of the patient at presentation. Patients with any alteration in mental status (confusion, lethargy, or obtundation) fare worse than patients with normal mentation. Other factors that appeared predictive of worse outcome in various studies include a higher CSF cryptococcal antigen titer, a low CSF leukocyte count (<20 cells/mm³), and positive extraneural cultures for *C. neoformans*.
5. **Maintenance therapy.** The risk for recurrence after induction therapy is nearly 100% after 1 year if suppressive therapy is not provided. Fluconazole (200 mg per day p.o.) is 98% effective for prevention of recurrence and is well tolerated (Powderly et al. *N Engl J Med* 1992;326:793). Amphotericin B (1 mg per kg i.v.) weekly is less effective (18% relapse)

and poorly tolerated (Powderly et al. *N Engl J Med* 1992;326:793). Itraconazole, 200 mg/day also is inferior to fluconazole (24% relapse) but may be an option in patients unable to take fluconazole.

6. **Prevention**. In a prospective trial, fluconazole (200 mg per day p.o.) reduced the occurrence of cryptococcal meningitis from 7.1% to 0.9% (Powderly et al. *N Engl J Med* 1995;332:700). Itraconazole 200 per day p.o. also reduces the occurrence of cryptococcal meningitis. Prophylaxis with fluconazole, but not itraconazole, also markedly reduces the incidence of oropharyngeal and esophageal candidiasis. Benefit is seen mostly in patients with CD4+ counts <50 per μL. However, prophylaxis does not reduce mortality, is expensive, and might select for resistant fungi. Routine prophylaxis for all patients is not recommended but may be appropriate in selected situations.

7. **Effect of potent antiretroviral therapy**. As with other opportunistic infections, the incidence of cryptococcosis has decreased significantly. Several recent reports have described cases suggestive of an immune reconstitution illness in patients with a history of cryptococcal meningitis, shortly after the initiation of potent antiretroviral therapy. These include the reappearance of meningitis and cryptococcal lymphadenitis. Although there is limited data on stopping suppressive treatment for cryptococcal infection, systemic fungal infections are unlikely to differ from other opportunistic infections, and it may be reasonable to cautiously stop suppressive treatment in patients with sustained rises in CD4+ counts and undetectable HIV RNA levels.

III. **Histoplasmosis.** Histoplasmosis is common in the Mississippi and Ohio River Valleys and is manifested as disseminated disease in 95% of cases (Wheat et al. *Medicine* 1990;69:361). In addition to the endemic area, histoplasmosis occurs in patients who have previously resided in the endemic area, which also includes much of Central America and the Caribbean. Most patients have fever, fatigue, and weight loss, and half have respiratory symptoms of cough and dyspnea. Skin, oral, and occasionally gastrointestinal ulcers also occur. Pancytopenia and abnormal liver-function tests (especially elevated serum alkaline phosphatase) are common, reflecting involvement of the bone marrow and liver.

A. **Diagnosis.** Cultures are positive in 85% of cases, and Histoplasma polysaccharide antigen can be detected in the urine or serum of 90% to 95%, permitting a rapid diagnosis and detection of relapse (Histoplasmosis Reference Laboratory, Indianapolis, IN, U.S.A.). Fungal stains of tissues (such as bone marrow or liver) also permit rapid diagnosis. Immunodiffusion or complement-fixation tests for antibodies are positive in ~70% of patients.

B. **Treatment.** Induction treatment to produce a clinical remission and maintenance treatment to prevent relapse are highly effective, with response rates of 85% to 95%.

1. **Induction**

a. **Severe or moderately severe**. Amphotericin B, 0.7 mg per kg per day, is 98% effective in patients who are not severely ill but only 40% to 50% effective in those with shock, respiratory failure, multiorgan failure, or central nervous system involvement (Wheat et al. *Medicine* 1990;69:361). Treatment can be changed to oral therapy with itraconazole after a few days in most cases.

b. **Mild infection** can be managed with itraconazole, 200 mg p.o. t.i.d. for 3 days and then b.i.d. for 12 weeks. This is 85% effective in those with mild to moderately severe histoplasmosis (Wheat et al. *Am J Med* 1995;98:336). Drug interaction with the medications that reduce gastric acidification (histamine-receptor antagonists, omeprazole) or induce hepatic cytochrome P-450 decrease blood concentrations of itraconazole and may cause treatment failure. Rifampin must be strictly avoided. Measurement of blood concentrations of itraconazole is recommended to document adequate therapeutic concentrations. Concentrations of ~1 mg per mL are regarded as therapeutic.

Fluconazole, 800 mg per day, is less effective (72% response) than itraconazole and should not be used unless itraconazole is contraindicated or not tolerated. Ketoconazole is not an acceptable treatment (10% response) for histoplasmosis in AIDS.

2. **Maintenance.** Chronic suppressive treatment is indicated to prevent relapse. Weekly or biweekly amphotericin B (50 to 100 mg) and itraconazole (200 to 400 mg per day) are >90% effective as maintenance therapy, and itraconazole is well tolerated (Wheat et al. *Am J Med* 1995;98:336; Wheat et al. *Ann Intern Med* 1993;118:610). Fluconazole is less effective; 31% of patients treated with 400 mg per day relapsed in a recent prospective trial.

3. **Prevention.** Prophylaxis may be indicated in cities with high prevalence rate (>10%). Itraconazole (200 mg per day p.o.) has been shown to prevent both histoplasmosis and cryptococcosis.

IV. **Coccidioidomycosis.** Coccidioidomycosis occurs in the southwestern United States and should be considered in patients who have resided in or have visited those areas (Wheat. *Clin Microbiol Rev* 1995;8:146). Patients usually have pulmonary illnesses, but dissemination is common, especially to skin, bone, and central nervous system.

A. **Diagnosis.** Diagnosis is made by fungal stain and culture. Spherules may be seen in respiratory secretions or tissues, and cultures are positive in 3 to 5 days in most cases. Serologic tests, positive in 80%, also are useful.

B. **Treatment**

1. **Induction.** Treatment is less effective than in cryptococcosis or histoplasmosis. Amphotericin B (0.5 to 1.0 mg per kg per day i.v.), however, remains the treatment of choice, and is effective in half of cases. Fluconazole (400 to 800 mg per day p.o.) and itraconazole (200 mg p.o. b:i.d.) also are effective and might be used in patients with mild manifestations (Catanzaro et al. *Am J Med* 1995;98:249; Graybill et al. *Am J Med* 1990;89:282). Fluconazole (400 to 800 mg per day p.o.) is the preferred therapy for coccidioidal meningitis.

2. **Maintenance.** Chronic maintenance treatment is needed to prevent relapse. Fluconazole or itraconazole, 200 to 400 mg per day p.o., or amphotericin B, 50 mg i.v. weekly, are alternatives.

3. **Prevention.** Travel to endemic areas poses risk for coccidioidomycosis. At-risk patients should try to avoid the desert in the late summer and fall when dusty conditions prevail.

V. **Penicilliosis.** Penicilliosis occurs in the Northern Thailand (Chiang Mai) and the southern part of China. It should be considered in patients who have resided in or have visited those areas. Patients usually have disseminated disease, with fever, hepatosplenomegaly and skin lesions.

A. **Diagnosis.** Diagnosis is made by fungal stain and culture of blood or tissue.

B. **Treatment**

1. **Induction.** Amphotericin B (0.5 to 1.0 mg per kg per day i.v.) is the treatment of choice for severe disease, as initial therapy. Itraconazole (200 mg p.o. b.i.d.) is effective and can be used in patients after initial amphotericin B or for patients with mild manifestations (Sirisanthana et al. *Clin Infect Dis* 1998; 26:1107).

2. **Maintenance.** Chronic maintenance treatment is needed to prevent relapse. Itraconazole, 200 to 400 mg per day p.o. is the agent of choice.

VI. **Aspergillosis** occurs in fewer than 1% of patients with AIDS, usually during the last 6 months of life (Khoo et al. *Clin Infect Dis* 1994;19(suppl 1):S41). Pneumonia, sinusitis, and otitis are common manifestation, but dissemination often is present at autopsy.

A. **Diagnosis** is usually made by fungal stains or cultures of biopsy material. Isolation from respiratory secretions does not definitively establish the diagnosis because Aspergillus may merely colonize the airways.

B. **Treatment.** The mean survival after diagnosis is only 2 to 3 months (Khoo et al. *Clin Infect Dis* 1994;19(suppl 1):S41). Fewer than one third of patients have responded to treatment with amphotericin B or itraconazole (Denning et al. *Am J Med* 1994;97:135). Amphotericin B, 1 mg per kg i.v., is the best choice for more severe cases. Although experience in patients with AIDS is limited, amphotericin B-lipid complex, 5 mg per kg per day i.v., or liposomal amphotericin B, 3 to 6 mg per kg per day i.v. are less-toxic alternatives for patients with aspergillosis. Itraconazole, 200 to 400 mg p:o. b.i.d., is indicated for those with mild manifestations and for maintenance therapy.

VI. Systemic antifungal agents

   A. Fluconazole is widely used in patients with fungal infection, because of its oral administration, high bioavailability, and low toxicity. Unlike other azoles, it does not require an acid milieu for absorption and does not affect testosterone levels or adrenal function. Major side effects include nausea, abdominal pain, and hepatotoxicity. Skin rashes occur, and Stevens–Johnson syndrome has been described.

   B. Itraconazole is orally available, but in the capsule formulation absorption is dependent on food and gastric acidity and thus may be erratic in patients with AIDS. Itraconazole as an oral solution has greater bioavailability and is better absorbed in the fasting state. It should not be used concomitant with rifabutin, rifampin, phenobarbitone, or phenytoin because serum levels of itraconazole are reduced and loss of therapeutic effect may occur. In addition, it should not be used concomitant with the antihistamines (terfenadine or astemizole) because of the risk of sudden cardiac events. Adverse effects include nausea, abdominal pain, rash, headache, edema, and hypokalemia.

   C. Ketoconazole is the least expensive azole antifungal, but its use is limited in HIV infection for several reasons. Normal gastric acidity is required for its absorption. Hypochlorhydria is frequently associated with AIDS. Concomitant use of histamine-2–receptor antagonists or proton-pump inhibitors also decreases the bioavailability of ketoconazole. Ketoconazole can increase the serum levels of several of the protease inhibitors. Adverse effects of ketoconazole include anorexia, nausea, increases of serum aminotransferase levels, decreased testosterone production, and hypoadrenalism.

   D. Amphotericin B deoxycholate is the drug of choice for seriously ill patients. Amphotericin B is given by intravenous infusion over a 4-hour period. Fever, chills, and nausea are common during infusion. Symptoms can be attenuated by premedication with aspirin, acetaminophen, hydrocortisone (25 mg i.v.), or meperidine (25 mg i.v.). Renal insufficiency, hypokalemia, and anemia may develop after several weeks of treatment.

   E. Amphotericin B–lipid complex, amphotericin B colloidal dispersion, and liposomal amphotericin B are newer formulation of amphotericin B. These formulations are designed to deliver more amphotericin B without the same degree of dose-limiting toxicity. There have been a limited number of randomized trials using these agents in comparison with amphotericin B deoxycholate; none have shown superiority of these agents although they tend to be less toxic. Generally, they are generally reserved for patients unable to tolerate amphotericin B deoxycholate. The usual toxicities of amphotericin B deoxycholate occur but at a lower frequency. Hepatotoxicity has also been described as a side effect.

25. VIRAL INFECTIONS

I. **Cytomegalovirus end-organ disease**
  A. **Background**. Latent cytomegalovirus (CMV) infection is prevalent in >98% of gay men and ~75% of heterosexuals with human immunodeficiency virus (HIV) disease. Nearly all patients with advanced HIV disease and latent CMV infection will have at least intermittent reactivation of CMV infection with viral shedding in urine, semen, blood, or respiratory secretions. Prior to the current era of antiretroviral therapy, the cumulative incidence of sight- or life-threatening CMV end-organ disease was 20% to 40% in patients with acquired immunodeficiency syndrome (AIDS). Like other opportunistic infections, the incidence has changed considerably with the use of highly active antiretroviral therapy for HIV. CMV end-organ disease occurs almost exclusively in patients with <50 CD4$^+$ cells per µL. Approximately 90% of patients with CMV end-organ disease have retinitis, 15% to 20% have gastrointestinal (GI) disease, and a small proportion have neurologic or pulmonary disease.
  B. **Clinical presentation**
    1. **Retinitis.** The clinical presentation of CMV retinitis is a function of the location of retinal lesions. CMV retinitis is painless, and the most common presenting symptom is the appearance of "floaters" that move across the visual field and result from necrotic retinal debris moving through the vitreous humor. Patients who have retinitis involving areas near the macula may complain of visual-field deficits, and those with disease involving the optic nerve may complain of a general loss of visual acuity in the involved eye(s).
    2. **Gastrointestinal disease.** Esophagitis and colitis are the most common manifestations of CMV GI disease and are seen with, respectively, odynophagia or substernal pain in the former and diarrhea, often with some hematochezia and abdominal pain, in the latter condition. Less common GI manifestations include painful gastric, rectal, anal, or oral ulcers.
    3. **Neurologic disease**. The two most common neurologic syndromes caused by CMV are polyradiculopathy and encephalitis. CMV polyradiculopathy is seen with lower extremity weakness and areflexia; in more severe cases, anal and bladder tone may be diminished. CMV encephalitis typically is seen with altered sensorium and fever. Both CMV polyradiculopathy and encephalitis often occur in patients already diagnosed with CMV retinitis or GI disease.
    4. **Pneumonitis.** CMV pneumonitis is a very rare complication of AIDS. The presentation is nonspecific and includes hypoxemia, diffuse interstitial infiltrates on chest radiograph, and fever. The disease is often more indolent than other infectious pulmonary complications of AIDS such as bacterial pneumonia or pneumocystosis.
  C. **Diagnosis**
    1. **Retinitis.** CMV retinitis is a clinical diagnosis that must be confirmed by an experienced ophthalmologist who can verify the presence of typical white opacified retinal lesions, often with associated hemorrhage (see Chapter 16). The vitreous and anterior chamber are typically clear. CMV retinitis cannot be excluded on the basis of an examination performed with a direct ophthalmoscope, even in a dilated eye, because direct ophthalmoscopy permits visualization of <50% of the retinal surface. Indirect ophthalmoscopy performed by a trained ophthalmologist

The author acknowledges the contribution of Mark A. Jacobson to the previous edition of this chapter.

permits visualization of the entire retina. Knowledge of the location in the retina of all CMV lesions is a key consideration in devising an optimal treatment strategy for an individual patient. The location of lesions are characterized as zone 1 if lesions are located within two disc diameters of the fovea or within one disc diameter of the optic nerve head, zone 2 if located between zone 1 and the equator of the globe, and zone 3 if located anterior to the equator (see Fig. 1, Chapter 16).

2. **Gastrointestinal disease**. Diagnosis of CMV GI disease requires all three of the following components:
   a. Presence of a cardinal symptom referable to a specific part of the GI tract, such as odynophagia for esophagitis or diarrhea for colitis.
   b. Gross macroscopic evidence of mucosal erythema, erosion or ulceration (e.g., determined by endoscopy or colonoscopy).
   c. Mucosal biopsy that confirms presence of typical CMV cytopathology (large intranuclear or intracytplasmic inclusions). Specificity can be achieved by staining the tissue section with a monoclonal or polyclonal antibody that is specific for CMV antigen.

3. **Neurologic disease**. Diagnosis is based on the presence of the typical clinical findings along with either cerebrospinal fluid polymorphonuclear pleocytosis for polyradiculopathy or computed tomography (CT) or magnetic resonance imaging (MRI) evidence of periventricular enhancement for encephalitis. A positive rapid cerebrospinal fluid test for CMV DNA [e.g., by branched-chain DNA or polymerase chain reaction (PCR) technique] can also confirm the diagnosis.

4. **Pneumonitis**. This diagnosis can be made when hypoxemia and interstitial infiltrates are present, and a bronchoalveolar lavage or bronchoscopy biopsy specimen demonstrates typical CMV cytopathology, if all other protozoal, fungal, mycobacterial, and bacterial pulmonary pathogens have been excluded in the histologic and microbiologic examination of bronchoscopy specimens.

5. **Viremia**. A number of different assays have been developed to detect CMV DNA or other antigens as rapid diagnostic tests. Data from various small studies suggest that CMV is detectable from blood using these assays, on average, four months before the onset of clinically evident disease. The results with quantitative PCR revealed that the risk of end organ disease increased with higher PCR levels. These assays may also be useful therapeutically in assessing response to therapy and/or prophylaxis.

D. **Treatment**
   1. **Systemic drugs for CMV disease**
      a. **Ganciclovir**
         (1) **Standard induction dosage** of ganciclovir is 5 mg per kg every 12 hours for 2 to 3 weeks. Doses must be adjusted for renal function (Table 1).
         (2) **Maintenance therapy** is 5.0 mg per kg per day. Doses must be adjusted for renal function. Alternatively, maintenance therapy can be used 1 g p.o. t.i.d. using the oral formulation. However, randomized trials suggest that, for retinitis, IV administration is more effective. The oral formulation is poorly bioavailable; it is likely to be supplanted by valganciclovir (see Section I.D.1.d): when the latter becomes available.
         (3) **Side effects**
            (a) **Myelosuppression** is dose limiting (i.e., absolute neutrophil count <500 cells per µl): in 15% to 20% of patients. Can be reversed with myeloid growth factors such as G-CSF or GM-CSF at doses (G-CSF): as low as 150 µg s.q. 3 times per week.
            (b) **Thrombocytopenia** is dose limiting in 5% of patients.
            (c) Azospermia and ovarian failure may be irreversible
            (d) Nephrotoxicity and altered mental status are rare.

Table 1. Ganciclovir: standard dosing and toxicities

Creatinine clearance (mL/min/kg)	Dose
INDUCTION	
≥1.1	5.0 mg/kg q12h
0.7–1.0	2.5 mg/kg q12h
0.4–0.6	2.5 mg/kg/d
≤0.3	1.25 mg/kg/d
MAINTENANCE	
≥1.1	5.0 mg/kg/d or 6 mg/kg 5 d/wk
0.7–1.0	2.5 mg/kg/d or 3 mg/kg 5 d/wk
0.4–0.6	1.25 mg/kg/d or 1.5 mg/kg 5 d/wk
≤0.3	0.625 mg/kg/d or 0.75 mg/kg 5 d/wk

    b. Foscarnet
        (1) Standard induction therapy is 90 mg per kg every 12 hours for 2 to 3 weeks (see the following). Dosages must be adjusted carefully for renal function (Table 2).
        (2) Maintenance therapy is 90 mg per kg per 24 hours. Doses must be adjusted for renal function (Table 2).
        (3) Side effects
            (a) Nephrotoxicity can be dose limiting in 10% to 23% of patients treated and manifests as increased serum creatinine. Cases of acute renal failure have been reported. To limit foscarnet-induced nephrotoxicity, clinicians are advised to keep patients well-hydrated while receiving this drug. Intravenous sodium loading with coadministered normal saline has been reported to reduce risk of nephrotoxicity in an uncontrolled study.
            (b) Ionized **hypocalcemia** is the second most common serious toxicity of foscarnet therapy. Foscarnet appears to complex with free, unbound serum calcium, resulting in transient ionized hypocalcemia associated with the high foscarnet plasma concentrations that occur during maintenance therapy. This latter phenomenon also may explain occasional arrhythmias and seizures reported in conjunction with foscarnet therapy, as well as the nausea, mental-status changes, and other forms of neurotoxicity reported to occur in some patients in temporal association with foscarnet infusions.
            (c) Renal losses of total body calcium, phosphate, magnesium, or potassium can result in hypocalcemia, hypophosphatemia, hypomagnesemia, or hypokalemia. These adverse effects can usually be managed easily by oral or intravenous electrolyte or mineral repletion. However, severe, fatal cases of hypocalcemia have been reported in individuals receiving foscarnet coadministered with parenteral pentamidine. Benign, self-limited, hyperphosphatemia has been described with foscarnet therapy, and mild worsening of anemia is common.
            (d) Rare toxicities include nephrogenic diabetes insipidus and acute penile ulcerations.
    c. Cidofovir. Cidofovir [(S)-1-(3-hydroxy-2-phosphonylmethoxypropyl)] cytosine, is a nucleotide analog with potent activity versus CMV that has poor oral bioavailability but does have a long *in vivo* duration of

Table 2. Foscarnet: standard dosing and toxicities

Creatinine clearance (mL/min/kg)	Dose
INDUCTION	
≥1.6	90 mg/kg q12h
1.4–1.59	85 mg/kg q12h
1.2–1.39	73 mg/kg q12h
1.0–1.19	62 mg/kg q12h
0.8–0.99	50 mg/kg q12h
0.6–0.79	80 mg/kg q24h
0.4–0.59	56 mg/kg q24h
MAINTENANCE	
≥1.6	90 mg/kg q24h
1.4–1.59	85 mg/kg q24h
1.2–1.39	73 mg/kg q24h
1.0–1.19	62 mg/kg q24h
0.8–0.99	50 mg/kg q24h
0.6–0.79	80 mg/kg q48h
0.4–0.59	56 mg/kg q48h
RECOMMENDATIONS FOR MINERAL/ELECTROLYTE REPLETION	
Hypokalemia	KCl, 20 mEq/d to 40 mEq p.o. t.i.d., depending on severity (or i.v. 10 mEq/h 1–4 times/d if very severe)
Hypomagnesemia	MgGluconate, 500 mg p.o. b.i.d.–q.i.d.
Hypophosphatemia	Neutra Phos i p.o. b.i.d.–t.i.d.
Hypocalcemia	$CaCO_3$, 650 mg i-ii p.o. t.i.d. (or i.v. CaGluconate if severe)

anti-CMV activity. Intravenous cidofovir infusions given just once every 1 to 2 weeks can control CMV disease.

(1) Cidofovir is typically administered at a 5 mg per kg dose, as a 1-hour i.v. infusion with 1 L normal saline before the infusion and a second liter of saline after the infusion. Probenecid, 2 g p.o., is administered 3 hour before and 1 g p.o. is administered 2 and 8 hours after the cidofovir dose. Initially cidofovir infusions are administered once weekly for 2 consecutive weeks and then subsequently at every-other-week intervals. Both serum creatinine and urine protein must be checked just before each cidofovir infusion. Cidofovir should be discontinued if persistent ≥3+ urine protein is detected or if the serum creatinine increases by >0.5 mg per dL above the baseline value after initiating treatment with this drug (see Table 3).

(2) The most important **toxicity** described with cidofovir has been nephrotoxicity, in particular a prolonged renal tubular toxicity that begins with proteinuria and subsequently can lead to azotemia and proximal renal tubular acidosis. Concomitant administration of probenecid and saline hydration with cidofovir appears to reduce the risk of nephrotoxicity, although probenecid may itself cause dose-limiting nausea, rash, or fever. Myelosuppression, alopecia, anterior uveitis, hypotony, and peripheral neuropathy also have been reported as side effects of cidofovir.

(3) In a randomized trial of immediate versus deferred cidofovir treatment for peripheral CMV retinitis, median time to retinitis progression was significantly longer for cidofovir-treated than

for untreated patients. However, approximately one third of cidofovir-treated patients had dose-limiting, but reversible, toxicity (13% proteinuria, 5% increased creatinine, and 5% rash).

   d. **Valganciclovir,** the valine ester of ganciclovir, is given orally and rapidly converted to ganciclovir after absorption. A dose of 900 mg p.o. achieves levels of ganciclovir equivalent to those seen with an intravenous dosage of 5 mg per kg. When given as induction therapy for CMV retinitis, rates of response and progression equivalent to intravenous therapy were seen in a randomized comparative trial. Toxicities were also similar. This formulation is likely to be available by 2001.

2. **Local therapy for CMV retinitis**

   a. An intravitreal sustained-release pellet of ganciclovir (**ganciclovir implant**) can be surgically implanted under the sclera. This implant delivers ganciclovir at the rate of a 1 µg per hour. For treated eyes with retinitis at baseline, the median times to retinitis progression are highly significantly longer for the implant than for the intravenous ganciclovir. With this intervention, reported time to retinitis progression has been longer than with any other treatment for CMV retinitis.

      (1) Although the efficacy of the implant is impressive, it has been associated with some serious, irreversible, ocular **adverse events** affecting vision. Endophthalmitis, early retinal detachment, and severe vitreal bleeding have occurred in implant-treated patients as complications of the surgical procedure. Overall, it appears that ~10% of patients who undergo this procedure may have such an adverse event, resulting in a permanent worsening of visual function, although less frequent side problems are seen with more experienced operators. In addition, most patients have a transient (up to 1 month) reduction in visual acuity caused by intraoperative bleeding into the vitreous. Also, there has been reported an ~30% risk of CMV disease developing outside the implant-treated eye (in the other eye or extraocular CMV end-organ disease), if no additional treatment is given.

      (2) Because CMV disease is systemic and because unilateral retinitis tends to progress to bilateral disease without systemic anti-CMV therapy, the ultimate role of this form of intervention remains uncertain. The implant seems to be a **reasonable treatment strategy for patients with zone 1 disease** (see Section C, Diagnosis) who are at high risk for losing visual function if retinitis progresses. **A combination of intravitreal and oral systemic therapy has been shown to be the optimal approach to treating sight-threatening CMV retinitis.**

   b. **Fomivirsen** is a novel agent (an antisense oligonucleotide complementary to the human CMV immediate early region 2 messenger RNA) which is used for intravitreal injection for patients who are can not take, are intolerant to or have failed other approved CMV therapies. Median times to progression of about 3 months in previously treated patients have been reported. Dosage is 330 µg every two weeks for first two doses and then monthly thereafter, given as an intraocular injection.

3. **Standard therapy for CMV retinitis**

   a. Patients who are diagnosed by an ophthalmologist as having CMV retinitis involving zone 1 of the retina (within two disc diameters of the fovea or one disc diameter of the optic nerve head) (see Chapter 16) in an eye that has potentially salvageable visual function should have **induction** therapy with foscarnet or ganciclovir initiated within 24 hours, and should be referred for a ganciclovir intraocular implant (see 2).

b. For all other patients, the decision regarding when to initiate therapy will require consideration of the individual's anatomic location of retinal lesions, underlying medical condition, social supports, and cognitive level.

c. **Choice of induction therapy**

(1) **Ganciclovir** is the drug of choice for those individuals whose estimated creatinine clearance (ClCr) is <1.2 mL per min per kg. Ganciclovir induction should consist of 5 mg per kg i.v. infusions administered over 1 hour b.i.d. for 14 days; an i.v. pump is not required for drug administration. Absolute neutrophil counts and platelets should be checked at least twice a week during induction. Outpatient induction is appropriate for individuals with no concurrent medical problems that require hospitalization. Ganciclovir therapy should not be interrupted as long as the absolute neutrophil count (ANC) is >500 cells per µL and platelets are >20,000 per µl. If dose-limiting neutropenia occurs, then G-CSF should be administered as an adjunctive agent (initially 150 or 300 µg s.q. 3 times per week, depending on the degree of neutropenia) and titrated to keep the trough ANC (obtained at the end of the longest interval between G-CSF injections) between 500 and 1,500 cells per µl. If dose-limiting thrombocytopenia occurs, the patient should be switched to foscarnet.

(2) **Foscarnet** is the drug of choice for those individuals whose platelet count is <20,000 per µL. Foscarnet should be administered as a 2-hours infusion (dose determined by estimated ClCr, see Table 2) administered every 12 hours by i.v. infusion pump for 14 days. Serum creatinine, calcium, potassium, phosphate, and magnesium should be checked at least 2 times/week and hemoglobin weekly during induction. Foscarnet therapy should be discontinued if the serum Cr increases to >2.9 mg per dL or if severe drug-related metabolic or neurologic toxicity occurs. Most patients with drug-related hypokalemia, hypocalcemia, hypomagnesemia, or hypophosphatemia can be managed by continuing foscarnet with appropriate oral or i.v. mineral repletion. Drug-related hyperphosphatemia is self-limited, and foscarnet can be continued without any specific intervention.

(3) **Either i.v. ganciclovir or foscarnet** may be appropriate induction therapy for all other patients. The optimal drug choice involves consideration of the individual's underlying medical condition. In addition, social supports and cognitive level are important considerations for outpatient induction.

(4) **Cidofovir** avoids the requirement for a chronic indwelling intravenous catheter: infusions are given weekly × 2 for induction, then bi-weekly for maintenance therapy. However, the median duration that patients can tolerate cidofovir has been reported to be only 3 to 4 months due to nephrotoxicity or other side effects of cidofovir or the concomitant probenecid that must be given to prevent serious, irreversible nephrotoxicity. Details of dosing and patient selection criteria are summarized in Table 3.

d. **Choice of maintenance therapy**

(1) **I.V. Ganciclovir** is the drug of choice for those individuals whose serum Cr at the end of induction therapy is >2.0 mg per dL. Ganciclovir maintenance therapy should consist of daily or, less preferably, 5 day per week 1-hour infusions with the dose adjusted to renal function; an i.v. pump is not required for drug administration. The dose should be reduced for patients with a reduced estimated ClCr (see Table 1). Absolute neutrophil

Table 3. Cidofovir: standard dosing and toxicities

	Induction	Maintenance	Monitoring
Cidofovir[ab]	5 mg/kg weekly × 2 doses	5 mg/kg q2wks	Check serum creatinine, urine protein, complete blood count before each infusion. If absolute granulocyte count is <500 cells/uL, co-administer granulocyte-colony stimulating factor, titrating dose to maintain absolute neutrophil count between 500 and 1,500 cells/μL. Monitor intraocular pressure monthly and discontinue cidofovir if pressure decreases below 50% of the baseline value. Symptomatic treatment for probenecid toxicity may include diphenhydramine or loritidine for rash, acetaminophen for fever, prochlorperazine or ondansetron for nausea.

[a] One hour intravenous fusion. Administer probenecid 2 g/3 h before and normal saline 1 liter 1 h before cidofovir infusion. Co-administer normal saline 1 L with cidofovir. Administer probenecid 1 g 2 h and 8 h after completing infusion.
[b] Cidofovir is contraindicated if baseline urine protein is ≥ 2+, serum creatinine is > 1.5 g/dl, or estimated creatinine clearance is ≤55 ml/min. Dose should be reduced from 5 mg/kg to 3 mg/kg if serum creatinine increases by 0.3 to 0.4 mg/dL over baseline value. Drug must be discontinued if serum creatinine increases by ≥0.5 mg/dl over baseline value or if ≥ 3+ proteinuria occurs. Cidofovir should not be administered concurrently, with or within 7 days of other nephrotoxic drugs (i.e., foscarnet, aminoglycosides, amphotericin, nonsteroidal antiinflammatory drugs, vancomycin, or parenteral pentamidine).

counts and platelets should be checked weekly. The patient should be weighed monthly. Management of ganciclovir-associated neutropenia or thrombocytopenia was described [see Section 2.c.(1)].

(2) **Foscarnet** is the drug of choice for those individuals whose platelet count is <20,000 per μL. Foscarnet should be administered as a 2-hour infusion (dose determined by estimated ClCr; see Table 2) administered daily by i.v. infusion pump indefinitely. Serum creatinine, calcium, potassium, phosphate, and magnesium should be checked weekly and hemoglobin every 2 weeks. The patient should be weighed monthly. Foscarnet therapy should be discontinued if the serum Cr increases to >2.9 mg per dL or if severe drug-related metabolic or neurologic toxicity or drug-related genital ulcers occur.

(3) **Either i.v. ganciclovir or foscarnet** may be appropriate maintenance therapy for all other patients. The optimal drug choice involves consideration of the individual's underlying medical condition and plans for concurrent antiretroviral therapy. In addition, social supports and cognitive level are key

considerations. The expected percentage of patients with dose-limiting toxicity (that cannot be controlled with adjunctive G-CSF) from long-term ganciclovir therapy is expected to be <5%. The expected percentage of patients with dose-limiting toxicity from chronic foscarnet therapy is expected to be ~20%.

(4) Cidofovir is another maintenance therapy option. See Section 2.C.i.v.

(5) **Oral ganciclovir for maintenance therapy** may be appropriate for certain selected patients. Oral ganciclovir should be used as adjunctive therapy in patients who receive the intravitreal ganciclovir implant to reduce the risk of disease in the contralateral eye or systemically. Oral ganciclovir is also reasonable therapy in patients who are initiating potent antiretroviral therapy. Patients who have progression occur while receiving oral ganciclovir should be reinduced with i.v. ganciclovir or foscarnet until complete regression of retinal lesions has occurred, after which it may be appropriate to reinstitute oral ganciclovir maintenance therapy.

e. Duration of therapy. If immunodeficiency persists, treatment must be given for life. However, patients with healed CMV retinitis who have both immunological and virological response to potent antiretroviral therapy can discontinue CMV-specific maintenance therapy. Therapy for CMV must be resumed if antiretroviral therapy fails as relapse will occur.

4. CMV gastrointestinal disease

a. When to initiate therapy. Therapy is indicated when (a) a patient has moderate or severe symptoms that are caused by CMV GI disease, (b) other causes of these symptoms have been excluded by appropriate microbiologic tests and direct GI mucosal visualization, and (c) GI mucosal biopsy shows evidence of typical CMV cytopathologic conditions.

b. Choice of therapy

(1) I.V. ganciclovir is the **initial** drug of choice for those individuals whose estimated ClCr is <1.2 mL per minute per kg. Ganciclovir therapy should consist of induction (5 mg per kg 1-hour infusions administered every 12 h) for a minimum of 21 days; an i.v. pump is not required for drug administration. Patients who have not had resolution of their symptoms at the end of 21 days of twice daily dosing may require ≤42 days of treatment. Patients who have not improved after 6 weeks of induction therapy should be considered to have failed and should receive a trial of foscarnet therapy. To accurately evaluate treatment response, repeated endoscopic visualization and biopsy may be necessary. Generally, patients should be treated with this regimen until they are symptom free or have endoscopic evidence of healing. Use of ganciclovir is described in Sections D.I.2 and D.2.c.(i).

(2) **Foscarnet** is the drug of choice for those individuals whose platelet count is <20,000 per μm. Foscarnet should be administered as an induction regimen (same as that for retinitis) for a minimum of 21 days. Patients who have not had resolution of their symptoms at the end of 21 days of induction dosing may require 42 days of treatment. To accurately evaluate treatment response, repeated endoscopic visualization and biopsy may be necessary. Generally patients should be treated with this regimen until they are symptom free or have endoscopic evidence of healing. Patients who have not improved after 6 weeks of therapy should considered the treatment to have failed and should be switched to ganciclovir. Serum creatinine, calcium, potassium, phosphate, and magnesium should be checked at least

2 times per week and hemoglobin weekly during induction. Foscarnet therapy should be discontinued if the serum creatinine level increases to >2.9 mg per dL or if severe drug-related metabolic or neurologic toxicity occurs. See Section 2.c.ii and Table 2 for guidelines on use of foscarnet.

(3) No published data demonstrate clinical benefit from administering long-term, indefinite maintenance therapy to patients with CMV GI disease who have completed an initial induction course of therapy with either drug. In fact, many patients have symptom-free intervals of considerable duration after completing an induction course of therapy. If, however, patients have a recurrence of CMV GI disease, again meeting the diagnostic criteria outlined, then a reinduction course of therapy is indicated. Generally patients should be treated with this regimen until they are symptom free or have endoscopic evidence of healing, and subsequently they should receive a long-term maintenance regimen as outlined. Some experts have suggested using oral ganciclovir maintenance therapy. As with any other opportunistic infection, optimal antiretroviral therapy improves outcome.

5. **Other CMV diseases** (polyradiculopathy, pneumonia, and so on)
   a. **When to initiate therapy.** A benefit of either ganciclovir or foscarnet therapy for these conditions has never been demonstrated in any prospective clinical trial. However, there are anecdotal reports that in rare cases therapy has ameliorated an individual's clinical course. Before initiating anti-CMV therapy for one of these diseases, the clinician should be confident that all other potentially responsible pathogenic processes have been excluded or adequately treated.
   b. **Choice of therapy.** There is no clinical database from which firm therapeutic guidelines can be made. The most rational course would probably be to follow the general recommendations outlined above.
   c. **CMV encephalopathy** tends to be seen in very advanced HIV disease, with over 90% of patients having prior CMV infection elsewhere. Prognosis is generally very poor with a median survival of only 12 weeks. A combination of both ganciclovir and foscarnet should be used, as well as optimal antiretroviral therapy.

6. **Salvage therapy with combination ganciclovir and foscarnet.** Results of a randomized prospective trial indicate that combining ganciclovir and foscarnet therapy can prolong the time to retinitis progression twofold in patients who have already had progression on standard antiviral monotherapy. Combination therapy could be particularly beneficial for patients who have active retinitis that is very close to critical structures such as the macula or optic nerve head and who still have good functional vision in the involved eye(s). The most commonly used combination regimen is to continue maintenance therapy with the antiviral drug (ganciclovir or foscarnet) that the patient is currently receiving and add standard induction and subsequent maintenance doses of the other agent.

E. **Prophylaxis for CMV end-organ disease**
   1. No definitive recommendations can be made regarding **prophylactic use of oral ganciclovir** to prevent CMV end-organ disease in patients with advanced HIV disease. Oral ganciclovir is effective in reducing the incidence of CMV disease when given to patients with CD4$^+$ counts <50 cells/mm^3. However, because of issues of cost and potential for resistance, Public Health Service Guidelines do not currently recommend routine prophylaxis for CMV infection.
   2. Because diagnosis is most commonly clinical, patients with HIV infection should be educated about the symptoms of CMV retinitis and advised to seek care in a timely manner after the onset of visual symptoms. The

importance of regular ophthalmologic and medical follow-up should be stressed and patients at high risk (CD4$^+$ counts < 50 cells/mm^3 or a history of other opportunistic infections) should have **ophthalmologic screening** (including indirect ophthalmoscopy) every 3 to 6 months. Patients with extraocular CMV disease should also have regular eye examinations and the diagnosis of CMV retinitis should trigger a search for extraocular CMV disease.

3. The role of **targeted prophylaxis** for patients with CD4$^+$ counts <50 cells/mm^3 and detectable plasma CMV DNA PCR is currently under investigation.

F. **CMV disease in the context of potent antiretroviral therapy.** Effective treatment of HIV has dramatic effects on the natural history of CMV infection.

1. Potent antiretroviral therapy is associated with **clearance of CMV viremia**, over a period of 3 to 6 months.

2. CMV disease can occur, especially in the first 3 months of therapy, before the immune benefit is secure. Patients may have CD4$^+$ T cell counts > 200 cells/mm^3 at the time of diagnosis of CMV retinitis and may develop **vitritis** which is rarely observed in AIDS related CMV retinitis. These findings seem consistent with the hypothesis that these patients had subclinical CMV retinal infection that was unmasked by the immune inflammatory response resulting from the use of HAART permitting reconstitution of CMV-specific, protective immunity.

3. **CMV-specific T cells** are restored with antiretroviral therapy, although their role in host immunity is less clear.

4. **Withdrawal of maintenance treatment** may be considered in patients with sustained increased of CD4$^+$ lymphocyte count to >100 to 150 cells/ mm^3 for >3 to 6 months on potent antiretroviral therapy and who have non-sight-threatening lesions. Vitritis may also be seen as a complication of stopping CMV suppressive therapy. Relapses with CMV retinitis occurred when HIV therapy failed and a consequent fall of CD4$^+$ T cell count.

II. **Herpes simplex virus infection**

A. **Background: prevalence of infection, pathogenesis, incidence of disease**. Most episodes of anogenital or nasolabial herpes are thought to be recurrences of latent infection. On the basis of serum antibody testing, latent herpes simplex virus (HSV) 1 and 2 infection has been reported to be prevalent in 66% and 77% of AIDS patients, respectively, with approximately two thirds of such patients having clinically apparent herpes recurrences. Clinical recurrences of anogenital or nasolabial herpes can occur at any CD4$^+$ count. Although, in the absence of specific antiviral treatment, recurrences tend to be more severe and prolonged in patients with <200 CD4$^+$ cells per μL, it appears that the frequency of herpes recurrences may not be more frequent than those in immunocompetent individuals.

B. **Clinical presentation**

1. **Anogenital herpes**. Anogenital herpes lesions are usually caused by HSV 2 and may be seen as clusters of small vesicles or as single or multiple small or large confluent ulcers of the buttocks, perineum, scrotum, vulva, or penis. Rarely herpes may involve the rectum and be seen as proctitis with rectal pain and tenesmus.

2. **Orolabial herpes**. Orolabial herpes lesions may be caused by HSV 1 or 2 and be seen as clusters of small vesicles or as single or multiple small or large ulcers of the lips, nose, or oral mucosa.

3. **Other manifestations**. Herpes esophagitis is a rare complication of AIDS and appears identical to CMV esophagitis with odynophagia. Esophageal ulcers are observed on endoscopy. HSV neurologic disease may be no more prevalent than that in the immunocompetent populations; very rarely cases of HSV myelitis, encephalitis, and retinitis have been reported.

C. **Diagnosis.** Mucocutaneous HSV disease can be diagnosed clinically by its typical location and appearance and rapid resolution after initiating oral acyclovir therapy. The diagnosis can best be confirmed microbiologically by culturing a swab taken from the base of an ulcer. Diagnosis of neurologic disease requires culture of cerebrospinal fluid or brain tissue.

D. **Therapy**

1. **Acyclovir.** Oral acyclovir, 200 to 400 mg p.o. 5 times per day, is very effective for the treatment of mucocutaneous herpes disease. Therapy may need to be continued for >1 week to heal large ulcers. In patients with very large ulcers, initial intravenous acyclovir treatment may be appropriate.

2. **Valacyclovir** is a valine ester of acyclovir that has much greater bioavailability than acyclovir and is rapidly and completely metabolized to acyclovir after absorption. Blood levels of acyclovir achieved by taking oral valacyclovir, 1,000 mg, greatly exceed levels achievable with maximal oral acyclovir dosing. Preliminary data from large multicenter controlled trials conducted in immunocompetent adults suggest that valacyclovir, 1,000 mg b.i.d., is at least as effective as acyclovir given 5 times per day in the treatment of recurrent genital herpes. Prolonged therapy with high doses of valacyclovir has been associated with hemolytic uremic syndrome/thrombotic thrombocytic purpura (HUS/TTP) syndrome and is not recommended.

3. **Acyclovir-resistant disease.** Large herpetic ulcers that do not resolve with oral or intravenous acyclovir and continue to grow HSV from ulcer swabs despite prolonged acyclovir therapy are likely caused by acyclovir-resistant HSV strains. Such acyclovir-resistant disease typically occurs only in patients with <100 CD4$^+$ cells per μL who have a history of long-term acyclovir exposure. The diagnosis can be confirmed by performing *in vitro* drug-susceptibility testing of HSV grown from the ulcer. Intravenous foscarnet (40 mg per kg t.i.d.) has been proven effective as treatment for acyclovir-resistant mucocutaneous disease. Reports indicate that topical treatment with trifloridine or cidofovir also may be effective.

E. **Prophylaxis.** Continuous oral prophylaxis with acyclovir (e.g., 400 mg b.i.d.) can effectively prevent HSV disease recurrences. However, in patients with <100 CD4$^+$ cells per μL, continuous oral acyclovir prophylaxis is associated with a small risk of acyclovir-resistant disease developing.

III. **Varicella-zoster virus infection**

A. **Background: prevalence of infection, pathogenesis, incidence of disease.** Disease caused by primary varicella zoster virus (VZV) infection is very rare in HIV-infected adults because of the high prevalence of latent VZV infection in the general adult population. The incidence of clinical VZV reactivation (i.e., as zoster) is clearly greater in HIV-infected patients than that in the general population and can occur at any CD4$^+$ count. Zoster incidence is estimated to be 5% to 10% per year in patients with advanced HIV disease who are not receiving antiherpesvirus prophylaxis.

B. **Clinical presentation**

1. **Cutaneous zoster** is the most common form of VZV disease in HIV and typically is seen as a painful, dermatomal eruption of vesicles, most frequently involving the head, chest, or arms or sacral nerve root distribution. Zoster can be multidermatomal or involve widespread cutaneous dissemination, and the lesions may be atypical-appearing papules. Often there is a prodrome of localized neuritic pain that precedes the rash. Typically lesions resolve without specific antiviral treatment, although persistence and recurrence are common in patients with more advanced HIV disease. Also, persistent pain (postherpetic neuralgia) may complicate episodes of zoster. Rare cases of primary varicella infection in adults with HIV can be seen with visceral dissemination and may progress to chronic skin involvement.

2. **Ocular zoster**. Zoster ophthalmicus [involving the ophthalmic branch (V_1) of the trigeminal nerve] has a propensity to result in conjunctival, corneal, anterior chamber, or retinal disease that can be sight threatening. Zoster retinitis preferentially involves the peripheral retina but tends to progress circumferentially and result in retinal detachment in most cases, even with antiviral treatment. Blindness is a common complication of zoster retinitis (see Chapter 16).

3. **Zoster meningoencephalitis**. Cases of viral meningitis, myelitis, and encephalitis, including cases with one or more of these manifestations combined, have all been reported as caused by VZV in patients with AIDS. As with retinitis, the prognosis is poor.

C. **Diagnosis: DFA, culture, clinical**. Cutaneous zoster is usually an obvious clinical diagnosis; however, if the presentation is atypical, the diagnosis can best be confirmed by testing a smear of a swab of the base of a skin lesion for the presence of VZV antigen by a direct fluorescent antibody (DFA) method. Viral culture is less sensitive than that for HSV skin infection. VZV retinitis is a clinical diagnosis made by the typical clinical appearance of the retina and confirmed by a history of concurrent or recent cutaneous zoster. VZV neurologic disease usually requires viral culture or antigen testing of cerebrospinal fluid to confirm the diagnosis.

D. **Therapy**

1. **Acyclovir and valacyclovir**. Acyclovir at a dose of 800 mg 5 times per day has been reported to reduce the time to pain resolution in elderly adults with localized zoster. Valacyclovir is a valine ester of acyclovir, which has much greater bioavailability than acyclovir and is rapidly and completely metabolized to acyclovir after absorption. Blood levels of acyclovir achieved by taking oral valacyclovir, 1,000 mg, greatly exceed levels achievable with maximal oral acyclovir dosing. Based on data from multicentered clinical trials showing shorter overall duration of dermatomal pain, the Food and Drug Administration (FDA) has approved valacyclovir at a dose of 1,000 mg t.i.d. for the treatment of zoster in elderly immunocompetent individuals. Convincing data that acyclovir or valacyclovir is clinically beneficial for HIV-associated zoster does not exist. On the other hand, treatment of zoster ophthalmicus with oral acyclovir, 800 mg q.i.d., has clearly been shown to reduce serious ocular complications in immunocompetent individuals. Thus acyclovir or valacyclovir would certainly be recommended for zoster ophthalmicus in HIV-infected patients. With respect to VZV neurologic disease, there are case reports of clinical improvement with intravenous acyclovir. Intravenous acyclovir also is indicated for VZV retinitis.

2. **Famciclovir** is another new nucleoside agent, also recently approved by the FDA for the treatment of zoster in the immunocompetent elderly. At a dose of 500 mg p.o. t.i.d., famciclovir resolves postherpetic neuralgia sooner than does placebo. Data from patients with HIV-disease is lacking.

3. **Acyclovir-resistant disease (foscarnet, cidofovir)**. Persistent hyperkeratotic lesions at the site of an initial zoster outbreak that do not resolve with oral or intravenous acyclovir and continue to grow VZV from swabs despite prolonged acyclovir therapy are likely caused by acyclovir-resistant VZV strains. Such acyclovir-resistant disease typically occurs only in patients with <100 CD4$^+$ cells per μL who have a history of chronic acyclovir exposure. The diagnosis can be confirmed by performing *in vitro* drug-susceptibility testing of VZV grown from skin swabs or biopsies. Intravenous foscarnet (40 mg per kg t.i.d.) has been reported to be effective as treatment for acyclovir-resistant mucocutaneous disease. Intravenous cidofovir might also be effective.

E. **Prophylaxis**. Continuous oral prophylaxis with acyclovir (e.g., 400 mg b.i.d.) may prevent VZV disease recurrences. However, in patients with <100 CD4$^+$ cells per μL continuous oral acyclovir prophylaxis may potentially lead to acyclovir-resistant disease developing.

26. PYOGENIC INFECTIONS

Bacterial infections are an important cause of morbidity and mortality during the course of human immunodeficiency virus (HIV) infection. With successful prophylaxis for opportunistic infections, bacterial infections emerged as a significant clinical problem. In 1993 recurrent bacterial pneumonia was added as an acquired immunodeficiency virus (AIDS)-defining condition in the expanded AIDS case definition.

I. **Epidemiology.** The incidence of bacterial infections during the course of HIV infection varies by stage of disease and risk group. Among injection-drug users (IDUs), incidence of sepsis and bacterial pneumonia in one series was 8.0 episodes per 100 person-years (Selwyn et al. *N Engl J Med* 1992;327:1697). Risk increases with lower $CD4^+$ count, injection-drug use, smoking drugs (but not cigarettes), and possibly neutropenia. **Upper respiratory infections, sinusitis, and pneumonia** are the most common bacterial infections reported in most series. Bacterial pneumonia and sepsis were associated with excess morbidity and risk of progression to AIDS among HIV-infected IDUs. HIV-infected persons are 4 to 8 times more likely to have bacterial pneumonia than are control populations followed up prospectively (Wallace et al. *Am Rev Respir Dis* 1993;148:1523; Selwyn et al. *N Engl J Med* 1992;327:1697).

II. **Pathogenesis**
  A. **Host defects**
    1. **Neutrophils.** HIV can infect neutrophils, and this may explain the depressed superoxide production and reduced phagocytic function noted in neutrophils from patients with advanced HIV disease.
    2. **B lymphocytes.** Abnormalities of B-cell function include the spontaneous secretion of antibody and lack of response to signals for activation). A reduction in the density of complement receptors has been described, which may also contribute to the impaired function.
    3. **Disruption of mucous-membrane and skin integrity.** Chronic dermatitis and mucosal ulcerations caused by HIV or other opportunistic pathogens may provide a portal of entry for bacteria.
    4. **Respiratory tract.** A reduction in the production of salivary immunoglobulin A (IgA) may lead to colonization with pathogenic bacteria. Impaired neutrophil function and reduced production of opsonizing antibody by B lymphocytes have been implicated as important factors predisposing to bacterial pneumonia. In addition, impaired function of alveolar macrophages may predispose to pneumonia.
  B. **External factors.** The use of broad-spectrum antibiotics for prophylaxis may promote colonization with resistant organisms and increase the risk for infections from these pathogens. Indwelling intravascular catheters used especially for treatment of cytomegalovirus (CMV) retinitis disrupt skin integrity and increase the risk of bacteremia.

III. **Specific syndromes**
  A. **Bacterial pneumonia.** Bacterial pneumonia is an important cause of morbidity and mortality for all patients with HIV infection but particularly among IDUs. The clinical presentation, etiologic agents, and outcome from bacterial pneumonia depend on the stage of disease and on whether the infection is community or nosocomially acquired. The most common pathogens are *Streptococcus pneumoniae, Haemophilus influenzae, Staphylococcus aureus,* and *Pseudomonas aeruginosa.* Higher rates of bacteremia, higher relapse rates, and higher mortality have been associated with episodes of pneumonia in HIV infection.

1. **Diagnosis.** The approach to the workup of respiratory symptoms in persons with HIV infection (see Chapter 11) includes a **chest radiograph, arterial blood gas, sputum for Gram stain, acid-fast bacilli (AFB) stain, and if appropriate, stains for *Pneumocystis carinii*** pneumonia (PCP; see Chapter 22), and blood cultures. The chest radiograph appearance of bacterial pneumonia ranges from lobar consolidation to a diffuse interstitial appearance indistinguishable from that of PCP. Bacterial pathogens (in addition to tuberculosis) also should be suspected when cavitary disease is present. An etiologic agent can usually be identified by sputum culture, bronchoscopy, or fine-needle aspiration in cases of cavitary disease.

2. **Empiric therapy.** The choice of initial therapy depends on the findings on Gram stain and chest radiograph and the clinical presentation. The following clinical factors may be helpful in determining which patients can be treated with oral therapy and who should be hospitalized: severe hypoxemia, hypotension, tachypnea, multilobar disease, and impaired renal or hepatic function all warrant hospital admission. If PCP has been excluded or is not a consideration based on the stage of HIV infection (i.e., CD4+ >300), it may be reasonable to treat with oral therapy with a macrolide such as azithromycin, a second-generation cephalosporin, trimethoprim–sulfamethoxazole (TMP/SMX; unless the patient takes it for prophylaxis), or amoxicillin/clavulanic acid. For patients for whom PCP is being considered, therapy with TMP/SMX will cover most bacterial pathogens and PCP. Patients with any of the clinical factors mentioned that suggest more severe pneumonia should be hospitalized for parenteral therapy with a third-generation cephalosporin. If *Pseudomonas aeruginosa* is suspected (see the following), an antipseudomonal-lactam plus an aminoglycoside should be used.

3. **Specific pathogens**
   a. *Pseudomonas aeruginosa* **pneumonia.** *P. aeruginosa* is an emerging pathogen in advanced HIV infection, and pulmonary disease is the most common syndrome. The **clinical presentation** ranges from **fulminant multilobar pneumonia to cavitary disease** to a more **indolent respiratory infection** that tends to recur (Baron et al. *Am Rev Respir Dis* 1993;148:992). Risk factors for developing Pseudomonas infections include a prior diagnosis of AIDS, prior hospitalizations, and recent antibiotic use (Fichtenbaum et al. *Clin Infect Dis* 1994;19:417). *Pseudomonas aeruginosa* infections are frequently community acquired, and the classic risk factors such as use of corticosteroids and neutropenia are usually absent.

   b. **Nocardia.** Although it is a infrequent pathogen, Nocardia bears mention because of the delays in diagnosis in most reported cases. The **radiographic appearance** is variable and can include lobar and multilobar consolidation, pleural effusions, pulmonary masses, and cavitary disease. The **diagnosis** is suspected by the finding of beaded or branching filaments organisms on **modified acid-fast stain. TMP/SMX** is the standard therapy for Nocardia. However, species with reduced sensitivity to TMP/SMX have been identified in patients with AIDS who are receiving chronic prophylaxis. For this reason, susceptibility testing should be performed by a reference laboratory.

   c. *Rhodococcus equii* is an aerobic, gram-positive, nonmotile pleomorphic bacillus that can cause **pulmonary cavitary** disease in patients with HIV infection. The organism can easily be overlooked as a contaminant in the laboratory. Extrapulmonary disease including **brain abscess, enteritis, and regional adenitis** have all been reported. **Therapy** includes the use of a **macrolide in combination with rifampin** and should be prolonged (i.e., 3 to 6 months). Lifelong therapy to prevent relapse may be required.

B. Sinusitis is a growing problem among HIV-infected adults. The role of bacteria in the pathogenesis of this problem remains uncertain; however, bacterial superinfection is common. The **symptoms of nasal discharge and facial pain** with or without fever should suggest the diagnosis of sinusitis. The most common pathogens are *S. pneumoniae*, *H. influenzae*, *S. aureus*, and in chronic cases, *P. aeruginosa*. Initial **therapy includes TMP/SMX (unless the patient has been receiving it), amoxicillin/clavulanic acid, cefaclor, or cefuroxime axetil in combination with a decongestant.** The role of surgical therapy for recurrent disease remains unclear. Fungal organisms such as Aspergillus or Mucor may be pathogens in patients with advanced disease and chronic sinusitis, and should be considered in more refractory cases.

C. Bacteremia. Injection-drug use, permanent indwelling intravascular catheters, and lower CD4+ counts appear to increase the risk of developing bacteremia. The most common organisms are *S. aureus*, coagulase-negative staphylococcal species, *P. aeruginosa*, *Salmonella enteritidis*, *Streptococcus pneumoniae*, and other streptococcal species.

    1. Catheter infections. The risk of catheter-related bacteremia is estimated to be **0.20 infections per 100 patient days of use** (Stanley et al. *J Acquir Immune Defic Syndr* 1994;7:272). A higher rate of infection has been seen with tunneled catheters compared with percutaneously placed lines.

        a. The diagnosis should be suspected any time a patient with an indwelling catheter has a fever, regardless of whether local erythema or tenderness are seen at the catheter site. The **diagnosis** is made by obtaining **blood cultures** from both the catheter and a peripheral site.

        b. Empiric therapy should include **vancomycin** (1 g i.v. every 12 hours to cover staphylococcal species) and an **aminoglycoside** or third-generation cephalosporin (to treat gram-negative organisms). **Therapy** can be made more specific once the organism is identified from blood cultures. It is usually possible to treat coagulase-negative staphylococcal infections with 14 days of vancomycin without removing the catheter; however, successful therapy for *S. aureus* and gram-negative organisms is less common if the catheter is not removed, but it can be attempted if the patient responds to parenteral therapy.

    2. Endocarditis. *Staphylococcus aureus* remains the most common pathogen causing endocarditis in HIV-infected patients. Although the clinical presentation of endocarditis is not influenced by HIV infection, higher recurrence rates and higher in-hospital mortality has been noted. Recommendations for therapy for endocarditis depend on the infecting organism and are not affected by concurrent HIV infection.

D. Skin and soft-tissue infections

    1. Folliculitis is an infection of the hair follicles and apocrine regions. The lesions are small (2 to 3 mm) erythematous papules with a pustular center and are sometimes pruritic. The most common origin is *S. aureus*. The most **common locations are the buttocks, hips, and axillae.** *Pseudomonas aeruginosa* has been known to cause folliculitis acquired from hot tubs and swimming pools. Treatment includes local measures such as saline compresses or topical antibacterials, and systemic oral antibiotics (e.g., dicloxacillin, 500 mg p.o. q.i.d.) may be required in severe cases.

    2. Furuncles are deep nodules, and **carbuncles** extend into the subcutaneous fat. The most common etiologic agent is *S. aureus*. Furuncles usually drain spontaneously or after the application of local heat. Carbuncles develop into a more serious infection, causing cellulitis around the lesion and possibly bacteremia. Intravenous therapy with **oxacillin** (2 g per 6 hours i.v.); **clindamycin** (900 mg per 8 hours i.v.) or vancomycin

(1 g per 12 hours i.v.) in a penicillin-allergic patient should be given when a carbuncle is complicated by cellulitis or systemic toxicity. Surgical drainage is required for fluctuant lesions. **Recurrence** is not uncommon and may be alleviated by **eradication of nasal staphylococcal carriage** by using either rifampin (600 mg per day p.o. for 10 days) or topical mupirocin. Eradication of nasal staphylococcal carriage should be considered in patients with AIDS who require long-term intravascular catheters in the hopes of reducing the risk of catheter-related bacteremia.

3. **Pyomyositis** is an uncommon but important bacterial infection of the skeletal muscles that may occur in HIV-infected patients. *Staphylococcus aureus* is the most common pathogen; streptococci are rarely involved. The most common **symptoms** are **localized muscle pain, tenderness, and swelling**, although the findings may be subtle initially. The most common sites are the **lower limbs**, and the clinical presentation may mimic thrombophlebitis or septic arthritis. Blood cultures are rarely positive. **Surgical drainage** is essential for successful treatment.

IV. **Specific pathogens**

A. **Bartonella species**, formerly known as *Rochalimaea*, are small gram-negative bacilli that cause **bacillary angiomatosis** (BA), fever and bacteremia, lymphadenitis, osteomyelitis, neurologic disease, and visceral parenchymal bacillary peliosis of the liver and spleen in HIV-infected and other immunocompromised patients. The **causative agents** are *Bartonella henselae* and *B. quintana*; these organisms have been cultured and identified by polymerase chain reaction (PCR) from the blood, skin lesions, and visceral organs of patients with Bartonella infections.

1. **Clinical manifestations** include friable vascular skin lesions that may resemble Kaposi's sarcoma, deep subcutaneous nodules, or pedunculated lesions. Other presentations include fever, lymphadenopathy, bone pain with lytic lesions seen on radiograph, elevations in alkaline phosphatase with hypodense lesions in the liver and spleen seen on computed tomography (CT) scan, as well as pancytopenia.

2. **Risk factors** for developing infection with Bartonella include a very low CD4$^+$ count (<50), owning a pet cat, and being homeless.

3. **The diagnosis** can be established by the histologic appearance and by staining with **Warthin–Starry** stain or by culture of the organism from blood by using the lysis–centrifugation method. An indirect immunofluorescence antibody (IFA) test also is available from the Centers for Disease Control.

4. **Therapy.** The drug of choice is **erythromycin**. For cases of bacteremia or peliosis hepatis, therapy should be given intravenously initially at a dosage of 500 mg to 1 gm i.v. every 6 hours. Doxycycline (100 mg per day i.v. or p.o.) can be used as an alternative. For severe or refractory disease, rifampin or gentamicin may be added. Other drugs that may have activity include clarithromycin, azithromycin, and rifabutin. Therapy should continue for a minimum of 3 months; lifelong maintenance therapy may be needed.

5. **Specific prophylaxis** for Bartonella infections is not indicated. As with other opportunistic infections, the incidence has decreased dramatically with potent antiretroviral therapy.

B. **Salmonella.** Invasive infection with nontyphoidal Salmonella species were recognized as a common problem early in the HIV epidemic. Infection can recur or be difficult to eradicate. Intravenous therapy with TMP/SMX, ceftriaxone, or a quinolone should be initiated pending results of susceptibility testing. Long-term suppressive therapy (with TMP/SMX if the isolate is sensitive) will usually prevent recurrences. Patients should be counseled to avoid eating raw eggs or undercooked meats to avoid Salmonella infection.

V. **Prevention.** In the absence of more effective antiviral therapy for the underlying HIV infection, strategies are needed to reduce the impact of bacterial infections on morbidity and mortality during the course of HIV infection.

A. **Pneumococcal vaccination** is currently recommended for patients with HIV infection. Although response to the vaccine is more reliable at higher $CD4^+$ counts, patients with $CD4^+$ counts <100/mm^3 should still receive the vaccination. Vaccination may be delayed for a short period of time in patients who have $CD4^+$ counts <100/mm^3 and who are initiating potent antiretroviral therapy, as $CD4^+$ cell count increase may occur, thus increasing the likelihood of a response to the vaccine. Pneumococcal vaccination is not contraindicated during pregnancy.

B. **Antibiotic prophylaxis.** TMP/SMX, when used for PCP prophylaxis, reduces the risk of bacterial infections (Hardy et al. *N Engl J Med* 1992; 327:1842). It is important to consider that patients receiving long-term antibiotic prophylaxis may be at risk for development of infections with resistant organisms when infection occurs. For this reason, patients receiving long-term therapy with TMP/SMX should not use this antibiotic to treat intercurrent bacterial infections. Patients receiving macrolide therapy as prophylaxis for *Mycobacterium avium* complex (MAC; see Chapter 23) have a lower incidence of bacterial pneumonia and sinusitis.

C. **Intravenous immunoglobulin (IVIG).** Monthly administration of IVIG at a dose of 400 mg per kg has been shown to reduce the incidence of serious and minor bacterial infections in **children** with HIV infection (Mofenson et al. *JAMA* 1992;268:483). The use of IVIG is not recommended for adults.

D. **Impact of potent antiretroviral therapy.** As with other infections, the incidence of bacterial infections has decreased significantly in patients receiving potent treatment of HIV infection. Furthermore, stopping antimicrobial prophylaxis in such patients has not been associated with an increase in bacterial infections.

27. TREPONEMAL INFECTION IN HIV DISEASE

I. Overview of syphilis

A. Definition. Syphilis is a systemic infection caused by *Treponema pallidum*. Recognition and management of infectious syphilis continues to play an important role in the care of human immunodeficiency virus (HIV)-positive patients. Dual infection with syphilis and HIV is confounded by the likelihood that genital-ulcer disease enhances transmission and acquisition of HIV. Syphilis continues to be the "great imitator" in the HIV era, and a high index of suspicion for testing and treating of syphilis in HIV patients is warranted.

B. Biological factors. *Treponema pallidum* is a spirochetal bacterium measuring 6 to 15 mm in length, and 0.15 mm in width. It replicates slowly *in vivo*, with a doubling rate between 30 and 33 hours. *Treponema pallidum* grows poorly in laboratory settings, requiring live rabbit models for replication. Consequently the diagnosis of syphilis depends on clinical and serologic data, rather than on direct culture of the organism. The lack of exposed cell-surface proteins of *T. pallidum* also limits the potential to develop effective vaccines against the organism.

C. Transmission

1. **Sexual contact.** Direct sexual contact accounts for >90% of all cases of syphilis. Exposure to an active chancre or secondary skin lesions leads to direct inoculation of the uninfected skin or mucosal membrane surface. Infection occurs through direct intradermal implantation of treponemes through microscopic abrasions in squamous and columnar epithelial layers. This local route of entry stimulates both cell-mediated responses at the site of infection and systemic humoral immune responses. The immune reactions are incomplete and protect poorly, if at all, against reinfection.

    a. **Efficiency of transmission.** Overall efficiency of transmission (likelihood of transmitting disease on exposure) is estimated at 25% to 30% per partnership. Transmission efficiency is likely to vary by specific sexual activities, duration of exposure to lesions, size of primary or secondary lesions, and other factors. Condoms reduce efficiency of transmission to <5% when they are used correctly.

    b. **Synergistic transmission of HIV and syphilis.** Several clinical studies confirm that presence of genital-ulcer disease is an independent cofactor for HIV acquisition.

        (1) The presence of active genital lesions allows a **portal of entry for HIV** through the disrupted mucosal barriers and local cellular defenses. This phenomenon has been termed epidemiologic synergy and may account for higher rates of HIV transmission among persons with active genital-ulcer disease resulting from syphilis, chancroid, herpes, or other ulcerative conditions.

        (2) Presence of HIV infection also may facilitate acquisition and transmission of syphilis (raise efficiency of transmission) through impairment of cellular immune responses, which limit the number of treponemes replicating at sites of dermal infection.

2. **Prenatal/congenital.** Syphilitic infection of infants during the prenatal and perinatal period accounts for nearly all remaining cases. Infection occurs by way of transplacental transfer of infectious organisms from mother to child.

3. **Other routes.** Transfusion-associated cases of syphilis have been reported but are quite rare. These generally occurred before the advent

of intensive blood-product screening. Accidental direct inoculation with treponemes has also been reported in laboratory personnel working with infectious materials.

D. Epidemiology

  1. General. 16,500 cases of primary and secondary syphilis were reported in the United States in 1995, yielding a per capita rate of infection of 6.3 per 100,000 population. Major cities throughout the country and rural areas of southern states continue to be particularly affected. Historically, syphilis peak infection rates follow a somewhat cyclical nature, with intervals of ~10 to 12 years between epidemics.

  2. Demographics. Surveillance data suggest that disadvantaged, urban, lower socioeconomic level populations are disproportionately affected by syphilis. 85% of cases in the United States are in members of ethnic minorities. Gender ratio among reported infections is ~1:1, suggesting a predominantly heterosexual transmission pattern. Higher rates of sexual activity, commercial sex work (prostitution), and the exchange of sex for drugs sustain infection in populations at highest risk.

  3. Epidemiology of syphilis and HIV. Populations affected by syphilis and HIV increasingly overlap, as HIV rates continue to increase among adolescents, women, and minorities. Common routes of transmission, along with the likelihood of epidemiologic synergy between syphilis and HIV, attest to the need for enhanced surveillance and screening activities among populations at risk. With genital-ulcer disease acting as an independent cofactor for HIV acquisition, aggressive treatment of syphilis is warranted to limit further extension of the HIV epidemic into populations at greatest risk.

E. Diagnosis. Syphilis is diagnosed based on the presence of signs and symptoms of disease, coupled with a history of possible exposure to active disease. In effect, all persons who are sexually active are at risk for exposure to syphilis, so the diagnosis generally rests on clinical and laboratory findings. Elicitation of sexual contact with a syphilis patient is an important component of the evaluation. Absence of reported contact to an active case does not rule out syphilis, because patients may not be aware of their partners' STD status or may conceal this information at the time of examination. However, confirmation of contact increases the likelihood that particular signs and symptoms may represent syphilis infection.

II. Clinical manifestations of syphilis. Clinical disease is divided into early and late infection. Early syphilis includes all infections of <1 year's duration. Late syphilis includes all infections of 1 year's duration. In general, early disease is characterized by the onset of primary and secondary symptoms and a robust serologic response. Left untreated, these clinical symptoms resolve, leading to the latent infectious state. Persons with latent disease are at risk for the development of tertiary disease, including neurosyphilis. A number of case reports have described unusual presentations of syphilis in patients with HIV infection, particularly when immunosuppression was markedly advanced. A study of the clinical presentation of syphilis in Baltimore suggested that HIV-infected patients were more likely to have secondary disease (Hutchinson et al. *Ann Intern Med* 1994;121:94). Most patients with HIV disease are likely to develop typical signs, symptoms, and serologic responses consistent with those of non-HIV-infected populations. HIV patients with latent infection may be at increased risk for developing symptomatic neurosyphilis as a consequence of treatment failure, although prospective studies have yet to document the likelihood of this occurrence.

A. Early disease (<1 year)

  1. Primary syphilis. Infection with *T. pallidum* generally occurs after direct exposure to active syphilitic lesions. After infection, the organisms incubate in the host for ~3 weeks (range, 9 to 90 days) before the onset of clinical manifestations.

  a. Chancre. The hallmark of primary syphilis is the chancre, most commonly identified as a painless, indolent ulcer at the site of infection.

The lesion begins as a papule, which then erodes and ulcerates over several days. The ulcer is characterized by a hard, granular base with scant yellow serous discharge and is often described as having a "punched-out" appearance with smooth, raised, and sharply defined borders. The chancre is often solitary, but multiple chancres may be present in the same individual.

  (1) **Sites affected**. Sites commonly affected include the coronal sulcus, glans, frenum, prepuce, and shaft of the penis in males, the fourchette, vulva, and cervix in females, and the anorectal area in both sexes. Oropharyngeal lesions affecting the lip, tongue, posterior pharynx, or tonsil also may occur in either sex after orogenital exposure.

  (2) **Natural history.** The chancre generally resolves completely within 3 to 6 weeks of appearance without treatment. At this point, the infection enters the secondary stage.

  b. **Regional lymphadenopathy.** Enlargement of regional lymph nodes also may occur in primary infection. Unilateral or bilateral inguinal adenopathy may be present in genital infection, and cervical adenopathy may be seen in oropharyngeal infection.

  c. **Differential diagnosis**. Chancre should be distinguished from any other cause of nontreponemal genital-ulcer disease, including chancroid (*H. ducreyi*), genital herpes infection [herpes simplex virus type 1 (HSV-1) or HSV-2], varicella-zoster virus (VZV), Behçet's disease, or benign aphthous ulcers.

2. **Secondary syphilis**. Left untreated, primary infection enters the secondary stage an average of 6 weeks after initial exposure. Secondary syphilis manifestations are commonly referred to as "rash," but this description does not capture the full range of skin and systemic findings in patients with secondary disease. Rather, a number of distinct rashes, as well as systemic responses to infection, may occur.

  a. **Systemic signs and symptoms.** These include general malaise or "flu-like" syndrome with myalgias, arthralgias, low-grade fever, weight loss, low-grade anemia, and elevated erythrocyte sedimentation rate (ESR). Generalized lymphadenopathy and hepatosplenomegaly also may be seen.

  b. Dermatologic manifestations

  (1) **Macular or erythematous eruption** may occur anywhere on the trunk, shoulders, upper arms, or forearm flexor areas. It is characterized by the development of nonindurated, nonblanching light red macular eruption that is most intense at the center and then fades toward the periphery.

  (2) **Maculopapular eruption** commonly occurs on the face, chest, back, abdomen, forearm flexors, palms, and soles. It is described as having a copper-red color, in contrast to the macular rash. Patients may have maculopapular lesions on oropharyngeal and genital mucosal areas, known as "mucous patches." These oval lesions possess a raised border and often have a gray–white membrane overlying the surface.

  (3) **Papular lesions.** These deep-seated, flat-topped, scaly lesions are found primarily on the palms and soles and may also involve the scalp or other areas. Persons with scalp involvement develop a "moth-eaten" nonscarring alopecia caused by follicular invasion.

  (4) **Annular lesions.** These macular, maculopapular, or papular lesions primarily affect mucocutaneous borders of the face and genital regions. Lesions may have a round or oval appearance ("nickel and dime lesions") and may appear and disappear with intervals of quiescence. Recurrent lesions tend to be larger, darker, and more discrete.

(5) **Condylomata lata**. Papular lesions that develop on moist body areas, especially the anogenital area, may coalesce to form hypertrophic, granulomatous, or condylomatous-appearing lesions. These may be confused with genital warts (condylomata acuminata), owing to their verrucous appearance. Condylomata lata lesions are often gray or red—brown, moist, and flat-topped. Postinflammatory pigmentation or depigmentation also may be present.

(6) **Pustular lesions.** This infrequent manifestation of secondary syphilis is characterized by papules that have softened, ulcerated, and crusted. The distribution is generalized and includes the fingernails, toenails, palms, and soles.

    b. **Natural history**. Dermatologic and systemic manifestations of secondary syphilis resolve in ~4 to 8 weeks without therapy. At this point, the infection enters a latent phase, which may progress to tertiary disease.

    c. **Differential diagnosis**. Secondary syphilis must be distinguished from a number of other exanthemous conditions. Macular lesions, with or without postinflammatory pigmentation, may resemble measles, rubella, pityriasis rosea, tinea versicolor, seborrheic dermatitis, or drug eruption. Papular lesions may resemble lichen planus, impetigo, or drug eruption.

   3. Early latent syphilis. Infections of <1 year's duration, in the absence of primary or secondary signs or symptoms, are termed early latent infections. In the absence of evidence confirming recent infection (e.g., negative blood test within the past year), patients should be treated as for late latent disease.

B. Late disease (≥1 year). Persons with syphilis of long-standing duration are at increased risk for complications of tertiary disease. Whereas infection may remain latent for life, persons with HIV may have accelerated progression of disease to include neurologic involvement.

   1. Late latent syphilis. This describes latent infection of ≥1 year, in the absence of signs and symptoms. HIV patients with latent syphilis may have asymptomatic neurologic involvement at the time of diagnosis. The implication of this finding and its significance for clinical management are not clear.

   2. Tertiary syphilis. Tertiary manifestations (other than neurosyphilis) are not often seen today. Systemic involvement of multiple organ systems can occur in tertiary disease, most commonly, mucocutaneous, bone, or cardiovascular, and typically 10 to 30 years after initial infection.

C. Neurosyphilis. Central nervous system (CNS) involvement in syphilis may occur at any time after initial infection. In particular, syphilitic meningitis may be seen within the first few weeks of infection or as a primary presenting symptom. Additionally, manifestations of CNS involvement in HIV patients may be accelerated, including progression to meningovascular disease.

   1. Signs and symptoms. Any of a variety of signs and symptoms can indicate CNS involvement in syphilis.

    a. **Meningeal and meningovascular involvement** may be suggested by changes in mental status, auditory or other cranial nerve dysfunction, ocular abnormalities, signs of meningeal irritation (meningismus), or stroke.

    b. **Parenchymatous involvement** of the brain tissue may lead to generalized paresis (dementia paralytica) or tabes dorsalis. The latter condition is characterized by lightning pains and paresthesias (particularly affecting the lower extremities), diminished deep tendon reflexes, Argyll–Robertson pupils, visceral pain crises affecting gastric, rectal, and laryngeal structures, impaired gait, or Charcot joint.

   2. Differential diagnosis. Any condition that may impair mental status should be included in the differential diagnosis of neurosyphilis. For patients with HIV infection, distinguishing neurosyphilis from other complications can be challenging. The differential diagnosis should include toxoplasmosis, lymphoma, progressive multifocal leukoencephalopathy (PML), cytomegalovirus (CMV), other bacterial infections (such as *Nocardia*), and HIV encephalopathy. Laboratory data are generally required to secure the diagnosis, although cerebrospinal (CSF) findings in neurosyphilis may be nonspecific.

III. **Laboratory findings.** Laboratory testing is an essential component of the clinical examination for syphilis. Serologic detection of an antibody response, coupled with direct observation of lesion exudate by dark-field microscopy, forms the basis of laboratory confirmation of syphilis in most cases. Other diagnostic modalities such as direct fluorescent antibody testing also may be used, especially when clinical suspicion for syphilis is high. The question of whether HIV infection systematically modifies the serologic response to syphilis continues to cloud the field. Available data suggest that exaggerated or attenuated responses may be seen in some circumstances.

A. **Direct examination of lesion exudate**

1. **Dark-field microscopy.** The dark-field microscopic examination of serous fluid taken from the surface of genital ulcers or moist skin lesions permits observation of treponemal structure (characteristic "corkscrew" appearance) and movement. Direct observation of motile treponemal organisms by dark-field microscopy essentially confirms the diagnosis of syphilis. The dark-field examination is generally not appropriate for evaluating oral lesions, because nonpathogenic spirochetal organisms that form part of the normal oral flora may be confused with pathogenic treponemal organisms. The dark-field examination is highly specific for syphilis, but sensitivity of the test is dependent on a number of factors, including the density of organisms present in the lesion, technique of slide preparation, and experience of the examiner. Consequently, a positive examination confirms but a negative examination does not necessarily rule out infection with *T. pallidum*.

2. **Direct fluorescent antibody examination for *T. pallidum* (DFA-TP).** Exudate or secretions from genital ulcers, oral ulcers, and skin lesions may be tested for the presence of *T. pallidum* antigens by using a DFA technique. The test has relatively high sensitivity and specificity. Tissue specimens from biopsy also may be tested with monoclonal antibody in the DFA tissue test for *T. pallidum* (DFAT-TP).

B. **Serologic testing for syphilis (STS)** is a mainstay of the diagnosis and management of syphilis. Serologic tests are used to screen for syphilis infection, to confirm suspected infection, and to monitor response to therapy. Serologic responses to syphilis infection may be modified by HIV infection, with HIV patients developing higher or lower antibody titers than expected. However, most HIV patients develop reliable and predictable serologic responses to infection with *T. pallidum*. Screening for infection is generally carried out through the sequential use of a nontreponemal test, followed by confirmation of infection by using a specific treponemal test if the nontreponemal screening test is positive.

1. **Nontreponemal tests.** These tests are used to diagnose new or previously undetected cases and also to monitor adequate response to therapy. The basic principle of testing involves identification of antilipid IgG and IgM antibodies, which are formed in response to lipid from treponemal cell surfaces. The addition of a standardized sample of cardiolipin–cholesterol–lecithin antigen causes a flocculation reaction that may be read and reported qualitatively (positive or negative) or quantitatively as a serial dilution titer. The titer reflects the lowest serum dilution at which flocculation is seen to occur (1:2, 1:4, etc.). A number of different nontreponemal tests are available, although the RPR (rapid plasma reagin) test and the VDRL (Venereal Disease Research Laboratory) test account for the vast majority of syphilis-screening examinations. Owing

to the nature of specimen preparation and visual interpretation of results, reported titers for nontreponemal tests are accurate only to within plus-or-minus one serial dilution. Additionally, RPR titers are generally one dilution higher than VDRL titers for the same level of reactivity, and so serial comparisons should use the same testing method to provide a more accurate basis for assessing longitudinal change in a patient's seroreactive status.

a. **False positive reactions**. False positive responses to nontreponemal testing occur at a rate of 1% to 2% in the general population (Table 1). **Transient biologic false positive (BFP)** reactions for syphilis are well described and may occur in acute febrile illness episodes, in immunization, or in pregnancy. These responses generally last <6 months before resolving to seronegative status. **Chronic BFP** reactions are seen in a number of chronic medical conditions, including immune-mediated and autoimmune disorders (lupus, psoriasis, and arthritis), and can be seen in the normal aging process (senescence). Studies of injection-drug users (IDUs) have documented false positive nontreponemal rates of 10%. The majority of false positive tests have titers of 1:8, although higher titers are not uncommon.

b. **False negative reactions**. A number of factors contribute to the insensitivity of nontreponemal tests. Typically, nontreponemal tests become reactive within 1 to 2 weeks of the onset of chancre, such that persons with incubating syphilis will test negative even in the face of true infection. Additionally, published reports suggest that 15% to 41% of patients with primary syphilitic lesions exhibit a nonreactive nontreponemal test at the time of clinical evaluation. In secondary syphilis, nontreponemal tests are nearly always reactive. However, prozone reactions may be seen in ~2% of patients with secondary syphilis, where undiluted serum samples may exhibit a granular negative flocculation pattern owing to excessive levels of antibody. Sample reactivity increases with subsequent dilutions and then decreases as the end-point titer is approached. Finally, persons with late syphilis may have false negative reactions owing to a general diminution of antibody response over time (Table 2).

c. **Monitoring response to therapy**. Nontreponemal tests are valuable for assessing adequate response to therapy. With appropriate therapy for primary or secondary disease, nontreponemal test titers should decrease fourfold within 6 months of treatment (e.g., 1:64

Table 1. Causes of false-positive nontreponemal syphilis serologic findings

BACTERIAL INFECTIONS	VIRAL INFECTIONS
Endocarditis	Measles
Pneumococcal pneumonia	Varicella
Mycoplasma pneumonia	Mononucleosis
Leptospirosis	Hepatitis
Chancroid	
Relapsing fever	NONINFECTIOUS CAUSE
Trypanosomiasis	Malignancy
Psittacosis	Pregnancy
Lymphogranuloma venereum	Injection drug use
Rickettsial disease	Autoimmune disease
Leprosy	Senescence
Tuberculosis	Myeloma
Scarlet fever	Chronic liver disease
Malaria	Multiple transfusions

Table 2. Nontreponemal test sensitivity by stage of disease

Test	Primary	Secondary	Early latent	Late latent
VDRL (%)	78	100[a]	95	71
RPR (%)	86	100	98	73

VDRL, Venereal Disease Research Laboratory; RPR, rapid plasma reagin.
[a] One case reported of secondary syphilis with negative VDRL at time of presentation.

decrease to 1:16). Serologic response to therapy has been noted to be attenuated in some HIV patients, although most persons exhibit a normal pattern of titer diminution. Failure to develop a significant titer decline, or a increase in titer, may indicate treatment failure or reinfection with syphilis. Patients with HIV infection should be monitored with quantitative nontreponemal serologies at intervals of 1, 2, 3, 6, 9, and 12 months to ensure appropriate serologic declines in nontreponemal test titers. Most patients with early disease revert to seronegative status within 1 year of treatment, although 50% of persons treated in late or latent stages may remain serofast 2 years after therapy, regardless of HIV serostatus.

2. **Treponemal tests.** Serologic tests to confirm syphilis infection measure IgG and IgM immunoglobulin directed against cellular antigens of *T. pallidum*. These tests are specific for treponemal infection, and their use is generally reserved to confirm infection with a positive nontreponemal test. The most commonly used treponemal tests are the fluorescent treponemal antibody absorption test (FTA-ABS) and the microhemagglutination assay for *T. pallidum* (MHA-TP). A reactive treponemal test generally indicates current or past infection with syphilis. Most patients remain serofast for life; however, 14% of persons treated with early disease will revert to seronegativity within 2 years of treatment. Treponemal tests exhibit a false positive rate of ~1% in the general population. Conditions known to cause a false positive treponemal response include other spirochetal infections (Lyme disease, relapsing fever, or leptospirosis), leprosy, malaria, mononucleosis, and lupus. Use of the test as a confirmatory rather than a screening modality substantially reduces the likelihood of a false positive result. As with nontreponemal tests, the treponemal tests are generally negative in incubating disease (false negative). Treponemal tests may be used to confirm syphilis infection in late disease when nontreponemal tests are negative.

3. **Serologic abnormalities in HIV infection.** Some investigators have reported unusually high titers of nontreponemal tests (>16,834) in HIV patients, although follow-up studies by the CDC have not confirmed these findings. Elevated immunoglobulin levels may occur in HIV infection, although the relation of this finding to syphilis serologies is unclear. Additionally, some HIV-infected patients may show persistently elevated nontreponemal test titers after adequate therapy and in the absence of evidence of reinfection, whereas others may have a nonreactive treponemal test response after successful therapy for syphilis. Nevertheless, most patients with HIV infection demonstrate reliable serologic responses to syphilis infection and exhibit a normal, if somewhat attenuated, decrease in nontreponemal test titer after treatment. One case report described a patient with secondary syphilis who demonstrated markedly delayed nontreponemal and treponemal test conversions (Hicks et al. *Ann Intern Med* 1987;107:492), although this appears to be the exception rather than the rule.

C. **Cerebrospinal fluid.** Examination of the CSF, coupled with clinical signs and symptoms, provides the basis for **laboratory confirmation of neuro-**

syphilis. Current CDC recommendations call for lumbar puncture **to evaluate CSF in all HIV-infected patients with latent syphilis,** of >1 year's duration (late latent syphilis). Although invasion of the CSF by *T. pallidum* is common in early disease regardless of HIV status, this rarely leads to neurosyphilis in the normal host (Lukehart et al. *Ann Intern Med* 1988;109:855), suggesting that immune-system containment of infection is essential to limiting the progression of disease. CSF findings consistent with neurosyphilis include elevated protein (>50 mg per dl) and elevated white blood cell (WBC) count (>5 mononuclear cells/mm³). A reactive VDRL test on CSF is very specific for neurosyphilis but quite insensitive, so clinical judgment must be used in making the diagnosis. Other conditions that may cause low-grade protein elevations and pleocytosis should be considered (CMV, toxoplasmosis, or HIV encephalopathy), but it is necessary to bear in mind that clinical progression to neurosyphilis may be accelerated in HIV disease, even after adequate therapy for primary or secondary disease. Several case reports have suggested that standard doses of benzathine penicillin-G may be inadequate to prevent development of clinically significant neurosyphilis in HIV-infected patients. Clinical progression of syphilis was demonstrated in >20% of patients with HIV infection who were treated with either benzathine penicillin-G or high doses of ceftriaxone, with many patients developing neurosyphilis (Dowell et al. *Am J Med* 1992;93:481). In another study, high-dose penicillin therapy was not uniformly effective in curing neurosyphilis in HIV-infected patients (Gordon et al. *N Engl J Med* 1994; 331:1469). These data call into question whether antibiotic therapy alone, in the absence of an effective immune system, can prevent progression of disease. Recent studies suggest that a negative FTA-ABS test on CSF effectively rules out neurosyphilis, although confirmation of this finding is required in larger samples (Marra et al. *Arch Neurol* 1995;52:68).

IV. **Treatment.** Therapy for syphilis is determined by duration of infection. In general, early disease (duration, <1 year) is treated with single-dose i.m. or short-course oral therapy, whereas late disease (duration, 1 year) is treated with multiple-dose i.m. or long-course oral regimens. Neurosyphilis, regardless of duration of infection, requires i.v. therapy or other approved alternative regimens that penetrate the blood–brain barrier.

A. **Early disease. Treatment of choice for primary, secondary, and early latent syphilis is single-dose benzathine penicillin-G (2.4 million units) delivered intramuscularly into the gluteal region.** Some experts suggest provision of a second dose of benzathine penicillin-G 1 week later to ensure maximal coverage, although this is not routinely recommended by the CDC. Alternatively, aqueous procaine penicillin G (600,000 units) may be given intramuscularly every day for 8 to 12 days, although this is generally less well tolerated than the benzathine-penicillin regimen. **Patients who are allergic to penicillin, and who are not pregnant,** may be offered one of the following alternative regimens:

1. tetracycline, 500 mg orally 4 times per day for 14 days;
2. doxycycline, 100 mg orally twice daily for 14 days; or
3. ceftriaxone, 250 mg intramuscularly daily for 8 to 10 days.

   Treatment failures in HIV-infected patients, as documented by increasing serologic test titers and progression of clinical disease, have been described with all of the recommended regimens. However, a recent CDC-sponsored trial demonstrated no advantage of additional dosage or duration of therapy in HIV-infected patients, despite plausible theoretic foundations. Although erythromycin (500 mg orally 4 times per day for 14 days) is approved by the CDC as an alternative treatment regimen, it has unacceptably high treatment-failure rates in HIV-infected populations and is not recommended for routine use. Regardless of HIV status, **pregnant patients** who are penicillin-allergic must be desensitized and treated with penicillin, because alternative agents do not effectively treat the fetus.

Extreme vigilance in **patient follow-up** is required after treatment for early syphilis, and providers should have a high index of suspicion for signs and symptoms of neurosyphilis after adequate therapy for primary or secondary disease.

B. **Late disease. Treatment of choice for syphilis of 1 year's duration (or of unknown duration) is three weekly injections of benzathine penicillin-G (2.4 million units) delivered intramuscularly into the gluteal region.** In latent and tertiary infection, spirochetal replication is substantially slower, and prolonged antiinfective therapy is required to ensure successful eradication. Patients should be counseled to adhere to the weekly regimen as closely as possible, because receipt of follow-up injections off-schedule may contribute to treatment failure. Patients who are **allergic to penicillin**, and who are not pregnant, may be offered one of the following alternative regimens:

1. tetracycline, 500 mg orally 4 times daily for 28 days; or
2. doxycycline, 100 mg orally twice daily for 28 days.

Ceftriaxone and erythromycin have not been adequately evaluated for treatment of late disease but are not recommended because of the likelihood of unacceptable high treatment-failure rates. Use of ceftriaxone to treat latent syphilis was associated with a 23% failure rate, as evidenced by progression to neurosyphilis (Dowell et al. *Am J Med* 1992;93:481). As in primary disease, **pregnant patients** who are allergic to penicillin must be desensitized and treated with penicillin, because alternative medications will not treat the fetus.

C. **Neurosyphilis. Treatment of choice for neurosyphilis is intravenous administration of aqueous crystalline penicillin-G (12 to 24 million units) daily for 14 days.** Initiation of therapy generally requires hospitalization, but many patients may be treated at home or an extended-care facility after placement of long-term peripheral or central venous access. If i.v. penicillin cannot be given, an alternative regimen for treatment of neurosyphilis may be used: procaine penicillin-G (2.4 million units) intramuscularly once daily for 10 to 14 days, PLUS probenecid, 500 mg orally 4 times daily for 10 to 14 days. Some experts follow these treatment regimens with one additional i.m. injection of benzathine penicillin-G (2.4 million units) to ensure prolonged antispirochetal activity. In general, the i.v. treatment regimen for neurosyphilis is preferred to the i.m. regimen, but as noted previously, treatment failures have been reported in HIV patients even when high-dose i.v. penicillin therapy is used. Experience with ceftriaxone for treatment of neurosyphilis is limited, but may be considered (Marra et al. *Clin Infect Dis* 2000;30:540). Patients allergic to penicillin should be desensitized, because there is currently no adequate non–penicillin-based therapy for neurosyphilis.

V. **Follow-up.** HIV-infected patients may be at increased risk for progression of syphilis despite adequate therapy. Clinical follow-up is essential to ensure early detection of possible signs and symptoms. **Regardless of stage of disease** or treatment regimen, patients should undergo clinical examination 1 week after initiation of therapy and should obtain follow-up nontreponemal serologic tests at 1, 2, 3, 6, 9, and 12 months, and then yearly for life, even if the nontreponemal test reverts to negative. Failure of the nontreponemal titer to decrease fourfold (e.g., 1:64 to 1:16) within 6 months of therapy suggests either treatment failure or reinfection. Lumbar puncture is recommended if serologic or clinical evidence of disease progression are evident. Patients treated for **neurosyphilis** require a high index of suspicion for relapse. Lumbar puncture should be performed at 6-month intervals after treatment until CSF values are normal, and reassessment of CSF should be undertaken when recurrence of neurosyphilis is suspected.

VI. **Other management issues**

A. **Jarisch–Herxheimer reaction**. Patients receiving therapy for syphilis should be informed of the possibility of developing a Jarisch–Herxheimer reaction in response to treatment. The reaction occurs as a systemic manifestation of treponemal lysis, and patients may have transient fever, malaise, headache, musculoskeletal pain, nausea, or tachycardia. Symptoms commonly occur within 4 to 8 hours of treatment and generally resolve within 24 hours. The reaction is more common in early syphilis but can be more severe in late disease, with temporary aggravation or flaring of primary and secondary lesions. Treatment is supportive, with fluids and antipyretic/analgesic agents (e.g., acetaminophen). The Jarisch–Herxheimer reaction is self-limited and should be distinguished from a true hypersensitivity reaction to penicillin or other antibiotic therapy.

B. **Syphilis in pregnancy**. Adequate treatment of syphilis in pregnancy is essential to prevent congenital syphilis in the newborn. **All women should be screened serologically** for syphilis in the first trimester, and strong consideration should be given to repeated screening in the third trimester and at delivery. When syphilis occurs in pregnancy, **penicillin therapy** is required, because alternative treatments do not adequately cross the placenta or may be toxic to the fetus. Pregnant women who are allergic to penicillin must be desensitized and treated with penicillin-based regimens.

For treatment of early syphilis in pregnancy, standard therapy with benzathine penicillin-G is recommended. In addition, some experts recommend a second dose of benzathine penicillin-G (2.4 million units i.m.) 1 week after initial treatment if secondary disease is present, or if the diagnosis is made in the third trimester regardless of stage of disease (primary, secondary, or early latent). Late latent disease in pregnancy is treated with three weekly injections of benzathine penicillin-G as per the standard regimen.

C. **Evaluation and treatment of sex partners**. All patients with syphilis should be referred to a disease-intervention specialist (DIS) in liaison with the local health department for immediate counseling and interview. All partners with potential exposure must be referred for clinical evaluation.

D. **Indications for lumbar puncture in latent syphilis**. Given the high rate of asymptomatic neurosyphilis in HIV-infected populations, the CDC recommends performing lumbar puncture in all HIV patients with latent syphilis of >1 year's duration.

28. KAPOSI'S SARCOMA

Kaposi's sarcoma (KS) was the first malignant complication of HIV infection to be recognized and for a long time was the most common malignancy in human immune deficiency virus (HIV) infection. Initially it was seen as an early phenomenon in AIDS, but as the epidemic matured, KS was seen more frequently as a late manifestation of HIV infection rather than as an index AIDS diagnosis (Rabkin et al. *J Natl Cancer Inst* 1994;86:1711–1716). As with many opportunistic diseases, the incidence of KS has declined dramatically with the use of potent antiretroviral therapy.

I. **Epidemiology.** Epidemic KS occurs predominantly among homosexual and bisexual men, who account for >90% of all HIV-associated KS. The association of KS with a history of sexually transmitted diseases, level of sexual activity, and the recognition of KS in HIV-1 seronegative homosexual men strongly suggested a role for a sexually transmitted KS **cofactor** (Beral et al. *Lancet* 1990;335:123). Recent identification of a new human herpesvirus, **human herpesvirus 8 (HHV-8)** led to several well-performed studies that confirmed that this virus plays a pivotal role in the pathogenesis of KS (Antman et al. *N Engl J Med* 2000;342:1027). Viral sequences have been have been identified in greater than 90% of KS biopsies from HIV-infected individuals. HHV-8 antigens have also been detected in blood from patients before the development of KS.

II. **Pathology.** KS is a highly vascular tumor composed of bands of spindle cells, lymphatic channels, an inflammatory mononuclear-cell infiltrate, and extravasated red blood cells. The **spindle cell**, a key element of KS lesions, is probably a mesenchymal progenitor cell of either endothelial or monocyte–macrophage lineage (Uccini et al. *J Pathol* 1994;173:23). The KS spindle cells secrete paracrine factors that appear to mediate angiogenesis and the mononuclear-cell infiltrate (Ensoli et al. *Science* 1989;243:233). The mononuclear cells in turn may secrete cytokines that stimulate the growth of KS spindle cells, setting up an autocrine–paracrine growth loop (Barillari et al. *J Immunol* 1992;149(11):3727).

III. **Clinical features.** Epidemic KS has a variable clinical course. For the majority of patients, KS ultimately progresses and results in significant morbidity and mortality. Although KS has been identified in virtually every site at autopsy, clinically, KS most frequently involves the skin, oral cavity, gastrointestinal (GI) tract, and lungs.

   A. **Cutaneous KS.** The skin is the most frequent site of presentation of KS. Skin lesions appear commonly on the face, lower extremities, and genitalia, although they may occur anywhere. Lesions may be symmetric and follow Langer's lines. Lesions have a **varied appearance** at presentation ranging from faint macules or papules to indurated plaques or exophytic nodules. **Lesion color** also varies; early lesions are typically pink to red, becoming darker purple or brown with time. With progressive disease, lesions may be palpable as subcutaneous nodules even before they are visible. Yellow perilesional halos may be seen with lesion growth. **Lymphedema**, resulting from obstruction of dermal lymphatics, most frequently involves the lower extremities and, to a lesser degree, the external genitalia and periorbital soft tissues.

   B. **Oral cavity.** Oral-cavity lesions occur in ~45% of patients with concomitant skin lesions. It is the initial site of KS in ~15% of patients and may first be identified during a dental examination. Oral-cavity disease most frequently is seen on the **hard palate**, usually as pink to purple macules. Gingival disease occurs with the next greatest frequency. KS also may involve the soft palate, tongue, tonsils, floor of the mouth, and pharynx. Although oral-cavity disease is usually asymptomatic, it may become exophytic, bulky, or ulcerated (or a combination of these) and interfere with speech or oral intake.

C. **GI.** GI involvement occurs in >40% of patients with cutaneous KS and may occur anywhere in the GI tract (Danzig et al. *Am J Gastroenterol* 1991;86:715). GI KS is usually **asymptomatic** but may cause bleeding, pain, gastric stasis, or obstruction. **Endoscopy** is the procedure of choice to diagnose GI tract involvement. Biopsies may be nondiagnostic because of the submucosal location of the lesions. Contrast x-ray studies and computerized tomography rarely identify GI tract KS.

D. **Pulmonary.** Pulmonary KS occurs without mucocutaneous disease in 20% of patients (Cadranel et al. *Thorax* 1994;49:958). The symptoms and radiologic appearance of pulmonary KS are nonspecific and indistinguishable from those of opportunistic infections. **Bronchoscopy** is frequently necessary to establish the diagnosis. KS has a characteristic bronchoscopic appearance as erythematous submucosal plaques. Because of the risk of bleeding, biopsy is usually not performed. In the case of a nondiagnostic bronchoscopy, **thallium–gallium scanning** may be useful. Whereas infection is usually gallium-avid and thallium negative, KS is **thallium-avid** and **gallium negative** (Lee at al. *Radiology* 1991;180:409).

IV. **Natural history.** KS may be seen any time during the course of HIV infection. The rate of KS progression varies from patient to patient and is not related to the level of immunosuppression. Corticosteroid therapy (Guo et al. *Am J Pathol* 1995;146:727) and opportunistic infection may stimulate KS growth, presumably as a result of their effects on cytokines.

V. **Patient evaluation**

A. The **initial evaluation** of a patient with KS should include a complete history and physical examination. The history should focus on the rate of progression of new KS lesions, lesion-associated symptoms, HIV-related opportunistic infections, overall immune status, treatment history, and the presence of respiratory or GI symptoms. Physical examination should include careful inspection of the scalp, retroauricular area and ears, oral cavity, genitalia, perirectal area, and soles. The baseline CD4$^+$ lymphocyte count and complete blood count (CBC) are important for treatment decisions. A baseline chest radiograph is important to rule out asymptomatic pulmonary disease. Computed tomography (CT) scans and GI contrast radiographs are not indicated unless there are signs and symptoms of abdominal disease.

B. **A standardized evaluation of KS** response to treatment requires a reproducible assessment of disease. Repeated assessments include bidimensional measurements of five discrete cutaneous **marker** lesions, a **count** of the total number of cutaneous lesions (if this number is >50, then lesions on one or more representative anatomic areas of the body are counted), and qualitative descriptions of the lesions (e.g., height and pigmentation). Measurement of the circumference of extremities may be helpful for serial evaluations of edema. In the presence of unexplained GI or pulmonary symptoms, endoscopy/bronchoscopy are often necessary. **Biopsy** of at least one lesion is recommended to rule out other diagnoses, in particular, **bacillary angiomatosis** (Tappero et al. *J Am Acad Dermatol* 1993;28:371).

VI. **Staging.** The prognosis for patients with KS depends not only on characteristics of the tumor, but also on HIV-related factors. As a result, the tumor–node–metastases (TNM) classification used for most solid tumors is not suitable for staging KS. The most widely used staging system is the **AIDS Clinical Trials Group** (ACTG) **staging system** (Table 1). Patients are categorized as **good** and **poor risk,** on the basis of **tumor** burden and sites of involvement (T), **immune function** (CD4$^+$ count > or <200 cells per μL) (I), and severity of systemic illness (S).

VII. **Management of Kaposi's sarcoma.** The advent of the era of potent antiretroviral therapy has dramatically changed the natural history of KS. Prior to the development of effective antiretroviral therapy, treatment of epidemic KS was palliative and had never been shown to improve survival. However, the use of potent antiretroviral therapy, with suppression of HIV replication and the consequent improvement of immune function has led to a decrease in the inci-

Table 1. ACTG staging classification for Kaposi's sarcoma

	Good risk ($_0$) (all of the following)	Poor risk ($_1$) (any of the following)
Tumor (T)	Confined to skin and/or lymph nodes and/or minimal oral disease[a]	Tumor-associated edema or ulceration Extensive oral KS Gastrointestinal KS KS in other nonnodal viscera
Immune system (I)	CD4+ cells ≥200/µL	CD4+ cells <200 µL
Systemic illness (S)	No history of OI or thrush No "B" symptoms[b] Performance status ≥70 (Karnofsky)	History of OI and/or thrush "B" symptoms present Performance status <70 Other HIV-related illness (e.g., neurologic disease, lymphoma)

T_0, tumor confined to skin, lymph nodes and/or minimal oral disease; T_1, any tumor in the "poor risk" criteria; S_0, no history of OI or thrush, no "B" symptoms, and Karnofsky performance status ≥70; S_1, any "poor risk" systemic illness signs and symptoms; OI, opportunistic infection; KS, Kaposi's sarcoma; ACTG, AIDS Clinical Treatment Group.
[a] Minimal oral disease is nonnodular KS confined to the palate.
[b] "B" symptoms are unexplained fever, night sweats, >10% involuntary weight loss, or diarrhea persisting >12 wk.

dence of KS and, improvement and clearance of disease. Thus all patients with KS should receive **potent effective antiretroviral therapy** (see Chapter 6). In many patients, especially those with disease limited to the skin, this will be the only treatment needed.

Some patients may require additional **specific KS treatment**. Treatment planning requires consideration of the extent of disease and its rate of progression, the degree of underlying immune suppression, and patient priorities and goals. Specific treatment for KS should be planned in conjunction with appropriate management of HIV disease. In general, there are **four indications for specific KS treatment:** life-threatening disease (usually pulmonary), symptomatic KS (i.e., painful disease of the soles or bulky oral cavity lesions), cosmetically unacceptable lesions (e.g., on the tip of the nose), and to prevent progression. A patient with very limited disease may be best treated initially with local therapy, whereas a patient with more advanced or rapidly progressive KS is a candidate for systemic chemotherapy.

A. **Local therapies.** Local therapy directed at individual lesions is appropriate only for patients with indolent disease and a limited number of lesions. It is important to remember that local therapies will not forestall the development of new lesions, and KS frequently recurs after local treatment. Surgical excision may be useful for solitary nodular or pedunculated lesions. The mainstays of local therapy are liquid nitrogen cryotherapy, radiation therapy, and intralesional vinblastine injections.

1. **Cryotherapy** with liquid nitrogen is useful for palliation of small cosmetically unacceptable lesions. A complete response rate of 80%, lasting 6 weeks to 6 months, has been reported for cryotherapy (Tappero et al. *J Acquir Immune Defic Syndr* 1991;4:839). Cryotherapy may cause treatment-related blisters, superficial scarring, and hypopigmentation. The latter may lead to cosmetically unacceptable results in dark-skinned patients.

2. **Radiation therapy.** KS is a **radiosensitive** neoplasm. Electron-beam therapy, which has limited penetration beyond the dermis, is effective for superficial lesions and generally provides good cosmetic results. Deeper lesions require conventional-beam irradiation. Radiation therapy offers **palliation** for periorbital edema, disfiguring lesions (particularly of the head and neck), obstructing lesions of the extremities, anus, or rectum, and painful disease. The optimal dose of radiation is controversial (Piedbois et al. *Int J Radiat Oncol Biol Phys* 1994;30:1207). Although >80% of lesions regress with radiation therapy, recurrence within 4 to 6 months is common (Hill. *Semin Oncol* 1987;14:19). Treatment of plaque-like and nodular lesions commonly results in areas of posttreatment hyperpigmentation. Whole-lung radiation may provide prompt relief of dyspnea in patients with pulmonary KS (Meyer. *Am J Clin Oncol* 1993;16:372). The treatment of oral lesions with radiation is frequently complicated by significant mucositis and the appearance of opportunistic infections. Radiation therapy is well tolerated and effective for KS of the conjunctiva, eyelid, and genitals (Le Bourgeois et al. *Radiother Oncol* 1994;30:263).
   3. **Intralesional therapy.** Intralesional injections of vinblastine have been used to treat solitary lesions. The usual concentration of vinblastine is 0.2 mg per mL, and doses of ~0.1 mL/0.5 cm^2 are usually given for KS. Most **responses are partial,** and tumor regrowth within 4 to 6 months is common. The **toxicity** of intralesional therapy includes pain, hyperpigmentation, intense edema, and erythema.
B. **Systemic therapy.**
   1. **Interferon-α** (IFN-α) is an attractive therapeutic option for treatment of KS because of its known **antiviral, antiproliferative, antiangiogenic,** and **immune-modulating** effects.
      a. **Single-agent IFN-α.** When used as a single agent, IFN-α has been most effective when administered to good-risk patients (CD4+ count ≥ 200/mm^3, no history of opportunistic infections, absence of B symptoms) and used at high doses (Real et al. *J Clin Oncol* 1986;4:544). (The FDA approved doses of IFN-α2a and IFN-α2b are 36 million units daily and 30 million units/m^2 3 times per week, respectively.) The objective complete- and partial-response rate for this subset of patients with good-risk features is ~30% (Evans et al. *J Immunother* 1991;10:39). The duration of response with IFN-a is greater than that with any other treatment; ≤ 2 years for complete responders and 6 to 12 months for partial responders. The time to response is generally 4 to 8 weeks, although maximal response may not appear for 6 months. Treatment is generally continued indefinitely, although it may be decreased to 3 times per week once maximal response has been obtained.
      b. **Combination therapy with IFN-α** and a variety of chemotherapeutic agents has led to increased toxicity without therapeutic benefit. **IFN-α** in combination with **nucleoside reverse transcriptase inhibitors** has resulted in higher response rates in a more diverse KS patient population. A response rate >40% can be achieved with IFN- and zidovudine. Even using lower IFN-α doses (4 to 18 million units per day); (*Ann Intern Med* 1990;1121:80), combination therapy is more likely than single-agent IFN-α to benefit patients with poor risk features (history of opportunistic infections, B symptoms, CD4+ counts <200 cells per μL). The major dose-limiting toxicity of this combination, neutropenia, can be ameliorated by the use of colony-stimulating factors (Scadden et al. *J Clin Oncol* 1991; 9:802). Combination therapy with IFN-α and didanosine (ddI), is well tolerated, and regression of KS has been observed with low doses of IFN-α (1 million units per day).

c. There is a paucity of data on the combination of interferon with more potent antiretroviral therapy.

d. **Dose**. There is no clear dose–response relation for IFN-α and KS. Most practitioners begin with relatively low doses, 5 MU s.q. daily, and increase to 10 to 15 MU per day over a 1- to 2-week period. Gradual dose escalation may limit toxicity.

e. **Adverse effects**. The dose-limiting toxicity is a **flu-like syndrome** characterized by low-grade fever, fatigue, and myalgia. Toxicity is **dose related** and tends to decrease in severity with continued treatment.

2. **Systemic chemotherapy**. Systemic chemotherapy may provide rapid palliation of KS-related symptoms. Relief of KS-associated pain or disabling lymphedema may improve after only one to two cycles of combination chemotherapy. Patients with extensive mucocutaneous KS, rapidly progressive cutaneous lesions (>10 new lesions per month), symptomatic visceral disease, or pulmonary disease or lymphedema or both, are candidates for systemic chemotherapy. There is no clear evidence that response varies based on disease site (i.e., viscera versus cutaneous). A variety of chemotherapeutic agents, individually and in combination, have been evaluated in clinical trials. Response rates of KS to single agents have varied widely, ranging from 21% to 80%.

a. The most widely used single agents are etoposide, bleomycin, paclitaxel, and liposomal doxorubicin.

(1) **Etoposide**, an epipodophyllotoxin, is a topoisomerase II inhibitor available in oral and parenteral formulations. **Oral** etoposide, an easily administered outpatient regimen, has been evaluated as a palliative agent for KS. In general, the response rate is higher in patients without prior chemotherapy. Clinically significant benefit (decreased KS-associated pain and edema) occurs more frequently than a "technical" response (50% decrease in disease volume or lesion number or both, without new disease).

(a) **Toxicity. Neutropenia** is the dose-limiting side effect. This is usually easily managed with the administration of **granulocyte–colony-stimulating factor (G-CSF**; 5 μg per kg per day s.q.), beginning 24 hours after the completion of therapy until 24 hours before the initiation of the next treatment. Alopecia is frequent. **Nausea and vomiting** occur in 50% of patients receiving oral therapy, leading to the recommendation for administration of etoposide with antiemetics. **Peripheral neuropathy** is not common but occurs with greater frequency and severity in patients previously treated with vincristine.

(b) **Dose and administration.** Etoposide is available as a 50-mg capsule and can be administered with or without food. Therapy should be initiated as a single nightly dose of 50 mg per day for 7 days every 2 weeks. The dose may be escalated to 100 mg per day if there is no unacceptable toxicity.

(2) **Bleomycin,** an antitumor antibiotic, has some efficacy for KS as a single agent and as part of combination chemotherapy regimens. Significant KS regression has been achieved with bleomycin, even in heavily pretreated patients. In a poor-risk population, treated with intramuscular (5 mg per day for 3 days) or infusional bleomycin (6 mg per m^2 per day), 48% of patients responded (Lassoued et al. *Cancer* 1990;66:1869). A partial response rate of 65% has been reported with prolonged infusional bleomycin (20 mg per m^2 per day for 72 hours); (Remick et al. *J Clin Oncol* 1994;12:1130).

(a) **Toxicity.** Bleomycin is associated with **little myelo-suppression**. Dose-related **pulmonary** toxicity seen as a subacute or chronic pneumonitis that progresses to interstitial fibrosis is the most important side effect of bleomycin. As the total dose of bleomycin increases (particularly >250 mg), the carbon monoxide diffusion capacity decreases. **Cutaneous** toxicity is frequent and is characterized by generalized hyperpigmentation or desquamation. **Raynaud's phenomenon** also may occur. **Fever** and **chills** may be observed during the first 48 hours after treatment. **Hypersensitivity reactions** with urticaria and bronchospasm occur less frequently and should prompt initiation of antihistamines and steroids before treatment. **Alopecia** is common.

(b) **Dose.** The ideal dose for bleomycin is not defined. Either of the regimens described are reasonable for patients with refractory KS.

(3) **Paclitaxel**, a taxane, induces irreversible polymerization of microtubules. Although clinical experience with paclitaxel for KS is relatively limited, it appears to be an **active agent** in both previously treated and untreated patients. A partial response rate of 65% was achieved in patients with advanced KS treated with paclitaxel, 135 mg/m^2 over 3 hours every 3 weeks (Saville et al. *Lancet* 1995;346:26). An alternative dose and schedule of paclitaxel (100 mg/m^2 over 3 hours very 2 weeks) achieved an overall response rate of 59%, confirming the efficacy of paclitaxel for the treatment of both newly diagnosed and refractory advanced KS.

(a) **Toxicity. Neutropenia** is the dose-limiting toxicity, although with these doses and schedules, G-CSF is not routinely required. Onset is generally 8 to 10 days after therapy. **Hypersensitivity reactions** (type 1), characterized by dyspnea with bronchospasm, urticaria, and hypotension occur in 1% to 3% of patients in spite of premedication. A sensory **peripheral neuropathy** in a glove-and-stocking distribution may occur after multiple courses of paclitaxel at conventional doses (<250 mg/m^2). Previous treatment with other neurotoxic agents does not increase the likelihood of neurotoxicity. Paclitaxel may cause transient **myalgias** or **arrhythmias. Alopecia** is frequent and may be associated with loss of all body hair with cumulative therapy. Gastrointestinal side effects (nausea, vomiting, diarrhea) and mucositis are infrequent.

(b) **Dose and administration.** Paclitaxel should be administered as a **3-hour infusion** at a dose of 100 mg/m^2 every 2 weeks or 135 mg/m^2 every 3 weeks. Because hypersensitivity reactions may occur, patients should be premedicated with corticosteroids and histamine antagonists. The following **premedication is most frequently recommended**: dexamethasone, 20 mg orally or intravenously 12 and 6 hours before treatment; diphenhydramine, 50 mg intravenously 30 minutes before therapy; and an H2 antagonist (e.g., cimetidine, 300 mg, or ranitidine, 150 mg) intravenously 30 minutes before treatment (Rowinsky et al. *N Engl J Med* 1995;332:1004).

(4) **Liposomal-encapsulated anthracyclines**. Liposomal encapsulation of chemotherapeutic agents has resulted in a prolonged plasma half-life, increased drug accumulation in tumor tissue, and a decrease in drug uptake by the reticuloendothe-

lial system compared with the unencapsulated drug. **Pegylated liposomal-encapsulated doxorubicin** is a preparation of doxorubicin encapsulated in a liposome composed of phosphatidylcholine, cholesterol, polyethylene-glycol, distearoylphosphatidylethanolamine, and a-tocopherol (Gabizon et al. *Cancer Res* 1994;54:987). This liposome prevents binding of the drug to plasma proteins and inhibits its excretion. In addition, pegylated liposomal doxorubicin is preferentially taken up by KS tumor cells (Papahadjopoulos et al. *Proc Natl Acad Sci* USA 1991;1:11460). Liposomal doxorubicin has achieved major objective response rates of 50% to 70% even in previously treated patients. Because pegylated liposomal doxorubicin has an excellent side-effect profile and produces a high response rate with a rapid onset of response (often in two or three treatments), this agent is likely to become front-line therapy either alone or in a combination regimen for the treatment of advanced KS. Phase II trials of liposomal anthracyclines for KS have demonstrated response rates of 25% to 93% (Gill et al. *J Clin Oncol* 1995;13:996). These response data are in marked contrast to the reported partial response rate of 10% with the use of single-agent doxorubicin (Fischl et al. *J Acquir Immune Defic Syndr* 1993;6:259). Liposomal daunorubicin also appears to be more effective than free drug; 33% to 55% of patients achieve a response.

> (a) **Toxicity.** Pegylated liposomal doxorubicin and encapsulated daunorubicin have similar toxicities and produce **dose-related myelotoxicity.** Neutropenia occurs in ~40% of patients and appears to be progressive with succeeding cycles. G-CSF (5 µg per kg per day s.q.) usually prevents treatment delays. Often relatively short courses of G-CSF (3 to 5 days) are adequate to maintain the granulocyte count. Treatment can be safely administered if the granulocyte count is 750/mm^3. Thrombocytopenia is uncommon. **Nausea** and **vomiting** are generally mild and infrequent. **Alopecia** occurs in fewer than 10% of patients. Anthracycline-induced cardiomyopathy is a potential long-term toxicity. Acute **infusion-related reactions**, characterized by flushing and abdominal or back pain, are seen infrequently. The infusion reactions resolve rapidly with cessation of the infusion. Therapy can be resumed after a brief (minutes) delay at a slower infusion rate. **Palmar–plantar erythrodysesthesia** occurs infrequently, resolves with interruption of treatment, and has been reported only with the pegylated liposomal doxorubicin.

> (b) **Dose and administration.** Liposomal doxorubicin, 10 to 40 mg/m^2 every 2 to 3 weeks, should be administered by i.v. **infusion** over a 30- to 60-minute period. Premedication with antiemetics is not usually necessary. Liposomal daunorubicin is well tolerated at a dose of 40–60 mg/mm^2 every 2 weeks.

b. **Combination chemotherapy**. Overall, results with single-agent chemotherapy have been disappointing. Toxicity is often unacceptable, the complete response rate is low, and the duration of response is brief. Combination chemotherapy has been used in an attempt to improve the complete and overall response rate, as well as response duration. Recommendation of one treatment regimen over another is difficult because prospective large, randomized Phase III clinical trials using strictly defined response criteria comparing one regimen with another have never been performed. The response rates achieved with combination chemotherapy have varied from 43% to 88%. Differences in response rates are the result in part of differences in efficacy, differences in the patient populations studied (i.e., history of prior opportunistic infections, treatment history, level of immune dysfunction), or differences in the response criteria used. Currently the combination regimens most frequently administered are doxorubicin (Adriamycin), bleomycin, and vincristine (ABV) and bleomycin plus vincristine (BV).

    (1) ABV (adriamycin, bleomycin, and vincristine) administered i.v. every 2 weeks is associated with manageable toxicity with clear superiority over single-agent doxorubicin (Gill et al. *Am J Med* 1991;90:437). Reported response rates for ABV vary from 28% to 88%. The initial report of ABV chemotherapy for KS reported a major response rate of 88%, with 38% of patients achieving a complete response. Subsequent trials have been unable to reproduce this high response rate, and few or no complete responses have been noted.

        (a) Toxicity. The toxicity of ABV reflects the side-effect profile of the individual agents. **Neutropenia** is frequent but easily managed with short courses (3 to 5 days) of G-CSF (5 μg per kg per day) initiated 6 to 8 days after treatment. **Alopecia** is frequent, occurring in about two thirds of patients. Other treatment-related toxicities include mild to moderate **nausea** and **vomiting, mucositis,** and sensory **peripheral neuropathy.** The severity of, or risk of developing, a vincristine-induced peripheral neuropathy is not increased when ABV is delivered in combination with known neurotoxic nucleoside reverse-transcriptase inhibitors (ddI, ddC).

        (b) Dose and administration. ABV is administered intravenously every 2 weeks and consists of bleomycin (10 mg/m^2), Adriamycin (20 mg/m^2), and vincristine (1.4 mg/m^2; maximum, 2 mg). G-CSF is used to maintain the granulocyte count at 750/mm^3.

    (2) BV (bleomycin, 10 mg/m^2 and vincristine, 2 mg) is an alternate regimen, particularly for patients with significant concern about alopecia. BV achieved an overall response rate of 72% in the only trial that evaluated this regimen (Gill et al. *Am J Clin Oncol* 1990;13:315). The **side effects** are similar to those seen with ABV, although overall there is less myelosuppression, and alopecia and nausea are less frequent.

  c. Combining chemotherapy with antiretroviral therapy. All patients being treated for KS should receive the best available antiretroviral therapy. However, important interactions can occur.

    (1) Myelosuppression is a frequent problem for patients with advanced HIV disease and can be worsened with concomitant zidovudine or ganciclovir. Colony-stimulating factors to support neutrophil counts should be used.

    (2) Neuropathy can be HIV related or a complication of nucleoside analogs such as didanosine or stavudine (see Chapter 13).

    (3) The protease inhibitors, particularly ritonavir, should be used cautiously in combination with cytotoxic agents as there is, as yet, minimal data available regarding pharmacokinetic interactions between the protease inhibitors and chemotherapy, but theoretically the inhibition of hepatic metabolism by protease inhibitors and certain NNRTIs could lead to higher levels of chemotherapeutic agents and consequently greater toxicity.

VIII. Conclusions. Although there is no established standard therapy for AIDS-related KS, general principles of treatment provide a basis for rational clinical decision making. The selection of therapy for KS requires consideration of the potential toxicities of the treatment regimen, its interaction with other medications, and its potential impact on the underlying HIV infection. Prophylaxis and treatment of opportunistic infections is essential because uncontrolled infection may stimulate KS progression, possibly by increasing the production of angiogenic cytokines. Because treatment for KS is primarily palliative, it is important to understand the treatment goals of individual patients. For a patient with bulky or rapidly progressive disease or both, a response that decreases edema and improves functional status may be meaningful, even if a "technical" response, based on change in tumor dimensions, cannot be achieved. As with all palliative therapy, close attention to the patient's quality of life is mandatory, and it is perhaps the best measure of clinical benefit from therapy.

29. LYMPHOMAS

Non-Hodgkin's Lymphoma

The human immunodeficiency virus (HIV)-associated non-Hodgkin's lymphomas (NHLs) are a molecularly heterogeneous group of predominantly B-cell neoplasms of uncertain origin. As is the case with other opportunistic complications of HIV disease the incidence of lymphoma has declined in the era of more potent antiretroviral therapy. However, the decline seems to be less marked than with most infections and is also clearly less marked than with Kaposi's sarcoma. The reasons for this difference is unclear but suggests that clinicians need to be alert for the possibility of lymphoma even in patients who have apparent responses to potent antiretroviral treatment. Individuals with these disorders tend to be seen with aggressive advanced stage disease, which is often present at extranodal sites. Management is complicated by the presence of underlying immunodeficiency and poor hematologic reserve, which make difficult the administration of cytotoxic therapy. As a result, complete remission rates and median survival times are poor in comparison with those seen in non–HIV infected individuals with similar lymphomas.

I. **Epidemiology**
   A. **Risk for development of NHL** appears to be constant over time at ~1.6% per year (Moore et al. *JAMA* 1991;265:2208) and is not confined to a single risk group, as is the case for Kaposi's sarcoma. In the era prior to the use of potent antiretroviral therapy, 12% to16% of patients eventually died of lymphoma.
   B. **Systemic NHL** may occur at any level of immune function. The median CD4+ lymphocyte count at diagnosis is ~100/mm^3. Approximately 75% will have a CD4+ count >50/mm^3, and 25% have CD4+ >200/mm^3.
   C. **Primary central nervous system NHL** occurs almost exclusively in individuals who are severely immunocompromised. The median CD4+ level for this group is ~30/mm^3. Seventy-five percent of these individuals have CD4+ lymphocyte counts <50/mm^3, and most have had prior opportunistic infection.
   D. **The effect of potent antiretroviral therapy** has been mainly seen in the incidence of primary CNS lymphoma which has declined considerably. However, rates of systemic lymphoma have not decreased as dramatically.
II. **Pathology**
   A. **B-cell NHL** composes the vast majority of HIV-associated NHL. This is true of virtually 100% of the primary central nervous system (CNS) cases and ~90% of the systemic cases (Herndier et al. *AIDS* 1994;8:1025).
   B. **Large-cell lymphomas** including intermediate-grade **diffuse large-cell** lymphoma and high-grade large-cell **immunoblastic lymphoma** account for approximately two thirds of all NHLs seen in HIV-infected individuals (Herndier et al. *AIDS* 1994;8:1025).
   C. **Small noncleaved (Burkitt's-like) NHLs** account for an additional 25% of acquired immunodeficiency syndrome (AIDS) NHLs. This histologic subtype is rarely encountered in the CNS.
   D. **T-cell NHL** has been encountered in fewer than 10% of all HIV-NHL cases. Several cases of cutaneous T-cell lymphoma also have been reported.
   E. **Anaplastic large-cell lymphoma** (Ki-1+) has been observed occasionally in individuals with HIV disease but occur with lower frequency than do the other histologic subtypes of B-cell lymphoma.
III. **Pathogenesis/origin**
   A. **Polyclonal B-cell proliferation**, a condition present in most HIV-infected individuals, may give rise to B-cell NHL. Polyclonal B-cell proliferations with typical features of aggressive large-cell lymphoma have been reported in a significant number of cases (Shiramizu et al. *J Clin Oncol* 1992;10:383). If

histopathology indicates aggressive lymphoma and molecular characteristics indicate polyclonality, the **histopathology should be used as the gold standard for diagnosis.** Despite the absence of evidence for monoclonal tumor, these "polyclonal lymphomas" behave no differently from aggressive monoclonal lymphomas (Meeker et al. *AIDS* 1991;5:669).

B. **Epstein–Barr virus** is present in ~40% of systemic NHLs, but in 100% of primary CNS NHLs.

C. **Other viruses**, including HIV and human herpesvirus 8, may be involved in the pathogenesis of subtypes of AIDS-NHL.

D. **Most large-cell lymphomas** occurring in HIV appear to be associated with overexpression of the cytokines interleukin-6 and interleukin-10.

IV. **Clinical presentation and diagnosis**

A. **Extranodal disease** is present in the majority of patients at the time of diagnosis.

1. **Gastrointestinal (GI) disease** occurs frequently, and any site in the GI tract (especially the stomach) may be involved. Oral cavity and ano-rectal lymphomas, unusual in the non-HIV setting, occur with relative frequency in the HIV-infected population.

2. **Hepatic and biliary NHLs** occur frequently and may be seen as intra- or extrahepatic obstruction.

3. **Other extranodal sites** frequently involved include bone marrow, meninges, and lung.

B. **Symptoms** often reflect the site of extranodal involvement. A high index of suspicion is therefore important in a variety of clinical situations, including an enlarging mass lesion at any site, asymmetric lymphadenopathy, chronic unexplained GI symptoms, evidence of obstructive hepatic disease, or unexplained fever. Although none of these symptoms is specific for the presence of lymphoma, any or all may be associated with the presence of the disease.

1. **Serum lactate dehydrogenase (LDH)** may be helpful if markedly elevated (>1,000). In the absence of established hepatic disease, pulmonary disease, or systemic fungal or mycobacterial infection, a markedly elevated or rapidly increasing LDH level should greatly increase the suspicion for an underlying lymphoma.

2. **Computed tomography (CT) or gallium scanning** may be a helpful diagnostic tool in patients with chronic unexplained constitutional symptoms or diffuse lymphadenopathy and may direct the clinician to a previously unrecognized site for biopsy.

C. **Diagnosis.** Tissue biopsy for histopathology is the diagnostic method of choice and is the definitive diagnostic procedure. Fine-needle aspiration may be useful as an initial diagnostic step to rule out the presence of infection, and a cytologic diagnosis may be possible; this may be a particularly useful diagnostic tool if the site of disease would otherwise be accessible only by a highly invasive surgical procedure.

D. **Evaluation of intracerebral mass lesions**. Primary CNS lymphoma cannot be easily distinguished from CNS toxoplasmosis. This presents a frequent diagnostic dilemma in the patient with HIV infection and an intracerebral mass lesion.

1. **A solitary mass lesion** on magnetic resonance scanning of the brain occurred in only 21% of patients with toxoplasmosis, but in ~50% of individuals with primary CNS NHL (Ciricillo et al. *J Neurosurg* 1990;73:720). Therefore the finding of a solitary lesion makes the diagnosis of lymphoma somewhat more likely but is not diagnostic.

2. ***Toxoplasma* serologic studies** should be obtained in all HIV-infected individuals with intracranial lesions. The false seronegativity rate for Toxoplasma is low (3% to 16%); (Grant et al. *AIDS* 1990;4:519; Porter et al. *N Engl J Med* 1992;327:1643). **It is highly unlikely** that an individual with negative Toxoplasma serologic tests will in fact have toxoplasmosis, regardless of the magnetic resonance imaging (MRI) appearance. It is recommended that patients with negative toxoplasma serologic

tests undergo **early brain biopsy** for diagnosis. Those with positive serologic studies should receive an empiric course of anti-Toxoplasma therapy, and those patients without clinical or radiographic improvement after ~10 days of therapy or those who worsen at any time during therapy should undergo biopsy at that time.

3. Evaluation of **cerebrospinal fluid** for evidence of Epstein–Barr virus or toxoplasma by PCR (polymerase chain reaction) may be very helpful. A positive Epstein–Barr virus PCR in the CSF, with a negative test for toxoplasmosis and a compatible clinical and radiologic finding may allow for a presumptive diagnosis of primary CNS lymphoma.

4. Although not widely available, **thallium-201 SPECT scanning** has also been shown to be sensitive and specific for the diagnosis of primary CNS lymphoma.

V. **Staging**

A. **Staging evaluation** should include CT scans of the chest, abdomen, and pelvis; bone marrow biopsy; and lumbar puncture.

1. **Bone marrow biopsy** should include two core biopsies. This will allow a determination of bone marrow involvement as well as providing an assessment of bone marrow reserve, which may influence choice of chemotherapy.

2. **Lumbar puncture** should be performed in all patients regardless of the presence of bone marrow involvement. Meningeal involvement with lymphoma does not appear to be as closely related to the presence of bone marrow disease in HIV-NHL patients as it is in non–HIV-infected NHL patients (Kaplan et al. *JAMA* 1989;261:719).

B. **Gallium scanning** can be highly useful as an adjunct to the usual staging approach, as well as for monitoring the response to therapy. Rapid clearing of gallium uptake after initial chemotherapy may have significant prognostic value.

VI. **Therapeutic approaches for systemic NHL**

A. **Combination chemotherapy** is virtually always indicated in the management of aggressive lymphoma, regardless of stage. Standard combination cytotoxic regimens commonly used in managing non-HIV lymphoma have been used in HIV-NHL as well.

B. **Major obstacles to therapy** have included the occurrence of opportunistic infections, especially *Pneumocystis carinii* pneumonia, during the course of therapy; and poor bone marrow reserve, which may result in prolonged episodes of neutropenia, febrile neutropenic episodes, and delays in chemotherapy administration. These complications have led to the frequent use of chemotherapy dose reductions in the management of these patients (Levine. *Blood* 1992;80:8).

C. **Therapeutic outcome** from clinical trials using a variety of standard combination-chemotherapy regimens indicate complete response rates of ~50% and median survival times of ~6 months.

D. **Prognostic features.** Both retrospective and prospective data indicate that the absolute CD4+ lymphocyte count is the most important predictor of clinical outcome in this patient population. A CD4+ count of <100/mm³ is associated with a particularly poor prognosis (median survival, 3 months).

1. **Other poor prognostic features** identified in retrospective trials have included poor performance score, the presence of extranodal disease, and a prior AIDS-defining opportunistic infection. **Prospective data** from a recent multicentered clinical trial indicated that advanced stage (III or IV), age older than 35 years, and i.v. drug use also are associated with a poor prognosis. Primary CNS lymphoma is also associated with a poor prognosis.

E. **Poor hematologic reserve** can be overcome by the use of a colony-stimulating factor or by using a reduced-dose chemotherapy regimen. A large randomized trial showed that for most patients, **reduced-dose chemotherapy** is as effective as and less toxic than standard-dose therapy in terms of response and survival (Kaplan et al. *N Engl J Med* 1997;336:1641).

VII. Treatment administration for systemic NHL
  A. Pretreatment laboratory tests. All patients should have blood specimens for CBC, differential, platelet count, measurement of renal function, hepatic function, LDH, electrolytes, calcium, phosphate, and uric acid.
  B. If tumor bulk is low (bone marrow not involved, no single mass >10 cm, LDH <500, and renal function, calcium, phosphate, potassium, uric acid all within normal limits), the patient may receive chemotherapy in the out-patient setting. Otherwise, hospitalization is required to reduce the risk of tumor-lysis syndrome.
  C. Hydration and monitoring for and prevention of tumor-lysis syndrome.
    1. Management of hyperuricemia or hyperphosphatemia or both. Aggressive i.v. hydration should begin 12 hours before planned initiation of chemotherapy. For hyperuricemia, 50 mEq of sodium bicarbonate may be added to 1 L half-normal saline or 100 mEq to 1 L D5W at a rate sufficient to alkalinize the urine to pH 7 and to maintain urine output of >100 mL per hour. The uric acid should be rechecked before beginning chemotherapy. Ideally treatment should not be instituted until the uric acid has normalized. Once chemotherapy is instituted, urine alkalinization should be discontinued, and normal saline used to maintain a urine output of >100 mL per hour. Alkaline urine impairs phosphate excretion. **For isolated hyperphosphatemia,** administer normal saline at a rate sufficient to maintain a urine output of >100 mL per hour.
    2. If creatinine is >2 mg per dL before beginning therapy, i.v. hydration should be administered as long as urine output is maintained. If hyperuricemia or hyperphosphatemia or both are also present, consideration should be given to the use of prophylactic dialysis immediately after chemotherapy.
    3. Laboratory monitoring for hospitalized patients with bulky disease should include a full electrolyte panel with calcium, phosphorous, uric acid, and creatinine **at least** twice daily for 48 hours after administration of chemotherapy.
  D. Chemotherapy administration. Both standard-dose and low-dose chemotherapy have been used in the management of patients with HIV-associated NHL. A recent randomized prospective clinical trial (Kaplan et al. *N Engl J Med* 1997;336:1641) demonstrated no statistically significant difference in clinical outcome (response or survival time) between patients treated with low-dose chemotherapy and those receiving standard-dose chemotherapy with a colony-stimulating factor. Low-dose therapy was associated with less hematologic toxicity and a reduced need for myeloid colony-stimulating factor use.
    1. Low-dose chemotherapy is appropriate therapy for most individuals with HIV-associated NHL. This applies to any patient with a CD4+ lymphocyte count of <200/mm^3. Some individuals with pretreatment CD4+ counts >200/mm^3 may be candidates for standard-dose chemotherapy. Improved myeloid reserve in these patients make them more likely to tolerate standard-dose therapy. However, no existing data demonstrate a benefit to the use of more aggressive therapy in this setting. This decision must be made on an individual basis and may include other factors such as performance status and stage of disease. The more commonly used combination chemotherapy regimens in both standard-dose and low-dose form are illustrated in Table 1.
    2. Myeloid colony-stimulating factor use. Either granulocyte–colony-stimulating factor (rGCSF) or granulocyte macrophage–colony-stimulating factor (rGM-CSF) may be used to reduce the complications of myelosuppression. However, rGM-CSF may be associated with a higher frequency of toxicity and in some studies has been shown to enhance HIV replication both *in vivo* and *in vitro* (Kaplan et al. *J Clin Oncol* 1991;9:929; Pluda et al. *Blood* 1990;76:463). If rGM-CSF is used, it is recommended that antiretroviral therapy be included in the treatment regimen.

Table 29-1 Chemotherapy for HIV-NHL

LOW-DOSE mBACOD[a]

Methotrexate	200 mg/m^2 over 2 h/d 15
Cyclophosphamide	300 mg/m^2/d 1
Doxorubicin	25 mg/m^2/d 1
Vincristine	1.4 mg/m^2/d 1
Bleomycin	4 mg/m^2/d 1
Dexamethasone	3 mg/m^2/d, days 1–5
Leukovorin	25 mg q6h × 6 doses, beginning 24 h after start of methotrexate

CHOP[b]

Cyclophosphamide[c]	750 mg/m^2/d 1
Doxorubicin[c]	50 mg/m^2/d 1
Vincristine	1.4 mg/m^2 (maximum, 2 mg), day 1
Prednisone	50 mg/m^2/d, days 1–5

INFUSIONAL CDE[d] (28-DAY CYCLE)

Cyclophosphamide	187.5 mg/m^2/d continuous infusion for 4 days
Doxorubicin	12.5 mg/m^2/d continuous infusion for 4 days
Etoposide	60 mg/m^2/d continuous infusion for 4 days

CHOP, cyclophosphamide, hydroxydaunomycin, Oncovin, and prednisone; CDE, cyclophosphamide, doxorubicin, etoposide; HIV-NHL, human immunodeficiency virus–non–Hodgkin's lymphoma.
[a] From *J AMA* 1991; 266:84–88, with permission.
[b] From *J Clin Oncol* 1984; 2:898, with permission.
[c] Low-dose CHOP. Reduce cyclophosphamide and doxorubicin dosages by 50%.
[d] From *Blood* 1993, 81:2810–2815, with permission.

       a. **With low-dose chemotherapy**, it is recommended that a CSF factor not be administered at the time therapy is instituted unless the baseline absolute neutrophil count is <1,500/mm^3. CSF should be administered only as required in this patient population. Only about one third of patients receiving low-dose chemotherapy for HIV-NHL will require the use of a CSF.

       b. **With standard-dose chemotherapy**, all patients should receive a CSF from the start of cycle 1. The most frequently used regimen has been 5 μg per kg per day s.c., beginning day 2 to 4, and continuing to approximately day 13.

    3. **Restaging evaluation** should be repeated after the completion of two cycles of chemotherapy and every two cycles thereafter. This should include reevaluation of all previously established sites of disease.

    4. **Duration of therapy**. Chemotherapy should be continued for a minimum of four total cycles or two cycles beyond documentation of complete response. Follow-up evaluation should be performed again ~30 days after completion of chemotherapy.

  E. **Meningeal prophylaxis**. The precise frequency of meningeal relapse in HIV-associated NHL is not known. Although some have advocated meningeal prophylaxis with intrathecal chemotherapy for all patients with HIV-associated NHL, limited existing data are more supportive of the use of meningeal prophylaxis only for those with typical risk factors for meningeal disease including **bone marrow involvement, epidural disease, paranasal sinus lymphoma, or small noncleaved histologic characteristics involving any site.** The most commonly used prophylactic regimen in HIV-NHL clinical trials has been the administration of weekly intrathecal cytosine arabinoside, 50 mg, administered via lumbar puncture during the first 4 weeks of therapy

(Levine et al. *JAMA* 1991;266:84). Because there are no data demonstrating the efficacy of this or any other prophylactic regimen, it is recommended that 4 weekly doses be administered as a minimum in those patients requiring prophylaxis (Table 2).

F. **Treatment of active lymphomatous meningitis** includes the use of both intrathecal chemotherapy and radiotherapy. Treatment can reduce symptoms and induce remission in many cases. The most frequently used regimen in HIV-NHL is illustrated in Table 2. Whole-brain radiotherapy should be instituted as soon as the diagnosis has been made and may begin at the same time systemic chemotherapy is instituted. Intrathecal chemotherapy should begin concurrently. Treatment is generally administered 3 times weekly until the cerebrospinal fluid (CSF) cytology has cleared. It is important to remember that isolated meningeal disease occurs rarely, and most patients will require administration of systemic chemotherapy in addition to treatment of the meningeal disease.

G. **Antibiotic prophylaxis** for *Pneumocystis carinii* pneumonia (PCP) has significantly reduced the frequency of this infection in AIDS-NHL patients receiving chemotherapy (Kaplan et al. *JAMA* 1989;261:719). Before the routine use of antibiotic prophylaxis, close to one third of individuals developed PCP during the course of chemotherapy. Recommended prophylactic regimens are illustrated in Table 2 (see also Chapter 4). Prophylaxis should be administered **regardless of pretreatment CD4+ lymphocyte count.**

H. **Antiretroviral therapy during chemotherapy**. The effect of concurrent administration of antiretroviral therapy and chemotherapy for individuals with HIV-NHL is not known. However, because HIV replication undoubtedly continues in the presence of opportunistic disease, it is **advisable to continue antiretroviral therapy** during chemotherapy administration.

1. **Zidovudine** can cause significant bone marrow suppression and should not be used with combination chemotherapy.

2. The use of more potent regimens, including protease inhibitors has not been well studied. One small study suggested that the clearance rates of cyclophosphamide were reduced in patients receiving concomitant protease inhibitors, which might increase toxicity. However, definitive data are not available, and the benefits of potent antiretroviral therapy on decreasing the risk of opportunistic complications in patients on chemotherapy suggest that appropriate treatment for the underlying HIV disease should continue.

Table 29-2 Adjunctive therapy for HIV-NHL

Colony-stimulating factor	rG-CSF, rGM-CSF, 5 µg/kg/d s.c. days 2–4 through 11–13
Meningeal prophylaxis	Cytosine arabinoside, 50 mg i.t. days 1, 8, 15, and 22
Treatment of active meningeal disease	Cytosine arabinoside, 50 mg i.t. qod until CSF cytology negative and then 50 mg/wk × 4 and 50 mg/mo × 1 yr Radiotherapy, 2,400 cGy whole brain at 200 cGy/d, lower border of field to encompass C2
Pneumocystis carinii prophylaxis	Cotrimoxazole, DS p.o. qd or dapsone, 100 mg/d p.o. or pentamadine, 300 mg aerosolized every 4 wk

VIII. Special considerations in management of HIV-NHL
  A. Management of patients with early stage (stage I and II) disease.
  HIV-infected individuals with early stage lymphoma are not commonly
  encountered. Although no published data exist regarding therapies directed
  specifically to patients with early-stage HIV-NHL, non–HIV-infected individuals with early-stage aggressive lymphoma are frequently treated with an
  abbreviated course of combination chemotherapy followed by involved field
  radiotherapy (Connors et al. *Ann Intern Med* 1987;107:25–30). Four cycles of
  a chemotherapy regimen such as cyclophosphamide, hydroxydaunomycin,
  Oncovin, and prednisone (CHOP) are frequently used in treating these
  patients. A similar approach might be taken in HIV-infected individuals with
  stage I or II aggressive lymphoma by using a reduced-dosage regimen.
  B. Management of refractory lymphoma is an especially difficult clinical
  problem, as most individuals with refractory disease have already received
  extensive chemotherapy, are severely immunocompromised, and tend to
  have advanced bulky disease. For patients who relapse or fail to respond to
  initial chemotherapy, the prognosis is extremely poor. Although complete
  remission is possible in ~50% of these patients, these remissions are generally of short duration. There is no evidence that one regimen is more effective than another for refractory disease. Most of these regimens are highly
  myelosuppressive, and therefore, the use of a myeloid CSF is essential in all
  cases. Referral to an experienced oncologist is essential for treatment of
  refractory aggressive lymphoma in HIV-infected individuals.
IX. Management of primary central nervous system lymphoma
  A. Early institution of therapy is essential for the management of primary
  CNS lymphoma. Those individuals with less severe neurologic compromise
  are most likely to have a beneficial palliative effect from therapy. Because systemic lymphoma occurs rarely in conjunction with primary CNS lymphoma,
  extensive routine staging evaluation is unnecessary in most of these patients.
  However, lumbar puncture for cytology should be performed as long as it is
  not contraindicated based on CT or MRI scan.
    1. Decadron at 4 mg every 6 hours may be administered if there is evi-
      dence of significant edema.
    2. Whole-brain radiotherapy should be instituted as soon as possible
      after the diagnosis has been made.
    3. Intrathecal chemotherapy (cytosine arabinoside) should be ad-
      ministered if cerebrospinal fluid cytology is positive.
    4. Clinical trials are exploring a combined-modality approach to therapy
      in which patients receive one cycle of combination chemotherapy fol-
      lowed by whole-brain radiotherapy.
  B. Improvement in neurologic symptoms will occur in ~75% of treated
  individuals (Baumgartner et al. *J Neurosurg* 1990;73:206), often providing
  significant improvement in quality of life. However, median survivals in this
  patient population are short (3 months), with most of these severely
  immunocompromised patients dying of opportunistic infection rather than
  refractory CNS lymphoma.

Hodgkin's Disease
Although several series of cases of Hodgkin's disease occurring with HIV infection have
been reported (Serrano et al. *Cancer* 1990;65:2248; Unger et al. *Cancer* 1986;58:821;
Monfardini et al. *Cancer Detect Prev* 1988;12:237), the relation between the underlying
immunodeficiency disorder and the occurrence of Hodgkin's disease remains unclear.
If there is indeed an increased risk of Hodgkin's disease with HIV infection, this risk
appears to be relatively small.

  I. Clinical features
    A. The histopathologic spectrum of Hodgkin's disease in HIV-infected indi-
      viduals differs from that in the general population with a shift toward a
      greater number of cases classified as **mixed cellularity** and **lymphocyte
      depletion.** The majority of cases are in these two categories.

B. **The clinical presentation**, like that of HIV-associated NHL, is characterized by advanced-stage disease in a high proportion of cases. Hepatic involvement is common, but more unusual sites of extranodal disease are significantly less common than with non-Hodgkin's lymphoma.

II. **Staging**

Standard staging procedures that are used in HIV-negative patients with Hodgkin's disease should be used here as well and should include CT scans of the chest, abdomen, and pelvis, and bone marrow biopsy. Whole-body gallium scanning also may be helpful in identifying sites of disease and in monitoring response to therapy.

III. **Treatment**

As is the case for non-Hodgkin's lymphoma, treatment of HIV-associated Hodgkin's disease is complicated by the presence of poor myeloid reserve, making more difficult the administration of cytotoxic therapy or radiotherapy or both. Although some series indicated a favorable complete response rate and durable responses, this has been achieved at the expense of considerable hematologic toxicity, and high recurrence rates have been reported. In addition, there is concern regarding the potential development of severe mucous membrane toxicity caused by radiation therapy in this patient population. It is therefore recommended that **most** patients receive cytotoxic therapy alone for treatment of Hodgkin's disease at any stage in HIV infection.

A. **Standard combination chemotherapy** may be used for the treatment of HIV-HD but should always be administered with a myeloid CSF. If standard therapy is to be used, it is recommended that the doxorubicin (Adriamycin), bleomycin, vinblastine,and dacarbazine (ABVD) regimen be administered in most cases.

B. **The use of relatively nonmyelosuppressive combination chemotherapy** has been reported. The regimen containing bleomycin, 10 units/m^2 on day 1; vincristine, 1.4 mg/m^2 on day 1; streptozocin, 750 mg/m^2 on days 1, 3, and 5; and etoposide, 100 mg/m^2 on days 1, 3, and 5 has been associated with a high complete-response rate and almost no hematologic toxicity.

C. **Radiotherapy.** Because there are few published data on the use of radiotherapy in the treatment of HIV-HD, no firm recommendations for the use of radiotherapy can be made. However, standard mantle-field radiotherapy might be considered in patients with carefully staged I or IIA disease, particularly those with CD4$^+$ counts >200/mm^3, who are more likely to tolerate radiotherapy.

APPENDIX

Michael Royal and William G. Powderly

Appendix 1. Available antiretroviral therapy with usual doses and costs[a]

Medication	Usual adult dose (daily total)	Strength and form	Quantity per 30 days	Unit cost ($)	Monthly cost ($)
NRTIs					
Abacavir (Ziagen)	600 mg	300 mg tabs	60 tabs	6.11 per tab	366.60
	—	20 mg/mL syrup	3.75 × 240 mL	96.29 per 240 mL	361.09
Combivir	600 mg/300 mg	300 mg/150 mg tab	60 tabs	9.85 per tab	591.00
Didanosine (Videx)	400 mg/d	200 mg tabs	60 tabs	3.79 per tab	227.40
	—	100 mg tabs	120 tabs	1.89 per tab	226.80
	—	20 mg/10 mL suspension	3 × 4 g	75.78 per 4 g	227.34
	250 mg/d	200 mg + 50 mg tabs	30 tabs each	200 mg, 3.79 per tab; 50 mg, 1.26 per tab	151.50
	—	100 mg + 25 mg tabs	60 tabs each	100 mg, 1.89 per tab; 25 mg, 0.47 per tab	141.60
	—	20 mg/10 mL suspension	2 × 4 g	75.78 per 4 g	151.56
	500 mg	250 mg powder packet	60 packets	4.53 per packet	271.80
	334 mg	167 mg powder packet	60 packets	3.03 per packet	181.80
	200 mg	100 mg powder packet	60 packets	1.81 per packet	108.60
Lamivudine (Epivir)	300 mg	150 mg tabs	60 tabs	4.54 per tab	272.40
	—	10 mg/mL syrup	4 × 240 mL	72.70 per 240 mL	290.80
Stavudine (Zerit)	80 mg	40 mg caps	60	4.95 per cap	297.00
	—	1 mg/mL syrup	12 × 200 mL	57.85 per 200 mL	694.20
	60 mg	30 mg caps	60	4.77 per cap	286.20
	—	1 mg/mL syrup	9 × 200 mL	57.85 per 200 mL	520.65
	40 mg	20 mg caps	60	4.57 per cap	274.20
	—	1 mg/mL syrup	6 × 200 mL	57.85 per 200 mL	347.10
	30 mg	15 mg caps	60	4.40 per cap	264.00
	—	1 mg/mL syrup	4.5 × 200 mL	57.85 per 200 mL	260.33
Zalcitabine (Hivid)	1.5 mg	0.75 mg tabs	60 tabs	2.43 per tab	145.80
	0.75 mg	0.375 mg tabs	60 tabs	1.94 per tab	116.40
Zidovudine (Retrovir)	600 mg	300 mg tabs	60 tabs	5.31 per tab	318.60
	—	100 mg caps	180 caps	1.77 per cap	318.60
	—	50 mg/5 mL syrup	7.5 × 240 mL	42.48 per 240 mL	318.60

NNRTIs					
Delavirdine (Rescriptor)	1,200 mg	100 mg tabs	360 tabs	0.79 per tab	284.40
Efavirenz (Sustiva)	—	200 mg tabs	180 tabs	1.57 per tab	282.60
	600 mg	200 mg caps	900 caps	4.56 per cap	410.40
	—	100 mg caps	180 caps	2.19 per cap	394.20
Nevirapine (Viramune)	400 mg	200 mg tabs	60 tabs	4.64 per tab	278.40
	—	50 mg/5 mL syrup	5 × 240 mL	60.34 per 240 mL	301.70
PIs					
Amprenavir (Agenerase)	2,400 mg	150 mg caps	480 caps	1.26 per cap	604.80
Saquinavir (Soft gel) (Fortovase)	2,740 mg	15 mg/mL susp	23 × 240 mL	31.72 per 240 mL	729.56
	3,600 mg	200 mg caps	540 caps	1.15 per cap	621.00
	800 mg	200 mg caps	120 caps	1.09 per cap	130.80
Indinavir (Crixivan)	2,400 mg	400 mg caps	180 caps	2.58 per cap	464.40
	—	200 mg caps	360 caps	1.29 per cap	464.40
Saquinavir (Hard gel) (Invirase)	3,000 mg	333 mg caps	270 caps	2.14 per cap	577.80
	1,800 mg	200 mg caps	270 caps	2.14 per cap	577.80
Nelfinavir (Viracept)	2,250 mg	250 mg tabs	270 tabs	2.26 per tab	610.20
	—	50 mg/g granules	10 × 144 g bottles	59.45 per bottle	594.50
	2,500 mg	250 mg tabs	300 tabs	2.26 per tab	678.00
	—	50 mg/g granules	11 × 144 g bottles	59.45 per bottle	653.95
Ritonavir (Norvir)	1,200 mg	100 mg caps	360 caps	1.86 per cap	669.60
	—	80 mg/mL liquid	2 × 240 mL	311.65 per 240 mL	623.30
	800 mg	100 mg caps	240 caps	1.86 per cap	446.40
	—	80 mg/mL liquid	1.25 × 240 mL	311.65 per 240 mL	389.56

[a] Costs represent average wholesale prices (costs to pharmacy) as of February, 2000.
[b] Capsule and suspension do not have equal bioavailability. Dose for suspension increased by 14% over capsule formulation per manufacturer recommendations.

Appendix 2. Dose modifications: dual protease therapies[a]

	Amprenavir (APV)	Indinavir (IDV)	Nelfinavir (NFV)	Ritonavir (RTV)	Saquinavir (FTV)
APV	—	APV 1,200 mg b.i.d. IDV 800 mg t.i.d.	Standard doses of both	APV 450–600 mg b.i.d. RTV 400 mg b.i.d. OR APV 900 mg b.i.d. RTV 200 mg b.i.d.	APV 1,200 mg b.i.d. FTV 800 mg t.i.d.
IDV	APV 1,200 mg b.i.d. IDV 800 mg t.i.d.	—	IDV 1,200 mg b.i.d. NFV 1,250 mg b.i.d.	IDV 400 mg b.i.d. RTV 400 mg b.i.d. OR IDV 800 mg b.i.d. RTV 200 mg b.i.d.	Not recommended
NFV	Standard doses of both	NFV 1,250 mg b.i.d. IDV 1,200 mg b.i.d.	—	NFV 750 mg b.i.d. RTV 400 mg b.i.d.	NFV 1,250 mg b.i.d. FTV 1,200 mg b.i.d.
RTV	RTV 400 mg b.i.d. APV 450–600 mg b.i.d. OR APV 900 mg b.i.d. RTV 200 mg b.i.d.	RTV 400 mg b.i.d. IDV 400 b.i.d. OR RTV 200 mg b.i.d. IDV 800 mg b.i.d.	RTV 400 mg b.i.d. NFV 750 mg b.i.d.	—	RTV 400 mg b.i.d. FTV 400 mg b.i.d.
FTV	FTV 800 mg t.i.d. APV 1,200 mg b.i.d.	Not recommended	FTV 1,200 mg b.i.d. NFV 1,250 mg b.i.d.	FTV 400 mg b.i.d. RTV 400 mg b.i.d.	

[a] Ritonavir can be used as a second antiretroviral (in which case a dose of at least 400 mg b.i.d. should be used) or to augment the pharmacokinetics of other protease inhibitors (in which cases lower doses, 200 mg p.o. b.i.d. are reasonable).

Appendix 3. Dose modifications: PI/NNRTI combination therapies

	APV	IDV	NFV	RTV	FTV
DLV	No recommendations	IDV 1,200 mg b.i.d. DLV 600 mg b.i.d. OR IDV 800 mg t.i.d. DLV 400 mg t.i.d.	NFV 1,250 mg b.i.d. DLV 600 mg b.i.d.	RTV 300 mg b.i.d. DLV 600 mg b.i.d.	FTV 1,200 mg t.i.d. DLV 400 mg t.i.d. OR FTV 1,600 mg b.i.d. DLV 600 mg b.i.d.
EFV	APV 1,200 mg b.i.d. RTV 200 mg b.i.d. EFV 600 mg qd	IDV 1,000 mg q8h EFV 600 mg qd	NFV 750 mg t.i.d. EFV 600 mg qd	RTV 500 mg b.i.d. EFV 600 mg qd	FTV 800 mg b.i.d. RTV 200 mg b.i.d. EFV 600 mg qd
NVP	No recommendations	Standard doses of both	Standard doses of both	Standard doses of both	No recommendations

Appendix 4. Dose modifications of antiretroviral agents: effects of renal failure and hemodialysis

Medication	Usual adult dose	GRF >50mL/min	GRF 10–50mL/min	GRF <10 mL/min	After hemodialysis
Abacavir (Ziagen)	300 mg bid	300 mg bid	300 mg bid	300 mg bid	Not affected.
Didanosine (Videx)	400 mg qd wt >60kg	400 mg qd	200 mg qd	100 mg qd	Possibly dialysed[a]
	250 mg qd wt <60kg	250 mg qd	125 mg qd	75 mg qd	
Lamivudine (Epivir)	150 mg bid	150 mg bid	150 mg qd	50 mg qd	Possibly dialysed[a]
Stavudine (Zerit)	40 mg bid wt >60kg	40 mg bid	20 mg bid	20 mg qd	Possibly dialysed[a]
	30 mg bid wt <60kg	30 mg bid	15 mg bid	15 mg qd	
Zalcitabine (Hivid)	0.75 mg bid	0.75 mg tid	0.75 mg bid	0.75 mg qd	Possibly dialysed[a]
Zidovudine (Retrovir)	300 mg bid	300 mg bid	300 mg qd	300 mg qd	Not affected
Delavirdine (Rescriptor)	400 mg tid	400 mg tid	400 mg tid	400 mg tid	Not affected.
Efavirenz (Sustiva)	600 mg bid	600 mg bid	600 mg bid	600 mg bid	Not affected
	600 mg qd	600 mg qd	600 mg qd	600 mg qd	
Nevirapine (Viramune)	200 mg bid	200 mg bid	200 mg bid	200 mg bid	Not affected
Amprenavir (Agenerase)	1200 mg bid	1200 mg bid	1200 mg bid	1200 mg bid	Not affected
Indinavir (Crixivan)	800 mg q8hr	800 mg q8hr	800 mg q8hr	800 mg q8hr	Not affected
Nelfinavir (Viracept)	750 mg tid	750 mg tid	750 mg tid	750 mg tid	Not affected
	1250 mg bid	1250 mg bid	1250 mg bid	1250 mg bid	
Ritonavir (Norvir)	600 mg bid	600 mg bid	600 mg bid	600 mg bid	Not affected
Saquinavir (Fortovase)	1200 mg tid	1200 mg tid	1200 mg tid	1200 mg tid	Not affected

[a] Consider redosing after dialysis.

SUBJECT INDEX

Locators annotated with *f* indicate figures.
Locators annotated with *t* indicate tables.

A

Abacavir, 37–38, 52, 54*t*, 63*t*, 112, 157, 258*t*
ABT-378/r, 47
Acid-base disorders, 130, 133, 163
Acid-fast bacillus (AFB) smear, 195–196, 200–201, 225
Aclometasone dipropionate cream, 107
Acyclovir, 22, 87, 109, 124, 135, 140, 169, 223
   resistant diseases, 222–223, Colorplate 5, Colorplate 7
Adefovir, 133
Adolescent HIV infection, 22, 60, 64, 69
Adrenal disorders, 133, 165–166
Advance directives, 86, 92
AIDS
   cardiovascular disorders with, 144–148
   classification of, 14, 16*t*, 250
   HIV progression to, 7–8, 14, 18–19, 48, 61
   stages of, 48, 84–85, 250. *See also* Terminally ill AIDS patient
AIDS-defining conditions, 14, 16*t*, 18, 62, 72, 84, 123
   wasting syndrome as, 158–159
AIDS dementia complex (ADC), 17–18, 25, 113–115
AIDS-related complex (ARC), 15
AIDS wasting syndrome. *See* HIV-associated wasting
Albendazole, 128, 193
Allergic rhinitis, 173
Allupurinol, 132
Aluminum hydroxide, for hyperphosphatemia, 133
Alveolar-to-arterial oxygen difference
   (D$_{A-a}$O$_2$), 182
Amikacin, 136, 140, 197*t*, 202*t*
Aminoglycosides, 136, 146, 192, 226
Amitriptyline, 91, 116, 118–120
Amniotic membranes, rupture of, 79, 82
Amoxicillin/clavulanate, 170, 172, 226
Amphetamines, 90
Amphotericin B
   complications from, 131*t*, 162, 164, 180
   indications for, 67, 136, 142–143, 172, 208–211
Amprenavir, 46–47, 54*t*, 63*t*, 259*t*–261*t*
Anabolic steroids, 151, 161
Anal cancer, 74–75
Analgesics, 89–91, 124
Anemia, 116–117, 176, 180, 186
Angiotensin-converting enzyme inhibitors, 146
Anorexia, 88–89
Anthropomorphic changes, 154, 157–161, Colorplate 19–Colorplate 20, Colorplate 27–Colorplate 28
Anticholinergics, 127

Anticoagulants, 147, 179–180
Anticonvulsants, 90–91
Antihistamines, 111
Antimalarials, 67, 180
Antimetabolites, 111
Antimicrobials. *See specific agent or infection*
Antiretroviral agents. *See also* Protease inhibitors; Reverse transcriptase inhibitors; *specific agent*
   doses and costs of, 258*t*–261*t*
   investigational, 41–42, 47
   pediatric, 36–37, 42, 63*t*
Antiretroviral therapy
   adherence factors, 54–55, 57, 59, 64, 91
   body composition and. *See* Anthropomorphic changes
   combination, 8, 14, 42, 48, 51–54, 54*t*, 57, 261*t*
   pediatric, 63–64
   disorders from, 125, 142, 148, 150–153
      endocrine, 154–157, 163–167
      metabolic, 56, 154, 156–157, 156*t*, 161–163, 161*t*, 167
      neurologic, 115, 117, 121
   drug resistance in, 30*t*, 31, 48–49, 51, 57–58, 84
   early advantages of, 8, 51–52
   failure of, 51, 56–59, 64, 85, 87
   goals of, 17, 50–52, 62
   guidelines for
      acute infection, 5, 7–8, 49–50
      asymptomatic patient, 14–15, 51–56
      CD4 cells 50 to 200, 17–18, 56
      CD4 cells 200 to 500, 17, 53–56
      CD4 cells greater than 500, 15, 53
      CD4 cells less than 50, 18
      initiation, 5, 7–8, 15, 26, 29, 50–56, 63
      pediatric, 62–64, 63*t*
      pregnancy, 68, 75, 79–81, 83
      terminal patient, 58–59, 85–87
   highly active (HAART), 154, 156, 161, 167, Colorplate 19–Colorplate 20, Colorplate 27
   immunologic markers for, 49–50, 56, 64
   with infectious disease therapy, 207, 209, 221, 228
      mycobacterial, 196, 198, 201–203
      protozoal, 186, 188, 191–193
   for Kaposi's sarcoma, 241–243, 246–247
   limited option patients, 58–59, 253
   monotherapy, 52, 63, 80
   new regimen usage, 57–59, 64, 86–87
   potency considerations of, 52–53, 101, 111
   prophylactic, 8, 9*t*, 11–13, 63, 79, 81
   renal disease and, 133–134
   response markers for, 26–27, 50–51, 59
   strategies for, 54–57, 85

Antiretroviral therapy (*contd.*)
  surrogate marker testing for, 48–51
  toxicity with, 48, 51, 53, 58, 81
    per body systems, 117, 119, 129
    viral markers for, 48–49, 55, 58, 64
Anti-Rh(D) immune globulin, 178
Antispasmodics, opiate, 88
Antitumor necrosis factor-based therapy, for
    myopathies, 151
Anxiety disorders, HIV-associated, 25, 89,
    116
Appetite stimulants, 65, 89, 160–161
Arthritis, 149–150
Artificial tears, 136–137
Aspergillosis
  extrapulmonary, 132, 143, 168, 172
  pulmonary, 94, 99*t*, 102, 210
  treatment of, 210–211
Aspirin, 145, 178, 197*t*
Assays
  antigen, 1, 7, 21, 26, 213, 223
  for antiretroviral resistance, 49, 57
  branched chain DNA, 4–5, 48, 213
  diagnostic, 6–7, 20–21, 26–27, 182, 223
  quantitative, 4–5, 4*f*, 48–49
  susceptibility, 3
Astemizole, 111
Atovaquone, 31, 67, 183*t*, 184, 186, 188,
    190–191
Atropine, 127
Avascular necrosis, 167
Azathioprine, 152
Azidothymidine. *See* Zidovudine
Azithromycin, 31, 31*t*, 110, 128, 191, 225
  for *Mycobacterium avium* complex, 201,
    202*t*, 203

B
Bacillary angiomatosis (BA), 110, 227, 240,
    Colorplate 12
Bacille Calmette-Guérin (BCG) vaccine, 199
Baclofen, 117–118
Bacterial infections, 66, 110, 224, 227–228
  arthritic, 149–150
  cardiovascular, 144–146, 148
  gastrointestinal, 125–126, 128–129
  ophthalmologic, 140–143
  of oral cavity, 169–170
  renal, 132, 134
  specific syndromes of, 66, 224–227
Bacterial pneumonia, 82, 224–225
  community-acquired (CAP), 94, 96, 98–99,
    99*t*
Bartonella infections, 110, 227, 240, Color-
    plate 12
Basal cell carcinoma, oral, 171
B-cells, pathology of, 111, 122, 224, 248–249
Benzamides, 88
Benzodiazepines, 88, 90, 116
Benztropine, 116
Biliary disease, 128–129, 192, 249
Biopsies. *See specific anatomy or pathology*
Bipolar disorders, with mania, 25
Bleomycin, 243–244, 246, 252*t*, 255
Blepharitis, 136

β-Blockers, 120
Blood products, 14, 18, 69, 179–181
Blood sugar imbalance, 154–155
Body composition changes, 154, 157
  adipose tissue maldistribution, 156–158,
    Colorplate 19–Colorplate 20,
    Colorplate 27–Colorplate 28
  HIV-associated wasting, 158–161
Bone density, Colorplate 28
Bone disorders, 167, 194
Bone marrow studies, 175, 250
Bone marrow suppression, drug-induced,
    179–180
Brain imaging studies
  for encephalopathy, Colorplate 25–
    Colorplate 26
  for lymphomas, Colorplate 23,
    Colorplate24
  for neurologic disorders, 114, 116,
    120–122
  for toxoplasma encephalitis, 188–189,
    Colorplate 21–Colorplate 22
BRAT diet, 126–127
Breastfeeding, 12, 28, 60, 68–69, 78, 82
Bronchoscopy, diagnostic, 95*f*, 96, 101–104,
    182, 213, 240
Buspirone, 116
Butyrophenones, 88

C
Calcitriol, 165
Calcium carbonate, for hyperphosphatemia,
    133
Calcium channel blockers, 147
Calcium chloride, for hyperkalemia, 133
Calcium deficiencies, 133, 165
Candidiasis, 67, 132, 142, 206–207
  oropharyngeal, 17–18, 29, 81, 109, 123,
    168, 173, 206, Colorplate 3
  vaginal, 72–73, 81, 109, 206–207
Cannabinoids, 88, 90
Capreomycin, 197*t*
Capsaicin, 91
Carbamazepine, 90, 116
Carbuncles, 226–227
Cardiac arrhythmias, 145–148, 244
Cardiomyopathies, 144, 146–147
Cardiovascular system, 24, 77, 156, 156*t*
  HIV manifestations in, 144–148, 226
Case-manager referral, 29, 66, 76
Catheter-related infections, 224, 226
CD4+ cell counts
  antiretroviral therapy per, 5–9, 11–18,
    49–50, 53–56
  disease classification per, 5–6, 14–19, 16*t*,
    25–26, 55, 61
  infections and, 100–101, 153
  Kaposi's sarcoma staging per, 240, 241*t*
  as lymphocyte marker, 25–26, 48, 175
  in special populations, 61–63, 68, 71–72,
    79–83
CD4+ receptor, 1–3
CD4+ turnover, kinetics of, 3, 5
CD8+ cells, 152
Cefaclor, 226

Cefazolin, 136
Cefepime, 98
Ceftazidime, 136, 140, 172
Ceftriaxone, 96, 236–237
Cefuroxime, 96, 226
Cellulitis, 143, 172
Cephalosporins, 96, 136
Ceprofoxacin, 136
Cerebellar syndrome, 121
Cerebrospinal fluid (CSF)
    infectious disorders and, 189, 213,
        235–236
    lymphoma and, 250, 253–255
    in neurologic disorders, 114, 119–122
Cervical disorders, 17, 24, 70, 72, 74–75
Cetirizine, 111
Chemotherapy
    for gastrointestinal disorders, 128–129
    for Kaposi's sarcoma, 111, 137, 170, 173,
        243–247
    for lymphoma, 250–255, 252t
    toxicity of, 38, 148, 243–247
Chest tubes, 105–106
Chlamydia trachomatis, screening for, 24,
    72, 80
Chlorambucil, 153
Chlorhexidine gluconate 0.12%, 170
Cholesterol levels, 155–158, 156t
Cholestyramine, 126–127
CHOP therapy, for non-Hodgkin's lym-
    phoma, 252, 254
Cidofovir, 137, 139, 214–219, 218t, 223
Cimetidine, 156, 244
Ciprofloxacin, 98, 128, 172, 198–199, 201,
    202t
Circumcision, 70
Clarithromycin, 31, 31t, 128, 137, 201–204,
    202t
Clindamycin, 67, 170, 183t, 186, 190–191,
    226–227
Clofazimine, 128, 142
Clostridium difficile diarrhea, 125–126, 159
Clotrimazole preparations, 109, 124, 136,
    206–207
Coagulation disorders, 179–181
Coccidioidomycosis, 96, 99t, 102, 210
Code of ethics, caregivers', 92–93
Colony-stimulating factors (CSF), 177,
    242–243, 251–252, 253t
Colposcopy, 72, 74
Combivir, 258t
Complete blood count (CBC), 6, 25, 175, 240
Computed tomography scans (CT)
    for lymphoma staging, 249, 255, Color-
        plate 23
    for neurologic disorders, 114, 116,
        120–122, 188–189, 213
    for orbital disorders, 143
Condoms, 22, 71, 82
Condylomata lata, 232, Colorplate 9–Color-
    plate 10
Confidentially, 12
Consent issues, 20
Contamination, of food and water, 27, 29,
    187–188, 192, 227
Contraceptives, 12, 28, 71, 75, 82–83, 167
Corneal ulcers, 135–136

Corticosteroids
    for infectious diseases, 101, 183t, 184, 191
    for lymphomas, 252t, 254
    miscellaneous indications for, 67, 145,
        166, 171–173, 178, 244
    for neurologic disorders, 117, 122, 191,
        254
    for ophthalmologic disorders, 135–136,
        140–143
    for renal disease, 131, 134
    for rheumatic disorders, 149, 151–153
    for skin disorders, 107–108, 110–112, 171
Cortrosyn stimulation test, 164, 166
Counseling
    contraceptive, 12, 28, 71, 75, 238
    for HIV infection, 8, 12–13, 15, 20, 22, 69,
        71
    injecting drug use, 8, 12–13, 28
    pregnancy, 12, 22, 28, 72, 75, 77
    for women, 71, 75, 238
Cromolyn sodium, 111
Cryotherapy, 74, 108, 137, 170, 241
Cryptococcosis, 67, 208–209
    clinical features of, 129, 148, 168,
        207–208, Colorplate 13
    meningitis, 113, 120–121, 207–209
    ophthalmologic, 141–142
    pulmonary, 96, 99t, 102, 207
Cryptosporidiosis, 125–126, 128–129, 192
Cultures. *See specific anatomy or pathology*
Cushing's syndrome, 166
Cyclophosphamide, 152–153, 252t, 254
Cycloplegia, topical ophthalmologic,
    135–137, 140–141
Cycloserine, 197t
Cytochromes, protease inhibitors and,
    42–47, 196
Cytokines, 3, 114, 247, 249
Cytomegalovirus (CMV) infections
    diagnosis of, 212–213
    endocrine/metabolic, 154–155, 159, 164
    gastrointestinal, 123–124, 128–129,
        212–213, 219–220
    miscellaneous, 68, 80, 131–133, 148, 169,
        173
    neurologic, 117, 119, 121–122, 212–213
    pneumonitis, 100, 212–213
    prophylaxis therapy, 31–32, 220–221
    treatment of, 213–221, 214t–215t, 218t
    viremia, 213, 221
Cytomegalovirus retinitis
    diagnosis of, 138–139, 212–213, Color-
        plate 18
    lesion zones, 138, 138f, 216
    pathophysiology of, 18, 23, 124, 138, 142
    treatment of, 139, 213–219, 214t–215t,
        218t
Cytoprotection, 124

D
Dacarbazine, 255
Danazol, 117
Dapsone, 67, 180, 188
    for *Pneumocystis carinii* pneumonia, 183t,
        186, 186t
    prophylactic, 30t, 31, 81, 186, 186t

ddC. *See* Zalcitabine
ddI. *See* Didanosine
Death and dying, issues of, 25, 82, 86, 91–93
Dehydration, 125, 127–128, 162
Delavirdine, 40, 54*t*, 259*t*
Demeclocycline, 133, 164
Depomedroxyprogesterone acetate, 75, 82
Depression, HIV-associated, 24–25, 89, 113, 115–116
Dermatologic system, 24, 230–232
HIV manifestations in
infectious, 108–110, 226–227, Colorplate 13
malignancies, 110–111
miscellaneous, 14–15, 17–18, 111–112, 224
noninfectious, 107–108, 170–172, Colorplate 1
Desipramine, 91, 116, 118
Desmopressin (dDAVP), 164
Desonide 0.05%-acetic acid, 2% otic solution, 173
d4T. *See* Stavudine
Diabetes insipidus (DI), 162, 164
Diabetes mellitus, for antiretrovirals, 154–155
Dialysis, 34, 130, 132, 134
Diarrhea
etiology of, 15, 24, 88, 125–126
treatment of, 17, 88, 126–127
with wasting syndrome, 88, 159–160
Diazepam, 116–117
Dicloxacillin, 172
Didanosine (ddI), 142, 155, 242, 246
doses and costs of, 34–35, 52, 54*t*, 63*t*, 258*t*
Diffuse infiltrative lymphocytosis syndrome (DILS), 152–153
Digoxin, 146
Dinitrochlorobenzene (DNCB), 108
Diphenhydramine, 244
Diphenoxylate with atropine, 127, 192
Diphtheria vaccination, 28
Diuretics, 146–147, 164
DNA
branched assays of, 4–5, 48, 213
in HIV replication, 2, 4, 7, 163
DNA probe screening, for sexually transmitted diseases, 24, 72, 80
Dobutamine, 146
Do-not-resuscitate orders (DNRs), 92
Dopamine, 146
Doxorubicin, 148, 245–246, 252*t*, 255
Doxycycline, 105–106, 110, 236–237
Dronabinol, 90, 160
Drug holidays, 59
Drug recycling, 58
Drug resistance, 30*t*, 31, 48–49, 51, 57, 84.
See also specific agent or pathology
Dry-eye syndrome, 136–137, 152
Dual-energy x-ray absorptiometry (DEXA), for adipose tissue evaluation, 158, Colorplate 28
Durable power of attorney (DPOA), 29, 91–92
Dysphagia, 123

E
Ear disorders, 171–173
Echocardiogram (ECHO), indications for, 105, 145–146
Efavirenz, 40–41, 53, 54*t*, 55, 157, 259*t*
Electrocardiogram (ECG), diagnostic, 145–147
Electrolyte imbalance, 125, 127–128, 130, 133, 162–163
Electromyelogram (EMG), for myopathies, 151
Emtricitabine (FTC), 38
Encephalitis
cytomegalovirus, 121–122, 212–213, 220
toxoplasma, 113, 120, 188–191, 207–208, Colorplate 21–Colorplate 22
Encephalopathy, HIV-associated, 113–114
brain imaging studies for, Colorplate 25–Colorplate 26
progressive. *See* AIDS dementia complex
Endocarditis, 145–146, 226
Endocrine disorders
from antiretrovirals, 154–157, 163–167
infectious, 154–155, 163, 165–166
Endophthalmitis, bacterial, 140
Endoscopy, gastrointestinal
lower, 126, 213
upper, 124, 126, 128, 206, 213, 240
Entamoeba histolytica, gastrointestinal, 125, 128
ENT disorders, 171–173
Enteral nutrition, 65, 125, 159–160
Enzyme-linked immunosorbent assay (ELISA), 7, 20
Epiglottitis, 173
Epistaxis, 173
Epstein-Barr virus (EBV) infections, 7, 68, 129, 168–169, 249–250
Ergots, 119
Erythromycin, 99, 110, 136, 227
Erythropoietin, 180
Esophageal disease, 123–125, 206–207, 221
Estrogen, 167
Ethambutol, 128, 196, 197*t*, 198, 201, 202*t*, 204
Ethics committees, 93
Ethionamide, 155, 197*t*
Etoposide, 243, 252*t*, 255
Exercise therapy, 156
Eye disorders. *See* Ophthalmologic disorders
Eye examination, 23

F
Factor IX-replacement, 179
Factor VIII-replacement, 179, 181
Famciclovir, 109, 135, 223
Fanconi-like syndrome, 133
Fentanyl patch, 90, 118
Fetal HIV infection. *See* In utero HIV infection
Fever
diagnostic, 6, 15, 17, 23, 87
drug-induced, 243–244
Fiber, dietary, 126–127
Filgrastim, 177

First-aid, for HIV exposures, 9–10
Fluconazole, 67, 87, 136, 201, 206–211
Fludrocortisone, 166
Fluid replacement, indications for, 133, 162, 251
Fluid restrictions, indications for, 133, 156, 162, 164
Fluoroquinolones, 136, 198–199, 201, 202*t*
Fluoxetine, 116
Folate deficiency, 117
Folinic acid, 31, 188, 190–192
Follicle-stimulating hormone (FSH), 164, 167
Folliculitis, 111, 226
Follow-up office visits, guidelines for, 22–23
Fomivirsen, 216
Food preparation, 27, 29, 187–188, 192, 227
Fortovase, 42–43, 259*t*
Foscarnet
    complications from, 112, 162, 164
    doses and toxicities of, 122, 128, 214, 215*t*, 219–220
    indications for, 109, 119, 124, 139, 217–219, 223
FTC. *See* Emtricitabine
Fumagillin, 136
Fungal infections. *See also specific infection*
    gastrointestinal, 123–124
    ophthalmologic, 141–143
    oral cavity, 17–18, 29, 81, 168
    pulmonary, 101–102, 207, 210
    in special populations, 66–67, 67*t*, 87
    treatment of, 107, 109, 123–124, 136, 172, 206–207, 211
Furuncles, 226–227

G

Gallium scanning, 103, 240, 249–250, 255
Ganciclovir
    doses and toxicities of, 180, 213, 214*t*, 219–220
    indications for, 119, 124, 139, 142, 216–219
Gastrointestinal system, 24, 78, 249
    HIV manifestations in, 6, 123–129
Gemfibrozil, 156
Genes
    Env, 1, 3
    Gag, 1
    Pol, 1
    TAT, 3
Genetics, of HIV-1, 1–5, 14, 49
Genital ulcerations, 6, 73, 109, 221
Gentamicin, 136
Giardiasis, gastrointestinal, 125, 128
Gingivitis, 169–170
Glucocorticoids, 90, 203
Glucose-6-phosphatase deoxyhydrogenase (G6PD), 81, 180, 186
Glucose supplements, 128
Glycoproteins, of HIV-1, 1, 2*f,* 5, 115
Gonadotropin deficiency, 164
Granulocyte colony-stimulating factor (G-CSF), 177, 203, 243, 251
Granulocyte-macrophage CSF (GM-CSF), 177, 203, 251

Growth hormone deficiency, 164
Guillain-Barré syndrome, 113, 118
Gynecologic care. *See* Obstetrical practices

H

Haemophilus influenzae
    infections, 15, 96, 98, 99*t*, 172, 224, 226
    vaccinations, 28
Haloperidol, 116
Headaches, 119–120
Health care access, 21–22, 76
Hematologic disorders
    scope of, 6, 25, 125, 132, 175–180, 186, 250
    transfusions and, 14, 18, 69, 180–181
Hematologic toxicity, drug-induced, 179–180
Hemolytic uremic syndrome (HUS), 132
Hemophiliacs, 14, 18, 179
Hepatitis viruses
    infections, 128–129, 181
    prevention of, 7, 10–11, 13, 27–28
Hepatobiliary disease, 27, 128–129, 192, 249
Herpes simplex virus (VSV) infections, 87, 100, 135, 221–222
    acyclovir-resistant, 222, Colorplate 5
    anogenital, 73, 109, 221, Colorplate 4
    esophageal, 123–124, 221
    oropharyngeal, 169, 173, 221
    in special populations, 67–68, 80, 82, 87
Herpes zoster virus, Colorplate 6. *See also*
        Varicella-zoster virus (VZV) infections
    acyclovir-resistant, Colorplate 7
Histamine$_2$-receptor antagonists, 124, 156, 244
Histoplasmosis, 209–210
    extrapulmonary, 132–133, 142, 168, Colorplate 14
    pulmonary, 94, 96, 99*t*, 101
HIV-1
    genetics of, 1–3, 14, 49
    latency of, 4–5, 4*f,* 14, 19
    life cycle of, 1–3, 28
    molecular biology of, 3–5, 4*f*
    screening for, 7, 10, 13, 20–21, 60–61
    transmission routes of, 6, 9–11, 21
        heterosexual, 70–71
        maternal. *See* Perinatal transmission
        vertical, 11, 14, 60, 68, 75, 78
HIV-1 exposures
    prophylaxis therapy, 8, 9*t,* 11–13, 63, 79
    risk factors for, 8, 14, 18
    types of, 6–13, 9*t*
HIV-1 infection
    acute, 6–15
    asymptomatic, 14–15, 51–56
    classification of, 14–15, 16*t,* 17
    clinical features of. *See also* Body composition changes
        natural history of, 6, 14–15, 15*f,* 17–18, 22
        pediatric, 61–62, 62*t*
    counseling with, 8, 12–13, 15, 20, 69, 71
    diagnostic markers, 6–7, 20–22, 25–27
    end-stage. *See* Terminally ill AIDS patient

HIV-1 infection (*contd.*)
immunosuppression mechanisms, 3, 5–6, 14, 19, 153
management of, 7–8. *See also* Antiretroviral therapy
manifestations of. *See specific anatomy or pathology*
pathogenesis of, 1–5
pediatric, 60–69
primary care of, 20–32
prognosis with, 17–19, 48, 56, 106
progression to AIDS, 7–8, 14, 18–19, 48, 61
in women, 70–76
with pregnancy, 77–83
HIV-1 replication, 1–5, 4*f*, 14
HIV-2, transmission routes, 14
HIV-associated wasting
CDC case definition of, 158–159
in terminal AIDS patients, 88–89, 158
treatment of, 17–18, 23, 151, 159–161
HIV-specific antibody, 6–7, 10, 13, 20
HMG-CoA-reductase inhibitors, 156–157
Hodgkin's disease, 175, 254–255
Homosexual populations, 14, 18, 28, 71
Hormone replacement therapy, 166–167
Hospice care, 92
Human growth hormone, 151, 158, 161, 164
Human herpes-viruses, 111, 170, 239
Human papilloma virus (HPV), 73, 108, 111, 169, Colorplate 11
Human T-cell leukemia virus type 1 (HTLV-1), 117
Hydrocodone, 90
Hydroxydaunomycin, 254
Hydroxyurea, 58
Hypercortisolism, 166
Hyperprolactinemia, 164
Hyperuricemia, 132
with non-Hodgkin's lymphoma, 251
Hypoglycemic agents, 155
Hypogonadism, 160, 164, 166–167
Hypothalamus disorders, 163–164

I

Idiopathic HIV-related diseases, 51, 96, 99*t*, 104–106
Imipramine, 116, 118
Immune Fluorescent Antibody (IFA) test, 187–188, 227
Immune response, to HIV-1, 3, 6, 19, 48
Immunoglobulin A (IgA), 134, 224
Immunoglobulin G (IgG), 15, 27, 187, 189
Immunoglobulins, intravenous (IVIG), 152, 176–178, 181, 187, 228
Immunosuppressive therapy, 149, 151–153
Indinavir, 11, 44–45, 53, 54*t*, 55, 259*t*–261*t*
Indomethacin, 149, 164
Infection-control procedures, 9, 12, 82, 199
Infectious diseases. *See* Opportunistic infections; *specific anatomy or infection*
Initial office visit
history taking, 22–23
physical examination, 23–25
Injecting drug use (IDU)
counseling with, 8, 12–13, 28, 70–71

disease impact of, 12, 18, 100, 145–146, 150
infectious, 132, 142, 224, 226, 234
Insomnia, 25, 89, 116
Insulin resistance, 155–156, 158
Integrase, 1–2
Intensive care, 106
Interferon, 117, 170, 178, 202–203, 242–243
Intracranial hypertension, 207–208
Intralesional therapy, for Kaposi's sarcoma, 242
Intraocular implants, 139
Intraocular lymphoma, 142
Intravaginal insemination, 71
Intravitreal ISIS 2922, 142
In utero HIV infection, 60–61, 68, 78, 82
Invirase, 259*t*
Iodine, radioactive, 165
Isoniazid (INH), 155, 204
prophylactic, 30*t*, 31, 71, 199
resistance to, 194–195, 198
for tuberculosis, 27, 100, 196, 197*t*, 198
Isosporiasis, 125–126, 128, 192–193
Isotretinoin, 111
Itraconazole, 206, 208–211

J

Jarisch-Herxheimer reaction, 237–238
JC virus, 121

K

Kanamycin, 197*t*
Kaposi's sarcoma (KS)
clinical features of, 239–240, Colorplate 16–Colorplate 17
cutaneous, 110–111, 239–242
ENT, 170, 172–173, 239–240
management of, 111, 137, 170, 172–173, 240–247
miscellaneous manifestations of, 129, 132, 147
natural history of, 15, 17, 239–240
ophthalmologic, 137, 143, 242
pediatric, 62, 68
pulmonary, 99*t*, 103–104, 240, 242
staging of, 239–240, 241*t*
Ketoconazole, 67, 107, 109, 206, 210–211

L

Laboratory tests
for HIV diagnosis, 6–7, 10–11, 20–21, 62
for HIV infection progression, 15, 16*t*, 17–19, 61, 125–126
for HIV manifestations. *See specific anatomy or pathology*
primary care, 25–28, 71–72, 80
terminal care, 85–86
Lactate dehydrogenase (LDH), 249
Lactic acidosis, 163
Lactose intolerance, 159
Lamivudine (3TC), 37, 52, 54*t*, 63*t*, 180, 258*t*
Larynx disorders, 173
Laser therapy, 74, 111, 170, 172
Left ventricular (LV) dysfunction, 144, 147

Lentiviruses, 1, 2*f*
Leucovorin, 30*t*, 67, 252*t*
Leukopenia, 176–177
Lipid disorders, 155–158, 156*t*, Colorplate 19–Colorplate 20, Colorplate 27
Liposomal-encapsulated anthracyclines, 245
Loperamide, 127, 192
Lorazepam, 116
Lumbar puncture (LP), 114, 120, 208
   for lymphomas, 250, 252, 254–255
Luminal agents, 126–127
Lung cancer, 99*t*, 104
Luteinizing hormone (LH), 164, 167
Lymphadenopathy, 14, 19, 23
Lymphocyte count, 6, 25–26, 175–176. *See also* CD4+ cell counts
Lymphomas
   brain imaging studies for, Colorplate 23, Colorplate24
   cellular pathology in, 111, 122, 248–249
   Hodgkin's, 254–255
   miscellaneous manifestations of, 68, 99*t*, 104, 111, 128, 142–143, 170
   non-Hodgkin's. *See* Non-Hodgkin's lymphoma
   primary CNS, 113, 119, 122, 248, 254
   systemic, 248, 250–253
Lymphoproliferative syndromes, 68, 132–133

M
Magnesium disorders, 163
Magnetic resonance imaging (MRI)
   of adipose tissue redistribution, Colorplate 27
   for lymphoma, 249, 254, Colorplate 24
   for miscellaneous disorders, 143, 158, 164
   for neurologic disorders
      HIV-assoicated, 114, 116, 120–122, 249, Colorplate 25–Colorplate 26
      infectious, 188–189, 213, Colorplate 21–Colorplate 22
Malabsorption disorders, 159–160, 176
Malignancies. *See also specific anatomy or malignancy*
   natural history of, 17–18, 87
   in special populations, 62, 68, 72, 74–75
Mammography, 72
Mania, 25, 113
Mastoiditis, 172
Measles, 68
Mechanical ventilation, 106
Megestrol acetate, 160
Meningitis, 232
   cryptococcal, 113, 120–121, 207–209
   lymphoma and, 252–253, 253*t*
   mycobacterial, 113, 194–195
Menstrual disorders, 72, 166–167
Metabolic disorders, 115, 154. *See also specific disorder*
   drug-induced, 56, 156–157, 156*t*, 161–163, 161*t*
   HAART-associated, 154, 156, 161, 167, Colorplate 19–Colorplate 20, Colorplate 27
   infectious, 154–155

Methadone, 118
Methotrexate, 149, 152, 252*t*
Methylcellulose, 126
Methylphenidate, 90
Methysergide, 120
Metronidazole, 111, 128, 170
Mexiletine, 91
Miconazole 1% cream, 107, 136, 207
Microangiopathy, HIV-induced, 137, 142
β_2-Microglobulin, 26, 50, 114
Microsporidiosis, 125–126, 128, 136, 193
Minocycline, 105–106, 110
Minority populations, 20–21
Molluscum contagiosum, 108, 136, 208, Colorplate 8
Morphine, 90, 118
Motor cognitive disorder, HIV-associated, 113
Mucormycosis, orbital, 143
Myalgias, drug-induced, 243–244
Mycobacterial infections. *See also specific infection*
   antimicrobials for, 196, 197*t*, 201, 202*t*
   antiretroviral therapy with, 196, 198, 201–203
   drug-resistant, 194–195, 198, 202
   scope of, 29, 148, 204–205, 204*t*
Mycobacterium avium complex (MAC)
   epidemiology of, 66, 199–200
   gastrointestinal, 125–126, 128
   with HIV infection, 94, 99*t*, 101, 153, 176, 200
   pregnancy and, 81–82
   prophylaxis therapy, 31–32, 31*t*, 203
   treatment of, 200–203, 202*t*
Mycobacterium kansaii, 203–204
Mycobacterium tuberculosis (MTB). *See* Tuberculosis
Mycoses. *See* Fungal infections
Myeloid colony-stimulating factors, 251–252, 255
Myelopathies, 113, 116–117, 119, 121
Myopathies, 119, 150–151

N
Natamycin 5% solution, 136
Nausea/vomiting, 87–88, 160, 243–246
Necrotizing infections, 170
Needle-exchange programs, 28
Needlesticks, 6, 8–10, 12. *See also* Injecting drug use
Neisseria gonorrheae, screening for, 24, 72, 80
Nelfinavir, 11, 45–46, 54*t*, 63, 259*t*, 261*t*
Neopterin, 26, 50, 114
Nephrotic syndrome, 132–133
Nerve-conduction studies, 118–119
Neurodevelopmental intervention, pediatric, 64–66
Neurologic system
   examination of, 24–25, 27, 172
   HIV manifestations in
      assessment of, 24–25, 27, 114, 119–122
      pediatric, 62, 64–65, 114
      spectrum of, 17–18, 113, 172
   imaging studies for, 114, 116, 120–122
   lymphoma manifestations in, 248, 254

Neuropathy, 24, 91, 121
    drug-induced, 243–247
    peripheral, 113, 117–119, 121
Neuropsychologic testing, 114–115
Neutropenia, 176–177, 224, 243–246
Nevirapine, 39–40, 53, 54t, 63t, 79, 157,
    259t
Nitrogen mustard, 111
Nocardia pneumonia, 99, 99t, 225
Non-Hodgkin's lymphoma (NHL)
    diagnosis of, 175, 249–250
    pathogenesis of, 111, 122, 137, 248–249
    primary CNS, 113, 119, 122, 248, 254
    staging of, 250, 252, 254
    systemic, 248, 250–253
    treatment of, 143, 250–254, 252t–253t
Non-nucleoside reverse transcriptase
        inhibitors (NNRTIs)
    with antimycobacterials, 196, 198, 201
    combination therapies, 53–54, 54t, 57,
        63–64, 247, 261t
    complications from, 112, 154, 163
    doses and costs of, 38–41, 63t, 64,
        258t–259t, 261t
Nonsteroidal antiinflammatory agents
        (NSAIDs)
    indications for, 89–90, 118, 145, 149, 151
    renal disease with, 131, 131t
Nortriptyline, 91, 116, 118
Nose disorders, 173, 226
Nucleoside analog reverse transcriptase
        inhibitors, 41–42, 52–54, 54t, 63–64
Nucleoside reverse transcriptase inhibitors
        (NRTIs), 33–38, 63t, 64, 117, 163
    combination therapies, 52–54, 54t, 57,
        63–64, 242–243
Nutrition
    management of, 15, 65, 89, 116–117,
        127–128, 156
    supplements for, 23, 65, 89, 117, 125, 128,
        192
    with wasting syndrome, 159–160
Nystatin preparations, 124, 207

O
Obstetrical practices, 12, 22, 28, 69–72,
    76–79, 82. See also Pregnancy
Occupational HIV exposure, 6, 8–12, 9t
Octreotide, 88, 127, 192
Odynophagia, 123–124
Ofloxacin, 136, 198–199
One-stop health care, 21–22, 76
Ophthalmologic disorders
    of anterior segment, 135–138
    choroidal, 141–142, 191–192
    infectious, 18, 23, 124, 135–143, 212,
        216–219
    malignant, 137, 142–143
    miscellaneous, 137–138, 142–143
    of posterior segment, 138–142
    screening for, 23, 221
    surface diseases, 136–137
Opportunistic infections (OIs). See also spe-
        cific infection
    cardiovascular, 144–145, 147–148

classifications of, 6, 14–15, 16t, 17–18, 87,
    89
    endocrine, 154–155, 163, 165–166
    neurologic, 113, 120
    ophthalmologic, 18, 23, 124, 135–136,
        138–143
    pediatric, 61–62, 66–68, 67t
    prophylaxis therapy
        indications, 17–18, 26, 29, 30t–31t,
            31–32
        for special populations, 66–67, 67t,
            80–82, 87
    renal disease from, 131–133, 131t
Oral cavity
    HIV manifestations in, 6, 23, 170–171
    infections of
        bacterial, 169–170
        fungal, 17–18, 29, 81, 168, 206, Color-
            plate 3
        viral, 15, 18, 109–110, 168–169, 221
Oral hairy leukoplakia (OHL), 15, 18,
        109–110, 168–169, 206, Colorplate 2
Oral-rehydration formula, 127–128
Organ donation/transplants, 12, 134
Organic brain disease, 17–18, 25
Oxacillin, 226
Oxycodone, 90
Oxygen, supplemental, 147

P
Paclitaxel, 244–245
Pain
    management of, 89–91, 118–120
    neuropathic, 91, 116, 118–120
Painful articular syndrome, 150
Pancreatic disorders, 129, 154–156, 156t
Panhypopituitarism, 164
Panic disorders, 25
Pap smear, 24, 72
Parasites, 109, 125–126
Parathyroid dysfunction, 165
Parenteral nutrition, 159–160, 192
Paromomycin, 128, 192
Parotid gland enlargement, 152–153
Paroxetine, 116
Parvovirus B19, 176, 181
Patient history, with initial office visit,
        22–23, 65, 71, 159
Pediatric HIV infection
    adult versus, 61–62
    antiretroviral therapy for, 36–37, 42,
        62–64, 63t
    classification system for, 61–63, 62t
    diagnosis of, 60–62, 77
    multidisciplinary management of, 62–66
    noninfectious complications, 68, 82, 114
    opportunistic infections, 61–62, 66–68, 67t
    screening for, 60–61
    transmission of, 11–12, 14, 28, 60
Pelvic examination, 24
Pelvic inflammatory disease (PID), 73–74
Penicillin G, 141, 236–238
Penicilliosis, 102, 210
Penile condylomata, 232, Colorplate 10

Pentamidine
    complications from, 133, 155, 180
    for *Pneumocystis carinii* pneumonia, 183*t*,
        184–186, 186*t*
    prophylactic, 30*t*, 31, 67, 81
Perianal condylomata, 232, Colorplate 9
Pericarditis, 144–145
Perinatal transmission, 11–12, 14, 28, 60,
    68, 78–80, 82
Periodontal infections, 169–171
Permanency planning, 75–76
Permethrin cream, 109
Personality disorders, 25
Pets, 27–29, 188
Pharyngeal disorders, 173, 206
Phenothiazines, 88
Phenylbutazone, 149
Phenytoin, 90
Phosphate disorders, 163, 251
Photosensitivity, 112
Phototherapy, 108, 110–111
Physical examination, with initial office
    visit, 23–25, 72
Piperacillin, 172
Pituitary gland disorders, 163–164
Plasma transfusions, 178–179, 181
Platelet disorders, 177–179
Pleurodesis, 105–106
PMPA prodrug (tenofovir disoproxil
    fumarate), 41–42
Pneumocystis carinii, 141, 172, 182
Pneumocystis carinii pneumonia (PCP)
    complications of, 105–106, 144
    diagnosis of, 99*t*, 102–103, 182
    natural history of, 6, 16*t*, 17, 23, 94, 182
    prophylaxis therapy, 29, 30*t*, 31, 153, 182,
        184, 186, 186*t*, 253
    in special populations, 66–67, 67*t*, 80–81
    treatment of, 182, 183*t*, 184–186
Pneumonitis
    infectious, 100, 212–213
    noninfectious, 96, 99*t*, 104–105
Pneumothorax, 105–106
Podophyllin resin solution, 110, 169
Polymerase chain reaction (PCR)
    diagnostic applications of, 4, 7, 21, 189,
        250
    in neurologic disorders, 121, 213
    in ophthalmologic disorders, 137, 139
    reverse transcription (RT-PCR), 48
Polymyositis, 113, 119, 151
Polyradiculopathy, 212–213
Polysporin ointment, 136
Porphyria cutanea tarda, 112
Postexposure prophylaxis, 8, 9*t*, 11–13, 63,
    79
Potassium imbalance, 128, 130, 133, 162
Povidone-iodine 10% solution, 169
Power of attorney, 29, 91–92
Pregnancy
    counseling with, 12, 22, 28, 72, 75, 77
    HIV infection with
        antiretroviral therapy, 68, 75, 79–81, 83
        CD4+ cell counts, 68, 79–83
        delivery mode and, 12, 22, 28, 69,
            78–79, 82

    maternal health impact, 77–78, 82
    obstetrical care impact, 80–83
    transmission of, 11, 14, 60, 68, 78–80,
        82
    physiologic changes with, 77–78
    syphilis in, 236, 238
Primaquine, 67, 180, 183*t*, 186
Primary care
    antiretroviral therapy initiation, 5, 7–8,
        15, 26, 29
    follow-up guidelines for, 29–32
    initial assessment with, 20–24
    laboratory tests in, 25–28
    prophylaxis therapy as, 17–18, 26, 29,
        30*t*–31*t*, 31–32
    psychiatric component of, 24–25
    scope of, 20–22, 28–29
    for women, 21, 60, 71–72, 76
Primary pulmonary hypertension (PPH),
    144, 147
Progesterone, 167
Progressive multifocal leukoencephalopathy
    (PML), 113, 121, Colorplate 25
Propamidine isethionate 0.1%, 136
Prophylaxis therapy
    for HIV-1, 8, 9*t*, 11–13, 63, 79, 224
    with HIV infection, 17–18, 26, 29, 30*t*–31*t*,
        31–32
    for infections. *See* Opportunistic infec-
        tions; *specific infection*
Propranolol, 120
Protease, 1, 42
Protease inhibitors (PIs), 42–47, 125,
    154–157. *See also specific agent*
    with antimycobacterials, 196, 198, 201
    combination therapies, 52–57, 54*t*, 63–64,
        260*t*–261*t*
    doses and costs of, 11, 63–64, 63*t*,
        246–247, 258*t*–261*t*
Protein S deficiency, 179
Proton-pump inhibitors, 124
Protozoan infections, 125–129, 136,
    190–193. *See also specific infection*
    antiretroviral therapy with, 186, 188,
        191–193
    pulmonary, 99*t*, 102–103, 182–186,
        191–192. *See also Pneumocystis
        carinii* pneumonia
Provirus, 2
Pruritus, 107–108, 111
Pseudomonas aeruginosa, 224–226
Psoriasis, 108, 111, 150
Psychiatric disorders, 17–18, 24–25, 113,
    115–116. *See also specific disorder*
Psychosocial factors, of HIV-1 infection, 22,
    29, 66, 75–76, 83, 115
Psychotherapy, 115–116
Psyllium, 126
Pulmonary emboli, 146
Pulmonary system, 23–24, 77–78, 94
    HIV manifestations in, 94, 99*t*, 106
        diagnosis of, 94, 95*f*, 95*t*, 96, 97*t*–98*t*,
            99, 101–105
        idiopathic diseases, 104–106
        infectious, 96, 98–103, 182–186,
            191–199, 207, 210
        malignancies, 103–104

Pyogenic infections. *See* Bacterial infections
Pyomyositis, 227
Pyrazinamide, 128, 196, 197*t*, 198–199
Pyridoxine, 31, 199
Pyrimethamine, 31, 188, 190–192

Q

Quality of life, issues of, 62, 66, 75, 84, 126

R

Radiation therapy, 153, 171
    for Kaposi's sarcoma, 111, 137, 172–173,
        242
    for lymphoma, 43, 122, 253–255, 253*t*
Radionucleotide scanning, 103, 188, 240,
    249–250, 255
Ranitidine, 156, 244
Rectal examination, 24
Red blood cell disorders, 77, 125, 176, 186
Reiter's syndrome, 110, 137, 149
Renal disease, 78, 131*t*, 163
    causally related to HIV infection, 133–134
    coincidental with HIV infection, 130–133
    end-stage (ESRD), 130, 131*t*, 133–134
Renal-replacement therapy, 134
Respiratory infections, 68, 94, 224
Reticuloendothelial system, tuberculosis of,
    194–195
Retinal disorders, 139–140, 142
    infectious. *See* Cytomegalovirus retinitis
Retinoid 0.05% solution, 169
Reverse transcriptase (RT), 1–2, 4, 14
Reverse transcriptase inhibitors (RTIs), 33,
    112. *See also specific agent or class*
    combination therapies, 53–54, 54*t*, 57,
        63–64
    non-nucleoside, 38–41
    nucleoside, 33–38
    nucleotide analogs, 41–42
    pediatric, 63–64, 63*t*
Rheumatic disorders, 149–153
Rhodococcus equi pneumonia, 98–99, 99*t*,
    225
Rifabutin
    for *Mycobacterium avium* complex, 128,
        137, 201, 202*t*, 203
    prophylactic, 31, 31*t*
    for tuberculosis, 128, 196, 198
Rifampin
    for bacterial infections, 99, 225, 227
    for *Mycobacterium avium* complex, 128,
        202*t*, 204
    prophylactic, 30*t*, 31, 199
    resistance to, 194–195, 198
    for tuberculosis, 100, 128, 196, 197*t*
Right ventricular hypertrophy (RVH), 144,
    147
Ritonavir, 43–44, 53, 54*t*, 63, 246, 259*t*–261*t*
RNA levels, plasma viral
    antiretroviral therapy and, 48, 50, 57, 63
    assessment guidelines for, 17–19, 26–27,
        72
    in HIV replication, 2–5, 7, 15

S

Salivary gland disease, 171
Salmonella infections, 227
Saquinavir (FTV), 42–43, 54*t*, 260*t*–261*t*
Sargramastim, 177
Scabies, 109, Colorplate 15
Sclerosing agents, 170
Screening techniques and recommenda-
    tions. *See specific pathology*
Seborrheic dermatitis, 107, 136, 171–173,
    Colorplate 1
Selective serotonergic reuptake-inhibitors
    (SSRIs), 88, 116, 118
Semen, 71
Seroconversion, 7, 10
Serologic testing
    predictive value of, 4, 7, 20–21, 110
    in special populations, 71, 80, 132
    for syphilis (STS), 233–235, 234*t*–235*t*
    for toxoplasmosis, 27–28, 71, 187,
        249–250
Sertraline, 116
Serum chemistry, 26
Sexual dysfunction, from hypogonadism,
    160, 164
Sexually transmitted diseases (STDs). *See
    also* Syphilis
    HIV infection risk with, 7, 12, 24, 69, 71,
        110
    Kaposi's sarcoma and, 239
    screening for, 7, 15, 24, 27, 72, 80
    in women, 61, 70, 72
Sexual practices, 8, 12, 28, 70–71, 238
Sick euthyroid syndrome, 164–165
Single-photon-emission computed tomogra-
    phy (SPECT), 122
Sinusitis, 94, 120, 143, 173, 224–225
Smooth-muscle tumors, pediatric, 68
Social support. *See* Psychosocial factors
Social-worker referral, 29, 66, 76
Sodium supplements, 127–128, 133, 162
Soft-tissue infections, 226–227
Somatostatin, 127
Spinal cord myelopathy, 113, 116–117
Splenectomy, for hematologic disorders, 178
Squamous cell carcinoma, 111, 170–171
Squamous intraepithelial lesions (SIL), 74
Staphylococcal infections, 145–146, 172,
    224, 226
Stavudine (d4T), 36–37, 52, 63*t*, 246, 258*t*,
    564*t*
Steroids. *See* Anabolic steroids; Cortico-
    steroids
Stevens-Johnson syndrome, 190
Stool analysis, 125–126, 192
Streptococcus pneumoniae
    infections, 96, 98, 99*t*, 172, 224, 226
    vaccinations, 28, 31*t*
Streptomycin, 128, 196, 197*t*, 198
Streptozocin, 255
Substance abuse
    as comorbidity, 7, 12, 54, 71, 113
    primary care for, 21, 25, 28
Sucralfate, 124
Suicidal ideation, 115–116

Sulfadiazine, 190–191
Sulfadoxine, 180
Sulfamethoxazole, 99, 180
Sulfasalazine, 149
Sumatriptan, 119
Sustiva, 40–41
Syncytium induction, 3, 49
Syndrome of inappropriate antidiuretic hormone secretion (SIADH), 133, 162, 164
Syphilis
  clinical manifestations of, 141, 172–173, 230–236
  with HIV infection, 110, 113, 229–230, 238
  neurological, 230, 232–233, 235–236
  in pregnancy, 236, 238
  serologic testing for (STS), 7, 15, 27, 230–236, 234t–235t
  transmission routes for, 229–230, 238
  treatment of, 236–238
Systemic disorders, 110, 248, 250–253

T
T-cells, pathology of, 5, 111, 117, 248
Tenesmus, 125
Tenofovir disoproxil fumarate (PMPA prodrug), 41–42
Terminally ill AIDS patient
  antiretroviral therapy for, 58–59, 85–87
  care principles for, 76, 84–85
  diagnosis of, 84–86
  orchestrating death for, 91–93
  pain control for, 89–91
  symptom control for, 87–89
Testosterone, 160, 166
Tetanus vaccination, 28
Tetracycline, 110, 236–237
Thalidomide, 124, 171
Thioanomides, 165
3TC. See Lamivudine
Throat disorders, 173, 206
Thrombocytopenia, 6, 177–180, 213
Thrush, 17–18, 29, 81, 109, 123–124, 168, 173, 206
Thyroid dysfunction, 164–165
Thyroxine, 165
Tincture of opium, 127
Tobramycin, 136
Total parenteral nutrition (TPN), 65, 89, 128
Toxoplasma encephalitis (TE), 113, 120, 188–191, Colorplate 21–Colorplate 22
Toxoplasmosis
  epidemiology of, 67, 80, 148, 187
  latent, 187–188
  ophthalmologic, 141, 191–192
  prophylaxis therapy, 30t, 31, 87, 188
  pulmonary, 99t, 103, 191
  screening for, 27–28, 71, 187, 249–250
Transfusion therapy, 14, 18, 69, 180–181
Travel precautions, 29, 96
Treponema pallidum. See Syphilis
Triamcinolone preparations, 108, 172–173

Tricyclic antidepressants (TCAs), 90–91, 116, 118–119
Trifluorothymidine 1% drops, 135
Trimethoprim-sulfamethoxazole (TMP-SMZ)
  complications from, 112, 131, 131t, 133
  indications for, 128–129, 141
    bacterial infections, 96, 98–99, 225, 227–228
    pediatric, 66–67, 67t
    Pneumocystis carinii pneumonia, 182, 183t, 184–186
    protozoan infections, 188, 191–192
  prophylactic, 30t, 31, 66, 67t, 81
Trimetrexate, 67
  with leucovorin, 183t, 184–186
Tuberculin skin testing
  methods of, 195, 198
  recommendations for, 5, 15, 27, 71, 80, 101
Tuberculosis (TB)
  diagnosis of, 94, 101, 194–196
  epidemiology of, 62, 66, 71, 80, 194
  extrapulmonary, 125, 128, 132–133, 148, 172
  with HIV infection, 99t, 100–101, 194
  meningitis, 113, 194–195
  multiple-drug resistant (MDRTB), 194–196, 198
  prophylaxis therapy, 30t, 31, 199
  screening for, 15, 27, 198–199
  in special populations, 62, 66, 71, 80
  treatment of, 196, 197t, 198
Tumor-lysis syndrome, 132, 251

U
Ulcerations
  corneal, 135–136
  gastrointestinal, 6, 123, 128, 170–171
  genital, 6, 73
Uveitis, anterior, 137–138

V
Vaccinations
  bacterial, 28, 31t, 98, 228
  hepatitis virus, 10–11, 13, 28
  as primary care, 28, 31t, 65
  tuberculosis, 199
Valacyclovir, 135, 222–223
Valganaciclovir, 216
Valproic acid, 116, 118
Valvular heart disease, 146–147
Vancomycin, 99, 136, 140, 146, 226–227
Varicella-zoster virus (VZV) infections
  acyclovir-resistant, 222–223, Colorplate 7
  clinical presentation of, 15, 18, 109, 169, 222–223, Colorplate 6
  ophthalmologic, 135, 139–140
Vascular lesions, 142, 147
Vasculitis, HIV-associated, 151–152
Vertigo, 172
Vidarabine 3% ointment, 135
Vinblastine, 148, 170, 242, 255

Vincristine, 179, 243, 246, 252t, 254–255
Viral culture, 21, 49, 223
Viral diversity, of HIV-1, 4, 14
Viral infections, 67–68, 99t, 100, 249. See
  also specific infection
  antimicrobials for, 135, 140, 214t–215t,
    218t
  gastrointestinal, 123–125, 128–129
  ophthalmologic, 135–136, 138–140
  of oral cavity, 15, 18, 109–110, 168–169
Viral load, of HIV-1
  as antiretroviral therapy marker, 48–49,
    51, 55
  dynamics of, 4–6, 4f
  maternal, 78–79
  natural history of, 14, 18–19
Viral markers, for antiretroviral therapy,
  4–5, 4f, 48–49
Viremia, 4–6, 4f, 14, 213, 221
Virology, for HIV-1, 3–4, 14
Vitamin B$_{12}$ deficiency, 116–117, 176
Vitamin D supplements, 165

W
Wasting syndrome. See HIV-associated
  wasting
Weight loss
  management of, 17–18, 88–89, 159–161
  patterns of, 64, 82, 158–159
Weight monitoring, 23
Western Blot (WB) test, 7, 20–21
Women. See also Pregnancy
  HIV education for, 22, 69, 71
  HIV infection in, 21, 60, 70–76

Z
Zalcitabine (ddC), 35–36, 52, 180, 258t
Zidovudine (AZT, ZDV), 33–34, 63t
  complications from, 112, 119–120, 148,
    150–151
  doses and costs of, 11, 52, 54t, 246, 253,
    258t
  hematologic disorders and, 176–180
  pregnancy and, 68, 79–81